Contemporary Issues in Patients with Implantable Devices

Editors

AMIN AL-AHMAD
RAYMOND YEE
MARK S. LINK

CARDIAC ELECTROPHYSIOLOGY CLINICS

www.cardiacEP.theclinics.com

Consulting Editors
RANJAN K. THAKUR
ANDREA NATALE

March 2018 • Volume 10 • Number 1

ELSEVIER

1600 John F. Kennedy Boulevard • Suite 1800 • Philadelphia, Pennsylvania, 19103-2899

http://www.theclinics.com

CARDIAC ELECTROPHYSIOLOGY CLINICS Volume 10, Number 1
March 2018 ISSN 1877-9182, ISBN-13: 978-0-323-58146-2

Editor: Stacy Eastman
Developmental Editor: Donald Mumford

Cardiac Electrophysiology Clinics (ISSN 1877-9182) is published quarterly by Elsevier Inc., 360 Park Avenue South, New York, NY 10010-1710. Months of issue are March, June, September, and December. Subscription prices are $215.00 per year for US individuals, $344.00 per year for US institutions, $236.00 per year for Canadian individuals, $415.00 per year for Canadian institutions, $299.00 per year for international individuals, $415.00 per year for international institutions and $100.00 per year for US, Canadian and international students/residents. To receive student/resident rate, orders must be accompanied by name of affilliated institution, date of term, and the signature of program/residency coordinator on institution letterhead. Orders will be billed at individual rate until proof of status is received. Foreign air speed delivery is included in all Clinics subscription prices. All prices are subject to change without notice. **POSTMASTER:** Send address changes to Cardiac Electrophysiology Clinics, Elsevier Health Sciences Division, Subscription Customer Service, 3251 Riverport Lane, Maryland Heights, MO 63043. **Customer Service: 1-800-654-2452 (US and Canada). From outside of the US and Canada, call 314-477-8871. Fax: 314-447-8029. E-mail: JournalsCustomerService-usa@elsevier.com (for print support); JournalsOnlineSupport-usa@elsevier.com (for online support).**

Reprints. For copies of 100 or more of articles in this publication, please contact the Commercial Reprints Department, Elsevier Inc., 360 Park Avenue South, New York, NY 10010-1710. Tel.: 212-633-3874; Fax: 212-633-3820; E-mail: reprints@elsevier.com.

Cardiac Electrophysiology Clinics is covered in *MEDLINE/PubMed (Index Medicus)*.

Contributors

CONSULTING EDITORS

RANJAN K. THAKUR, MD, MPH, MBA, FHRS
Professor of Medicine and Director, Arrhythmia
Service, Thoracic and Cardiovascular Institute,
Sparrow Health System, Michigan State
University, Lansing, Michigan, USA

ANDREA NATALE, MD, FACC, FHRS
Executive Medical Director, Texas Cardiac
Arrhythmia Institute, St. David's Medical
Center, Austin, Texas, USA; Consulting
Professor, Division of Cardiology, Stanford
University, Palo Alto, California, USA; Adjunct
Professor of Medicine, Heart and Vascular
Center, Case Western Reserve University,
Cleveland, Ohio, USA; Director, Interventional
Electrophysiology, Scripps Clinic, San Diego,
California, USA; Senior Clinical Director, EP
Services, California Pacific Medical Center,
San Francisco, California, USA

EDITORS

AMIN AL-AHMAD, MD
Cardiac Electrophysiologist, Texas Cardiac
Arrhythmia Institute, St. David's Medical
Center, Austin, Texas, USA

RAYMOND YEE, MD, FRCPC, FHRS
Chair, Division of Cardiology, Gunton Professor
of Medicine, Schulich School of Medicine and
Dentistry, Western University, City-Wide Chief
of Cardiology, University Hospital, London,
Ontario, Canada

MARK S. LINK, MD
Professor of Medicine, Department of Internal
Medicine, Division of Cardiology, The
University of Texas Southwestern Medical
Center, Dallas, Texas, USA

AUTHORS

AMIN AL-AHMAD, MD
Cardiac Electrophysiologist, Texas Cardiac
Arrhythmia Institute, St. David's Medical
Center, Austin, Texas, USA

SANA M. AL-KHATIB, MD, MHS
Professor of Medicine, Division of Cardiology,
Duke Clinical Research Institute, Duke
University Medical Center, Durham, North
Carolina, USA

KHALID ALJABRI, MD
CardioVascular Center, Tufts Medical Center,
Tufts University School of Medicine, Boston,
Massachusetts, USA

FAHAD ALMEHMADI, MBBS, FRCPC
Division of Cardiology, Department of
Medicine, Western University, London,
Ontario, Canada

THARIAN S. CHERIAN, MD
Section of Cardiology, The University of
Chicago Medicine, Pritzker School of
Medicine, Chicago, Illinois, USA

GOPI DANDAMUDI, MD, FHRS
System Medical Director, Cardiac
Electrophysiology, Indiana University School of
Medicine, Indianapolis, Indiana, USA

JAMES DANIELS, MD
Assistant Professor, Department of Internal
Medicine, Division of Cardiology, The
University of Texas Southwestern Medical
Center, Dallas, Texas, USA

DOMENICO G. DELLA ROCCA, MD
Texas Cardiac Arrhythmia Institute, St. David's
Medical Center, Austin, Texas, USA

LUIGI DI BIASE, MD, PhD
Texas Cardiac Arrhythmia Institute, St. David's
Medical Center, Department of Biomedical
Engineering, Cockrell School of Engineering,
The University of Texas at Austin, Austin,
Texas, USA; Albert Einstein College of
Medicine, Montefiore Hospital, Bronx,
New York, USA; Department of Cardiology,
University of Foggia, Foggia, Italy

STEPHEN DUFFETT, MD, FRCPC
Cardiac Electrophysiology Fellow, Heart
Rhythm Program, Department of Medicine,
Western University, London, Ontario, Canada

IMANE EL HAJJAJI, MD
Cardiac Electrophysiology Fellow, Heart
Rhythm Program, Department of Medicine,
Western University, London, Ontario, Canada

CHRISTOPHER R. ELLIS, MD, FACC, FHRS
Associate Professor, Vanderbilt Heart &
Vascular Institute, Nashville, Tennessee, USA

FATIMA M. EZZEDDINE, MD
Clinical Assistant Professor, Indiana
University School of Medicine, Indianapolis,
Indiana, USA

DANIEL J. FRIEDMAN, MD
Electrophysiology Fellow in Training, Division
of Cardiology, Duke Clinical Research Institute,
Duke University Medical Center, Durham,
North Carolina, USA

ANN GARLITSKI, MD
Assistant Professor of Medicine,
CardioVascular Center, Tufts Medical Center,
Tufts University School of Medicine, Boston,
Massachusetts, USA

CAROLA GIANNI, MD, PhD
Texas Cardiac Arrhythmia Institute, St. David's
Medical Center, Austin, Texas, USA

NITIN KULKARNI, MD
Cardiac Electrophysiology Fellow, Department
of Internal Medicine, Division of Cardiology,
The University of Texas Southwestern Medical
Center, Dallas, Texas, USA

MARK S. LINK, MD
Professor of Medicine, Department of Internal
Medicine, Division of Cardiology, The
University of Texas Southwestern Medical
Center, Dallas, Texas, USA

MICHAEL LOGUIDICE, MD
Fellow, Department of Internal Medicine,
Division of Cardiology, The University of Texas
Southwestern Medical Center, Dallas, Texas,
USA

**CHARLES J. LOVE, MD, FACC, FAHA, FHRS,
CCDS**
Professor of Medicine, Director, Cardiac
Rhythm Device Services, The Johns Hopkins
Hospital, Baltimore, Maryland, USA

CHRISTOPHER MADIAS, MD
Assistant Professor of Medicine,
CardioVascular Center, Tufts Medical Center,
Tufts University School of Medicine, Boston,
Massachusetts, USA

JAIMIE MANLUCU, MD, FRCPC
Training Program Director, Heart Rhythm
Program, Assistant Professor, Department of
Medicine, Division of Cardiology, Western
University, London, Ontario, Canada

JOSE M. MARCIAL, MD
Department of Medicine, Division of Cardiology,
Cardiac Arrhythmia Center, MedStar Heart &
Vascular Institute, MedStar Washington
Hospital Center, Washington, DC, USA

NICOLLE MILSTEIN, BS
Research Study Coordinator, Valley Health
System, The Snyder Center for Comprehensive
Atrial Fibrillation, Ridgewood, New Jersey, USA

SUNEET MITTAL, MD
Director, Electrophysiology, Valley Health System, The Snyder Center for Comprehensive Atrial Fibrillation, Ridgewood, New Jersey, USA

JAY A. MONTGOMERY, MD
Assistant Professor, Vanderbilt Heart & Vascular Institute, Nashville, Tennessee, USA

DANIEL P. MORIN, MD, MPH, FHRS, FACC
Cardiac Electrophysiologist, Associate Professor of Cardiology and Medicine, Medical Director, Cardiovascular Research, John Ochsner Heart and Vascular Institute, Ochsner Clinical School, Faculty of Medicine, The University of Queensland, New Orleans, Louisiana, USA

DAN L. MUSAT, MD
Director, Electrophysiology Research, Valley Health System, Snyder Center for Comprehensive Atrial Fibrillation, Ridgewood, New Jersey, USA

ANDREA NATALE, MD, FACC, FHRS
Executive Medical Director, Texas Cardiac Arrhythmia Institute, St. David's Medical Center, Austin, Texas, USA; Consulting Professor, Division of Cardiology, Stanford University, Palo Alto, California, USA; Adjunct Professor of Medicine, Heart and Vascular Center, Case Western Reserve University, Cleveland, Ohio, USA; Director, Interventional Electrophysiology, Scripps Clinic, San Diego, California, USA; Senior Clinical Director, EP Services, California Pacific Medical Center, San Francisco, California, USA

MAKI ONO, MD, PhD
Department of Cardiology, Kameda General Hospital, Kamogawa City, Chiba, Japan; Cardiac Pacing and Electrophysiology, Heart & Vascular Institute, Cleveland Clinic, Cleveland, Ohio, USA

ROD S. PASSMAN, MD, MSCE, FACC, FHRS
Professor of Medicine, Division of Cardiology, Northwestern University Feinberg School of Medicine, Chicago, Illinois, USA

GILLIAN D. SANDERS, PhD
Professor of Medicine, Clinical Pharmacology, Duke Clinical Research Institute, Duke University Medical Center, Durham, North Carolina, USA

MERRILL H. STEWART, MD
Cardiology Fellow, John Ochsner Heart and Vascular Institute, Ochsner Clinical School, Faculty of Medicine, The University of Queensland, New Orleans, Louisiana, USA

GAURAV A. UPADHYAY, MD
Assistant Professor of Medicine, Director, Section of Cardiology, Center for Arrhythmia Care, Heart and Vascular Center, The University of Chicago Medicine, Pritzker School of Medicine, Chicago, Illinois, USA

NIRAJ VARMA, MD, PhD
Cardiac Pacing and Electrophysiology, Heart and Vascular Institute, Cleveland Clinic, Cleveland, Ohio, USA

JEREMIAH WASSERLAUF, MD, MS
Fellow, Division of Cardiology, Northwestern University Feinberg School of Medicine, Chicago, Illinois, USA

JONATHAN WEINSTOCK, MD
Assistant Professor, Department of Medicine, Division of Cardiology, Co-Director, New England Cardiac Arrhythmia Center, CardioVascular Center, Tufts Medical Center, Tufts University School of Medicine, Boston, Massachusetts, USA

SETH J. WORLEY, MD, FACC, FHRS
Director of the Interventional Implant Program, Cardiac Arrhythmia Center, Department of Medicine, Division of Cardiology, MedStar Heart & Vascular Institute, MedStar Washington Hospital Center, Washington, DC, USA

RAYMOND YEE, MD, FRCPC, FHRS
Chair, Division of Cardiology, Gunton Professor of Medicine, Schulich School of Medicine and Dentistry, Western University, City-Wide Chief of Cardiology, University Hospital, London, Ontario, Canada

NATH ZUNGSONTIPORN, MD
Fellow, Department of Internal Medicine, Division of Cardiology, The University of Texas Southwestern Medical Center, Dallas, Texas, USA

Contents

> Battery depletion is the most common reason for device reoperation, which is associated with significant patient morbidity and mortality. This article describes the history of pacing and defibrillation power supplies and the factors that determine the longevity of pacing and defibrillator generators with a special emphasis on factors that can be adjusted or controlled by the implanting and following physician. Optimization of longevity is attained through device selection; shock minimization; avoidance of prolonged radiofrequency telemetry; selection of higher impedance vectors; avoidance of long pulse duration when possible; and avoidance of unnecessary feature activation, such as continuous electrogram storage.

> The wearable cardioverter defibrillator has been shown to be effective in terminating ventricular arrhythmias in patients at risk for sudden cardiac death. There are numerous scenarios in which implant of a permanent implantable cardioverter defibrillator is temporarily contraindicated or not advisable and a wearable cardioverter defibrillator may be beneficial. There are no prospective randomized studies published that provide conclusive guidance toward the use of the wearable cardioverter defibrillator, and thus, patient management needs to be individualized based on the available data.

> Leadless pacemaker therapy is a new technology that aims at avoiding lead- and pocket-related complications of conventional transvenous and epicardial pacing. To date, 2 self-contained leadless pacemakers for right ventricular pacing have been clinically available: the Nanostim Leadless Pacemaker System and the Micra Transcatheter Pacing System. In addition, a new multicomponent leadless pacemaker for endocardial left ventricular pacing has been proposed as an alternative choice for cardiac resynchronization therapy. In this article, the authors describe the state of the art of leadless pacing and compare the currently available devices with traditional transvenous leadless pacemakers.

> Long-term right ventricular pacing is associated with electrical and mechanical dyssynchrony and ultimately development of pacing-induced cardiomyopathy (PICM) in

a subset of patients. Patients with a high degree of pacing burden and reduced left ventricular (LV) function before pacemaker implantation are at the greatest risk for developing PICM. Cardiac resynchronization therapy (CRT) has an established role in the treatment of patients with LV systolic heart failure and intraventricular delay and has been used to successfully treat PICM. This article evaluates predictors for PICM, as well as highlights the role for CRT in prevention and treatment in high-risk patients.

This article aims to cover the latest evidence of remote monitoring of cardiac implantable electronic devices for the management of atrial fibrillation and heart failure. Remote monitoring is useful for early detection for device-detected atrial fibrillation, which increases the risk of thromboembolic events. Early anticoagulation based on remote monitoring potentially reduces the risk of stroke, but optimal alert setting needs to be clarified. Multiparameter monitoring with automatic transmission is useful for heart failure management. Improved adherence to remote monitoring and an optimal algorithm for transmitted alerts and their management are warranted in the management of heart failure.

The historical preference for dual-coil implantable cardioverter defibrillator leads stems from high defibrillation thresholds associated with old device platforms. The high safety margins generated by contemporary devices have rendered the modest difference in defibrillation efficacy between single- and dual-coil leads clinically insignificant. Cohort data demonstrating worse lead extraction outcomes and higher all-cause mortality have brought the incremental utility of a superior vena cava coil into question. This article summarizes the current literature and reevaluates the utility of dual-coil leads in the context of modern device technology.

Use of implantable cardioverter-defibrillators as a primary prevention therapy has been shown to reduce mortality in patients after cardiac arrest and also with left ventricular systolic dysfunction. Yet, inappropriate shocks are variably reported and associated with a reduction in quality of life. Inappropriate shocks are the result of environmental causes leading to electromagnetic interference and inappropriate sensing of external noise, device-related causes from inappropriate sensing of physiologic or pathologic signals, and supraventricular arrhythmias. Strategies to reduce inappropriate shocks include aggressive treatment of supraventricular tachycardia, changes in device programming including prolonged detection time, programming antitachycardic pacing and using discriminator algorithms, and cardiac rehabilitation.

Device-detected atrial high-rate episodes (AHREs) are frequently encountered in patients with no history of atrial fibrillation (AF) and represent a challenge for clinicians because patients with device-only documented AF have not been included in clinical trials of anticoagulants and other AF therapies. For patients with a known history of AF, wireless continuous rhythm monitoring and rapidly acting oral anticoagulants offer the possibility of tailored anticoagulation in response to AHREs, with studies ongoing to evaluate the safety of this approach. This article provides an overview of the current evidence on device-detected AHREs and evolving areas of investigation.

controlled laboratory setting. Although the procedure is safe, complications can occur and DFT is associated with an increased procedural time and cost. DFT is useful in assessing device function when programming changes or patient characteristics raise concerns regarding ICD efficacy. DFT remains the standard of practice following implantation of subcutaneous ICDs and other specific circumstances. Implanting physicians should remain familiar with the process of DFT and situations in which it is useful for individual patients.

with antimicrobial therapy. Understanding the risks of CIED infection and using pre-ventive measures are critical. It is hoped that emerging technologies will mitigate CIED infection rates.

Venous System Interventions for Device Implantation

Jose M. Marcial and Seth J. Worley

 Video content accompanies this article at http://www.cardiacep.theclinics.com.

Subclavian obstruction is common after lead implantation and the need to add or replace a lead is increasing. Subclavian venoplasty (SV) is a safe and effective option for venous occlusion. Peripheral venography overestimates the severity of the obstruction. A wire can usually be advanced into the central circulation for SV. Compared with dilators, SV improves the quality of venous access, providing unre-stricted catheter manipulation for His bundle pacing and left ventricular lead implan-tation. SV preserves venous access and reduces lead burden. SV can easily be added to the implanting physicians lead management options.

CARDIAC ELECTROPHYSIOLOGY CLINICS

THE CLINICS ARE AVAILABLE ONLINE!
Access your subscription at:
www.theclinics.com

Foreword
Cardiac Implantable Electronic Devices

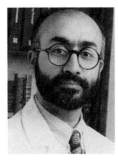
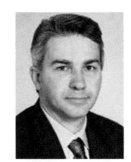

Ranjan K. Thakur, MD, MPH, MBA, FHRS   Andrea Natale, MD, FACC, FHRS

Consulting Editors

Care of patients with cardiac implantable electronic devices (CIED) comprises the bulk of time most cardiac electrophysiologists in clinical practice spend providing patient care. Thus it's appropriate to discuss current thinking on various issues related to management of patients with CIEDs. We are pleased that Drs Al-Ahmad, Yee, and Link have assembled a respected panel of contributors and put together this excellent issue of *Cardiac Electrophysiology Clinics* on contemporary review of CIED with future directions.

This volume is clinically oriented and covers many contemporary topics of interest to clinicians, such as the use of wearable defibrillators during the waiting phase before an implantable defibrillator is implanted, current status and future developments in leadless pacemakers, His bundle pacing, use of single- or dual-coil defibrillator leads, inappropriate implantable cardioverter defibrillator shocks, device-detected atrial fibrillation, procedural issues, technology issues, and controversies about contemporary practice issues.

This volume will be of interest to all clinical electrophysiologists as well as cardiology and electrophysiology fellows in training and lab and nursing personnel who help us take care of these complex patients. This volume is easy to read because it deals with subjects that are familiar to all of us, well presented, and clearly written. We hope you enjoy it.

Ranjan K. Thakur, MD, MPH, MBA, FHRS
Sparrow Thoracic and Cardiovascular Institute
1400 East Michigan Avenue
Suite 400
Lansing, MI 48912, USA

Andrea Natale, MD, FACC, FHRS
Texas Cardiac Arrhythmia Institute
Center for Atrial Fibrillation at
St. David's Medical Center
1015 East 32nd Street, Suite 516
Austin, TX 78705, USA

E-mail addresses:
thakur@msu.edu (R.K. Thakur)
andrea.natale@stdavids.com (A. Natale)

Card Electrophysiol Clin 10 (2018) xiii
https://doi.org/10.1016/j.ccep.2017.12.001
1877-9182/18/© 2017 Published by Elsevier Inc.

Preface

Contemporary Review of the Cardiovascular Implantable Electronic Devices with Future Directions

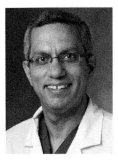   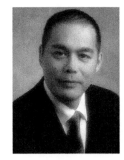   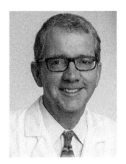

Amin Al-Ahmad, MD   Raymond Yee, MD, FRCPC, FHRS   Mark S. Link, MD

Editors

This issue of *Cardiac Electrophysiology Clinics* is focused on aspects of cardiovascular implantable electronic devices. The contributors are experts in the field who discuss the latest advancements and controversies and take a look toward the future.

We examine clinical issues, such as management of device infection, as well as management of device-detected atrial arrhythmias with respect to anticoagulation therapy. We also update the reader on issues relating to inappropriate implantable cardioverter-defibrillator (ICD) discharge and remote monitoring.

Procedural issues, such as device selection, lead extraction, venous system intervention, and perioperative anticoagulation, are also highlighted in this issue.

Device technology is discussed in several articles, including an article on device longevity, leadless pacing, His bundle pacing, and advances in subcutaneous ICD technology.

This issue also features articles that highlight areas of change and controversy in the field, for example, when is it safe to not reimplant an ICD; the role of CRT pacing in patients expected to have a high pacing percentage in the right ventricle; defibrillation threshold testing and the use of single versus dual coil leads as well as the use of the wearable defibrillator.

We are confident that this issue will be of value to cardiac electrophysiologists and cardiac electrophysiology trainees as well as any clinician interested in the modern management of cardiovascular implantable electronic devices.

Amin Al-Ahmad, MD
Texas Cardiac Arrhythmia Institute
5904 Waymaker Cove
Austin, TX 78746, USA

Raymond Yee, MD, FRCPC, FHRS
Division of Cardiology
Schulich School of Medicine and Dentistry
Western University
University Hospital
Room C6-004
339 Windermere Road
London, Ontario N6A 5A5, Canada

Mark S. Link, MD
Internal Medicine
UT Southwestern Medical Center
Professional Office Building 1, Suite HP8.110
5959 Harry Hines Boulevard
Dallas, TX 75390, USA

E-mail addresses:
aalahmadmd@gmail.com (A. Al-Ahmad)
ryee@uwo.ca (R. Yee)
mark.link@utsouthwestern.edu (M.S. Link)

Card Electrophysiol Clin 10 (2018) xv
https://doi.org/10.1016/j.ccep.2017.12.002
1877-9182/18/© 2017 Published by Elsevier Inc.

cardiacEP.theclinics.com

Preface

Contemporary Review of the Cardiovascular Implantable Electronic Devices with Future Directions

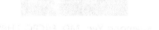

Amin Al-Ahmad, MD   Ranjan K. Thakur, MD, FHRS, FACC   Paul J. Wang, MD
Editors

This issue of *Cardiac Electrophysiology Clinics* is focused on advances of cardiovascular implantable electronic devices. The contributors are leaders in the field who discuss the latest advances, care, and controversies and take a look toward the future.

We address critical issues such as management of device infection, as well as management of cardiac arrhythmia with cardiac resynchronization therapy. We also address the future of leadless pacing in pacemaker therapy, subcutaneous or defibrillator (ICD) placement, and venous preservation.

Important issues such as device extraction, lead location, venous system intervention, and percutaneous procedures are now also highlighted in this issue.

Device technology is discussed in several articles...

Amin Al-Ahmad, MD

Ranjan K. Thakur, MD, FHRS

Toronto, ON, Canada

Sparrow Health System

Michigan State University

Radford House

East Lansing, MI

Paul J. Wang, MD

Stanford Heart Rhythm

London, Ontario N6A 4V2, Canada

Stanford University School of Medicine

300 Pasteur Drive, H2146

Stanford, CA 94305

We are confident that this issue will be of value to cardiac electrophysiologists and physicians interested in the newest advances in the field of cardiovascular implantable electronic devices.

Card Electrophysiol Clin 10 (2018) xv
http://doi.org/10.1016/j.ccep.2018.12.002
1877-9182/18/© 2018 Published by Elsevier Inc.

Longevity of Cardiovascular Implantable Electronic Devices

Jay A. Montgomery, MD*, Christopher R. Ellis, MD, FHRS

KEYWORDS

- Device longevity • Pacemaker longevity • Strength-duration curve • Pacing

KEY POINTS

- Cardiac implantable electronic device generator changes caused by battery depletion are a major source of morbidity and mortality.
- Modern pacemakers and defibrillators last much longer than their predecessors because of improvements in microcircuitry, capacitors, and battery chemistry and architecture.
- Device longevity is maximized through device selection; minimization of high-voltage shocks; avoiding prolonged radiofrequency telemetry; and avoiding unnecessary, energy-intensive features, such as continuous unfiltered electrogram storage.
- Optimal pacing parameters include choosing higher impedance vectors when feasible; avoiding unnecessarily long pulse duration (chronaxie is often near 0.25 ms); pacing near threshold where appropriate; and, in some devices, avoiding crossing voltage multiplication thresholds as able.

INTRODUCTION

Cardiac implantable electronic devices (CIEDs) require a continuous power source to function, and all currently available devices are powered by nonrechargeable batteries. Battery depletion is the most common reason for device reoperation, which is associated with at least a 4.0% risk of major complications.[1] This article describes the history of pacing and defibrillation power supplies and the factors that determine the longevity of pacing and defibrillator generators with a special emphasis on factors that can be adjusted or controlled by the implanting and following physician.

HISTORICAL PERSPECTIVE

In 1957, C. Walton Lillehei and Earl Bakken collaborated on the first wearable, transistorized pacemaker for use in patients with postoperative complete heart block after surgical repair of congenital heart malformations in Minneapolis, Minnesota.[2] One year later, Ake Senning implanted the first fully implantable pulse generator, which featured a rechargeable nickel-cadmium battery, in a 43-year-old man with heart block after a viral infection in Stockholm, Sweden.[3] Although the first unit failed within 6 hours, the second lasted 7 weeks, with recharging every 2 weeks via an external induction coil. At the same time,

Disclosure Statement: J.A. Montgomery has nothing to report. C.R Ellis reports research funding from Medtronic and Boston Scientific; advisory board for Boston Scientific and Medtronic; and Vanderbilt receives fellowship support from Medtronic, Boston Scientific, and St. Jude Medical (Abbott).
Vanderbilt Heart and Vascular Institute, Medical Center East, 5th Floor, 1215 21st Avenue South, Nashville, TN 37232, USA
* Corresponding author. 5429 Medical Center East, 5th Floor, 1215 21st Avenue South, Nashville, TN 37232.
E-mail address: jay.a.montgomery@vanderbilt.edu

Card Electrophysiol Clin 10 (2018) 1–9
https://doi.org/10.1016/j.ccep.2017.11.001
1877-9182/18/Published by Elsevier Inc.

Wilson Greatbatch was developing a pulse generator using a nonrechargeable zinc-mercury battery, which was first implanted by William Chardack in 1960 in Buffalo, New York.[2]

EARLY POWER SOURCES

Zinc-mercury batteries served as the primary energy source for implantable pulse generators for the first 15 years of the industry.[4] Early zinc-mercury batteries lasted up to 18 months but were plagued by unpredictable failure. Improvements in design led to a battery from a company named Ruben Mallory (which later became Duracell) with a projected longevity of greater than 5 years, although with unpredictable modes of failure and a clinical lifespan averaging less than 3 years.[4] Insurmountable problems with mercury cells arose mainly because of the need to vent hydrogen gas while maintaining water impermeability.

In the early 1970s, rechargeable cells were once again commercially produced, this time by Pacesetter Systems (later St. Jude Medical). These devices were limited by the need for weekly charging, high temperatures during charging, and excessive gas pressures.[4] While these problems were being addressed, other technological improvements in nonrechargeable CIED energy sources led to the decline of the rechargeable pacemaker battery.

In this setting of unreliable and short-lived pacemaker batteries, nuclear energy cells were developed in 1965, which converted heat energy from nuclear decay into electric energy via a thermopile.[5–10] Plutonium[238] was the most-used isotope.[7] Although nuclear energy sources had outstanding longevity and safety, concerns about long-term radiation exposure and extensive regulations and licensing limited the widespread adoption of nuclear energy sources for CIEDs.[5,9,10]

LITHIUM AS A POWER SOURCE

Lithium was first investigated as an anode for battery use in the late 1960s.[4] Iodine was the first of many cathodes paired with lithium, and this combination was developed as a pacemaker energy source by Catalyst Research Corporation in conjunction with Wilson Greatbatch and Greatbatch Inc.[4] The lithium-iodine (Li/I_2) battery was solid state and did not produce gas, allowing the battery to be hermetically sealed, unlike mercury batteries. Within a few years, Li/I_2 batteries were developed, which were similar to modern devices in terms of total charge, although they were large by today's standards.[4] Because lithium has the highest electrode potential of all elements, it has been used as the predominant anode material with various cathode combinations for CIEDs for the last 40 years. Throughout this time, the Li/I_2 cell has been a large part of the market and remains so in simple single- and dual-chamber pacemakers.[4] However, more energy-intensive multifunctional dual-chamber and biventricular pacemakers are now being powered primarily by lithium-manganese dioxide (Li/MnO_2), lithium-carbon monofluoride (Li/CFx), or lithium-carbon monofluoride/silver vanadium oxide laminate (Li-CFx/SVO), which have higher energy density. Currently available pacemakers use one of these four cell configurations (Li/I_2, Li/CFx, Li-CFx/SVO, and $LiMnO_2$) (**Table 1**).

BATTERY LONGEVITY

Batteries are the only component of modern CIEDs that do not theoretically last indefinitely. Therefore, the most common reason for patients with modern devices to undergo reoperation of a previously placed CIED is for battery replacement.[11,12] There are many factors that potentially affect longevity of a given device battery

Table 1
Battery chemistry by manufacturer

Company	Pacemaker	Leadless Pacemaker	CRT-P	ICD	ICD and CRT-D	ILR
Biotronik	Li/MnO_2, LiCFx/SVO	—	Li/MnO_2, LiCFx/SVO	Li/MnO_2, LiCFx/SVO	Li/MnO_2, LiCFx/SVO	Li/MnO_2
Boston Scientific	Li/CFx	—	Li/CFx	Li/MnO_2	Li/MnO_2	Li/MnO_2
Medtronic	Li/I_2, LiCFx/SVO	LiCFx/SVO	LiCFx/SVO	Li/SVO	LiCFx/SVO	Li/CFx
St. Jude Medical	LiCFx/SVO	Li/CFx[a]	LiCFx/SVO	Li/SVO	LiCFx/SVO	—

These data were obtained from the manufacturers and refer to the most recently released models of CIEDs.

Abbreviations: CRT-D, cardiac resynchronization therapy defibrillators; CRT-P, cardiac resynchronization therapy pacemaker; ICD, implantable cardioverter-defibrillator; ILR, implantable loop recorder.

[a] Currently not Food and Drug Administration approved.

(see **Fig. 2**). These include power-supply-side characteristics and demand-side requirements. Power-supply-side characteristics include overall battery capacity, battery chemistry, and battery architecture. Demand-side requirements include background current, radiofrequency (RF) telemetry transmission, electrogram storage, high-voltage capacitor reformation, pacing outputs, pacing burden, and usage of antitachycardia pacing and high-voltage shocks. Each of these factors plays a role in determining the length of time from device implant to the determination of the elective replacement interval (ERI) of the device.

SUPPLY-SIDE FACTORS
Battery Capacity

The capacity of a pacemaker or defibrillator battery has a direct effect on the projected lifespan of the device. Although the theoretic battery capacity is virtually limitless, an exceptionally large-capacity battery would have a large mass and volume, and at some point the battery capacity, which declines predictably over time, would likely exceed the lifespan of other CIED components, some of which could fail with less warning. Battery capacity is typically measured in ampere-hours (Ah, the electrical equivalent of 1 A delivered continuously for 1 hour) with modern implantable cardioverter-defibrillators (ICDs) generally having between and 1 and 2 Ah of usable capacity (**Fig. 1**). As might be expected, larger-capacity batteries, especially 2.0 Ah, have been associated with improved longevity across multiple studies.[11,13–15] For comparison, absolute capacity of most modern rechargeable smartphone batteries (typically between 1 and 3 Ah), meets or exceeds that found in all modern CIEDs. However, many other necessary characteristics of CIED batteries (eg, lack of self-discharge and need for intermittent high current in the case of ICDs) restricts current chemistry and architecture to a few

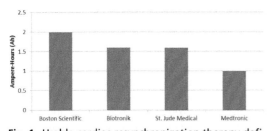

Fig. 1. Usable cardiac resynchronization therapy defibrillator (CRT-D) battery capacity by manufacturer. These data were obtained from the product manuals and refer to the highest capacity, currently available models of CIEDs.

specific types. Available data support the idea that current-generation 2.0 Ah devices are likely to outperform lower-capacity devices, keeping in mind that available real-world data apply generally to devices implanted 6 to 13 years ago.[11,13–16]

Battery Chemistry

All batteries consist of an anode and a cathode. Oxidation occurs at the anode, which is electrically connected to the cathode (where reduction occurs) by ions moving within an electrolyte (usually a liquid).[17] All CIED batteries currently use lithium as the anode with several different cathodes currently in use. Low-power pacemakers (specifically those without RF interrogation capability) are often Li/I$_2$. Power demands for defibrillation are vastly different from cardiac pacing. Although a pacemaker delivers a charge of a few volts, approximately the voltage of the pacemaker battery, a defibrillator is required to deliver a high-energy therapy up to 40 J at 700 to 800 V over 10 to 15 ms. This is accomplished through the use of capacitors, which have dramatically down-sized since the inception of ICDs in the 1980s, and through chemistries, which allow a high-current flow to rapidly charge the capacitor.[4] The early defibrillator was powered by lithium-vanadium pentoxide batteries. These cells were plagued by self-discharge and overall unreliable discharge characteristics and were replaced as better cells became available.[18]

Li-SVO became a dominant power source for ICDs after being unveiled in the mid-1980s.[19] These cells have a high energy density but are limited somewhat by a flat voltage profile and sharp increase in internal resistance, leading to long charge times, at around 70% discharge, where the ERI is typically set.[17] These problems are partially mitigated with Li/SVO CFx hybrid cells, which provides repetitive pacing discharges primarily from the CFx cathode but preferentially uses the SVO cathode for high-voltage discharges.[4] The Li/MnO$_2$ battery is also a popular power source in ICDs and pacemakers, given the high energy density and consistent discharge profiles. The Li/MnO$_2$ Enduralife battery (Boston Scientific, Natick, MA) maintains a stable internal resistance and relative high battery voltage, allowing ERI to be set at 90% discharge.[17] Currently available ICDs and cardiac resynchronization therapy defibrillators (CRT-Ds) all use one of these three cell types (Li/SVO, Li/SVO CFx, or Li/MnO$_2$).

Battery Architecture

The anode and cathode are ideally positioned with large surface areas physically close to, but not touching, one another. An electrolyte in between the two electrodes must allow free movement of ions while the separator does not allow the two electrodes to come into contact. During discharge of the battery, electrons pass from anode to cathode outside the battery, while internally ions flow from anode to cathode through the electrolyte. The lithium anode is typically a thin sheet or pressed onto a screen with the cathode coated over a separate screen.[17] These surfaces are arranged as stacked plates, folded plates, or spirals. There is a direct relationship between increasing complexity of manufacturing and increasing energy density, progressing from spiral wound (least energy dense) to stacked plate (most energy dense).[17] Unintended consequences of battery architecture design can include increased propensity to develop lithium cluster formation, such as because of uneven overlap of anode and cathode or increased areas of electrolyte pooling.[17]

DEMAND-SIDE FACTORS
Background Current

Every CIED has a background current that powers microprocessors. This is continuous and is in the microampere range. In general, these circuits are smaller and significantly more energy efficient than they were in the past, allowing device models to progressively have greater longevity and a lower volume.[17] Despite improvements in circuitry, most devices have a greater overall background current drain than all dynamic factors combined (including pacing). Therefore, background processes have a significant effect on device longevity. In addition, some patient-specific factors, such as the presence of frequent ectopy, can lead to increased microprocessor usage.

Radiofrequency Telemetry

RF telemetry requires power in the milliampere range, which is several orders of magnitude greater than the background current. The frequency of interrogation and the volume of transferred data have an effect on the total current drawn over time. Lau[17] estimates that approximately 4% to 8% of the usable battery capacity of a contemporary ICD/CRT-D is used on RF telemetry. However, if a programmer is used to interrogate a device but the RF telemetry session is not "ended," 0.6% to 1.0% of the battery capacity could be used in one setting. The same can occur during a prolonged device implantation or complex ablation if the device is activated several hours before telemetry is ended at the end of the case; repeated termination and reinitiation of RF telemetry or disabling RF telemetry

and using inductive telemetry during the procedure (as is done during ablations for ventricular tachycardia) is preferable in this circumstance. Newer-generation devices may be programmed to "timeout" after a period of inactivity, limiting the potential current drain of a prolonged RF telemetry session.

In addition, if the device is frequently "looking" for a telemetry hookup (as could be in the case of a misplaced or turned off home base station), unnecessary current drain can occur even without actual data transfer. The increased current drain posed by RF telemetry has led to the adoption of medium-power (rather than low-power) batteries in pacemakers.

Electrogram Storage

Capturing electrograms just before an episode of tachycardia for later review requires continuous electrogram storage. Continuous unfiltered electrogram storage can shorten device longevity by 16%.[20] This is a programmable feature and is programmed off by default. Alternatively, continuous filtered electrogram storage has a smaller effect on device longevity and is often programmed on and not able to be turned off in devices in which it is present (Boston Scientific and St. Jude Medical).[17]

Capacitor Reformation

A capacitor consists of two parallel conductive plates in proximity to, but electrically insulated from, one another. Modern ICDs typically have two aluminum or three tantalum capacitors. Relative miniaturization of modern capacitors is accomplished by maximizing surface area of the conductors via etching on aluminum foil or pressing tantalum powder into porous pellets. Rapid charging of capacitors requires a high-contact surface area between anode and cathode, often accomplished by interlacing of cathode and anode plates.[4] An oxide layer forms on the anode surface but can degrade over time. This is referred to as "deformation" of the capacitor and can lead to long charge time, heating, or even explosion of the capacitor when subjected to a high current load. The capacitor can be "reformed" by passing an electric current through it. This is typically only needed in aluminum capacitors, is typically required at least twice yearly, and uses approximately 5% to 8% of the overall battery longevity throughout the lifetime of the device.[17] Tantalum capacitors have a higher energy density, leading to a smaller size, but are still heavier and more costly to produce than aluminum capacitors. Currently, Boston Scientific and Biotronik defibrillators use tantalum capacitors, Medtronic uses a hybrid aluminum/tantalum capacitor, and St. Jude Medical uses aluminum capacitors.

Pacing Output

Pacing impulses greater than the battery voltage (typically >2.5 V) require voltage amplification. Traditionally, this has been accomplished with a voltage multiplier/charge pump. The voltage multiplier consists of a series of successive capacitors that can each charge (theoretically) to near the battery voltage. The primary drawback of this method lies in the need to charge multiple capacitors at higher voltages. If the output voltage is only slightly higher than the battery voltage, two capacitors are charged, and inherent inefficiencies cause a "step up" in the overall current drain. If the output is more than double the battery voltage, three capacitors charge, and inefficiency increases further. Because of this, there is some incentive to avoid increasing pacing output past certain thresholds when possible. These steps occur around 2.5 V and 5.0 V but can vary by manufacturer.

A switched mode power supply, as may be used in the future, uses an inductor to store energy in a magnetic field. The voltage amplification can be more precisely tuned with a smoother current drain curve and less wasted energy than is achieved in voltage multipliers at certain voltages. However, this type of power supply cannot operate in a strong magnetic field. Therefore, MRI-conditional CIEDs still need a voltage multiplier/charge pump to be used temporarily during MRI scanning.[17]

Pacing Impedance

For any given voltage and pulse duration, an increase in pacing impedance leads to a reduction in current and has been associated with increased device longevity in dual-chamber pacemakers and CRT-D devices.[13,21] In fact, for a given pacing output, an increase in impedance by 100% (ie, increase from 500 Ω to 1000 Ω) decreases current drain by 50% (**Fig. 2**). Although it is not possible to change the pacing lead impedance for a given vector once the lead is implanted, there are often large differences across the various pacing vectors available in left ventricular (LV) leads. Therefore, it is important to note pacing impedance (or note current drain, if available) rather than just voltage required for capture to make an informed decision about LV pacing vector selection.

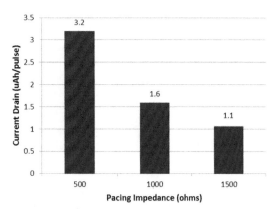

Fig. 2. Effect of changing impedance on current drain. As pacing impedance doubles, current drain is cut in half, all other things being equal. This is especially important to consider when choosing left ventricular pacing vectors, which typically have comparatively low impedance when using the pulse generator or right ventricular coil as anode. (Assumes 4.0-V output, 0.4-ms pulse duration, and disregards the inefficiences of voltage amplification for simplicity).

Practical Considerations in Choosing Pacing Vector and Output

Current drain (as measured in microampere-hours, μAh) by a single pacing stimulus is calculated as V*T/R, with V equal to voltage, T equal to the pulse duration (in milliseconds), and R equal to the impedance (in ohms). Therefore, a doubling of impedance decreases battery drain by 50%. Doubling the voltage output doubles battery drain, although this actually underestimates the true effect, because of the inefficiencies of charge amplification. Changing the pulse duration from 0.4 ms to 1.0 ms increases battery drain ×2.5.

When attempting to optimize device longevity while choosing pacing parameters, it is therefore prudent to determine whether the patient is pacing-dependent on a given lead, and if he or she is not, then pacing closer to threshold voltage is wise. Similarly, especially in the case of multipolar LV leads, choosing a vector with an equal pacing threshold but higher impedance reduces current drain. Finally, consideration of manipulation of pulse duration as needed to minimize output should be undertaken. A simplified visualization of the effect of changing each of these parameters is illustrated in three graphs (see **Fig. 2**; **Figs. 3** and **4**). Modern CRT devices are now increasingly coming equipped with automated algorithms to determine the lowest current drain vectors and may even provide a device longevity estimate from each pacing vector in a quadripolar CRT system.[22]

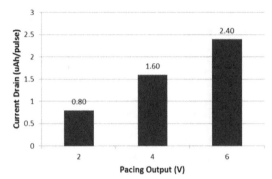

Fig. 3. Effect of changing pacing output on current drain. As pacing output voltage doubles, current drain theoretically doubles, all other things being equal. Crossing certain voltage output thresholds (often near 2.5 V and 5.0 V) may further amplify the current drain effect of increasing output voltage. (Assumes 1000-Ω impedance, 0.4-ms pulse duration, and disregards the inefficiences of voltage amplification for simplicity).

Strength-Duration Curves

In programming pacing output and pulse duration, it is important to keep in mind the expected strength-duration curves of myocardial capture. The lowest possible pacing output voltage that captures myocardium at a given site, with a given lead, in a given patient at an infinite pulse duration

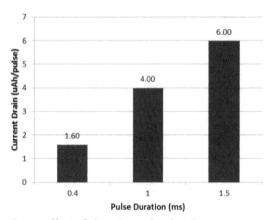

Fig. 4. Effect of changing pulse duration on current drain. Increasing pulse duration leads to a linear and proportional increase in current drain. Increasing the pulse duration from 0.4 ms to 1.0 ms, as is commonly done in the case of high capture threshold, increases current drain ×2.5. As discussed in the text, myocardial chronaxie rarely exceeds 0.4 ms and is likely often near 0.25 ms. However, small increases in pulse duration are helpful when attempting to avoid phrenic capture or to avoid crossing a voltage multiplication threshold. (Assumes 4.0-V output, 1000-Ω impedance, rectangular pacing pulse output, and disregards the inefficiences of voltage amplification for simplicity).

is known as the rheobase (**Fig. 5**). The energy required for cardiac stimulation varies with pulse duration as a U-shaped curve because capture threshold (in current or voltage) and pulse duration have an asymptotic relationship. Specifically, as pulse duration increases linearly, capture threshold approaches the rheobase hyperbolically, with progressive increases in pulse duration of the same size leading to smaller and smaller decreases in capture threshold. The minimum nadir point of this energy curve is known as the chronaxie and signifies the pulse duration with the minimal current drain for pacing. The chronaxie typically lies at ×2 the rheobase.[23] That is, if the lowest possible capture threshold is found (with long pulse duration), the lowest energy output is found by doubling the rheobase voltage and then lowering the pulse duration to just above threshold. Studies have previously shown that chronaxie values tend to be less than 0.5 ms for most pacing leads with standard electrode sizes.[24,25] Coates and Thwaites[24] showed chronaxie values of approximately 0.25 ms ± 0.07 ms for atrial and ventricular leads and noted that using default pulse durations of 0.4 ms or longer lead to significant energy waste in most patients. They recommended pacing at the chronaxie with a safety margin of ×2 capture threshold voltage.

It is most common for LV leads to have a higher pacing threshold and to consequently be programmed with a longer pulse duration. Is this rational? Most studies have found that LV leads have similar chronaxie values to right ventricular or right atrial endocardial leads.[25–27] In all of these studies, chronaxie, as measured by the Lapicque method, was at or lower than default programmed pulse duration. Therefore, it is generally not advisable to program a longer pulse duration to lower the pacing output of LV leads, except if small increases in the pulse duration can avoid voltage multiplication.

In addition, there is evidence that tuning the pulse duration may help to achieve LV capture while avoiding phrenic nerve capture.[28,29] A study by Hjortshoj and colleagues[28] observed in 11 patients with phrenic capture at the proposed LV site a longer chronaxie for the myocardium versus the phrenic nerve (0.47 ms vs 0.22 ms; $P = .017$). A study by Oh and colleagues[29] showed in a canine model a statistically significant longer chronaxie (Lapicque method) for the LV myocardium in both bipolar and unipolar configurations with a larger absolute difference in bipolar configuration (0.81 ms vs 0.19 ms; $P<.01$). Therefore, it is reasonable to increase the pulse duration to avoid phrenic nerve capture and sometimes to avoid crossing certain voltage thresholds of pacing

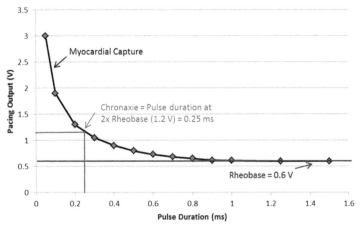

Fig. 5. Sample strength duration curve. The lowest possible pacing output voltage that captures myocardium at an infinite pulse duration is known as the rheobase. As pulse duration increases linearly, capture threshold approaches the rheobase hyperbolically, with progressive increases in pulse duration of the same size leading to smaller and smaller decreases in capture threshold. The minimum nadir point of this energy curve is known as the chronaxie and signifies the pulse duration with the minimal current drain for pacing. The chronaxie, which signifies the output and pulse duration of the minimum current drain that can capture myocardium, typically lies at ×2 the rheobase. That is, if the lowest possible capture threshold is found (with long pulse duration), the lowest energy output is found by doubling the rheobase voltage and then lowering the pulse duration to just above threshold. Chronaxie is typically near 0.25 ms in humans with standard pacing leads and rarely exceeds 0.4 ms.

amplitude output, but it is generally not advisable to increase the pulse duration reflexively because of high voltage output.

High-Voltage Therapy

Not surprisingly, delivery of high-voltage therapy can consume a much larger quantity of battery capacity than any other single process. A single high-voltage shock can consume approximately 0.5% to 1.0% of the total battery capacity of a defibrillator.[30] Irrespective of this fact, clinicians and patients generally strive, all other things being equal, to keep the number of high-voltage discharges to a minimum. Any strategy that reduces overall high-voltage discharges, therefore, leads to an increase in device longevity. In the MADIT-RIT study of patients receiving de novo primary prevention ICDs, high-rate-only therapy and delayed ICD therapy were associated with fewer shocks and improved mortality as compared with conventional settings.[31] Although these data cannot necessarily be extrapolated to other populations, it is reasonable to conclude that this programming strategy is also likely to lead to improved device longevity in these patients.

SPECIAL SCENARIOS
Leadless Cardiac Pacing and Subcutaneous Implantable Cardioverter-Defibrillator

The Micra (Medtronic, Minneapolis, MN) transcatheter pacemaker is the only Food and Drug Administration–approved leadless pacing system available at the time of this writing.[32] Although real-world device longevity remains to be seen, a 12-month follow-up study projects device longevity of 12.1 years, approximately equivalent to modern pacing systems.[33] Notably, the nominal pulse duration in the Micra pacemaker is 0.24 ms, consistent with the approximate human myocardial chronaxie.[24–27]

Boston Scientific's first-generation fully subcutaneous ICD has a median longevity of 5.0 years.[34] The second-generation device carries a projected longevity from the manufacturer of 7.3 years, although this device has been commercially available less than 2 years. There are few programmable features to affect this longevity in a meaningful way.

Lithium Cluster Formation

The most recent device recall with significant implications for generator longevity has come in the form of lithium cluster formation leading to an increased risk of abrupt discharge of stored battery charge among a large group of ICD and CRT-D devices from St. Jude Medical (now Abbott). This was first described by Pokorney and colleagues[35] and has now been observed at many (if not most) centers with a large group of patients with St. Jude ICDs and CRT-Ds.[36] This phenomenon can theoretically occur in any lithium battery and is favored by intermittent high-power discharges, uneven overlap between anode and cathode as is present in folded-plate architecture, and open space within the battery case.[17] Modifications to the battery architecture may help protect against lithium cluster formation.[17] When lithium clusters create a bridge between anode and cathode, battery often drains from baseline voltage to end-of-life in less than 24 hours. For this reason, many centers have opted to perform prophylactic generator replacements on pacemaker-dependent patients and have deployed various strategies in nondependent patients, including consideration of generator replacements for patients who have relied on life-saving tachyarrhythmia therapies. For primary prevention, nonpacing patients, most centers have opted for targeted patient education and reprogramming vibratory alerts to increase the likelihood that a patient will be alerted and subsequently seek urgent treatment in the event of an abrupt battery discharge. Any recall that causes physicians to replace a large proportion of a manufacturer's devices obviously decreases the effective device longevity drastically, irrespective of how long each device may have lasted without intervention.

SUMMARY

A significant amount of patient morbidity and mortality is spared through optimization of parameters and behaviors to extend device longevity. It is expected that each generation of CIEDs will, on average, outperform their predecessors, with many patients never requiring a generator change.[14,37] Physicians and allied health professionals following CIEDs can improve device longevity through device selection; minimization of high-voltage therapies; avoidance of prolonged RF telemetry; choosing higher impedance vectors; avoiding long pulse duration when possible; and avoidance of unnecessary feature activation, such as continuous electrogram storage.

REFERENCES

1. Poole JE, Gleva MJ, Mela T, et al. Complication rates associated with pacemaker or implantable cardioverter-defibrillator generator replacements and upgrade procedures: results from the REPLACE registry. Circulation 2010;122(16):1553–61.
2. Jeffrey K. Machines in our hearts: the cardiac pacemaker, the implantable defibrillator, and American health care. Baltimore (MD): Johns Hopkins University Press; 2001.
3. Elmqvist RS, Senning A. Implantable pacemaker for the heart. London: Iliffe and Sons; 1960.
4. Mond HG, Freitag G. The cardiac implantable electronic device power source: evolution and revolution. Pacing Clin Electrophysiol 2014;37(12):1728–45.
5. Chauvel C, Lavergne T, Cohen A, et al. Radioisotopic pacemaker: long-term clinical results. Pacing Clin Electrophysiol 1995;18(2):286–92.
6. Norman JC, Sandberg GW Jr, Huffman FN. Implantable nuclear-powered cardiac pacemakers. N Engl J Med 1970;283(22):1203–6.
7. Parsonnet V. Power sources for implantable cardiac pacemakers. Chest 1972;61(2):165–73.
8. Parsonnet V. Cardiac pacing and pacemakers. VII. Power sources for implantable pacemakers. Part II. Am Heart J 1977;94(5):658–64.
9. Parsonnet V. Cardiac pacing and pacemakers VII. Power sources for implantable pacemakers. Part I. Am Heart J 1977;94(4):517–28.
10. Smyth NP, Millette ML. The isotopic cardiac pacer: a ten-year experience. Pacing Clin Electrophysiol 1984;7(1):82–9.
11. Zanon F, Martignani C, Ammendola E, et al. Device longevity in a contemporary cohort of ICD/CRT-D patients undergoing device replacement. J Cardiovasc Electrophysiol 2016;27(7):840–5.
12. Thijssen J, Borleffs CJ, van Rees JB, et al. Implantable cardioverter-defibrillator longevity under clinical circumstances: an analysis according to device type, generation, and manufacturer. Heart Rhythm 2012;9(4):513–9.
13. Ellis CR, Dickerman DI, Orton JM, et al. Ampere hour as a predictor of cardiac resynchronization defibrillator pulse generator battery longevity: a multicenter study. Pacing Clin Electrophysiol 2016;39(7):658–68.
14. von Gunten S, Schaer BA, Yap SC, et al. Longevity of implantable cardioverter defibrillators: a comparison among manufacturers and over time. Europace 2016;18(5):710–7.
15. Alam MB, Munir MB, Rattan R, et al. Battery longevity in cardiac resynchronization therapy implantable cardioverter defibrillators. Europace 2014;16(2):246–51.
16. Landolina M, Curnis A, Morani G, et al. Longevity of implantable cardioverter-defibrillators for cardiac resynchronization therapy in current clinical practice: an analysis according to influencing factors, device generation, and manufacturer. Europace 2015;17(8):1251–8.
17. Lau EW. Technologies for prolonging cardiac implantable electronic device longevity. Pacing Clin Electrophysiol 2017;40(1):75–96.
18. Takeuchi ES, Quattrini PJ, Greatbatch W. Lithium/silver vanadium oxide batteries for implantable defibrillators. Pacing Clin Electrophysiol 1988;11(11 Pt 2):2035–9.
19. Holmes CF, Visbisky M. Long-term testing of defibrillator batteries. Pacing Clin Electrophysiol 1991;14(2 Pt 2):341–5.

20. Medtronic. Viva quad XT CRT-D manual. Minneapolis (MN): Medtronic; 2016. p. 31.
21. Berger T, Roithinger FX, Antretter H, et al. The influence of high versus normal impedance ventricular leads on pacemaker generator longevity. Pacing Clin Electrophysiol 2003;26(11):2116–20.
22. Medtronic. Claria MRI quad CRT-Ds manual. Minneapolis (MN): Medtronic; 2017. p. 376.
23. Irnich W. The chronaxie time and its practical importance. Pacing Clin Electrophysiol 1980;3(3):292–301.
24. Coates S, Thwaites B. The strength-duration curve and its importance in pacing efficiency: a study of 325 pacing leads in 229 patients. Pacing Clin Electrophysiol 2000;23(8):1273–7.
25. Huizar JF, Kaszala K, Koneru J, et al. Disparity in left ventricular stimulation among different pacing configurations in cardiac resynchronization therapy. Circ Arrhythm Electrophysiol 2012;5(1):140–6.
26. Dhar SK, Heston KJ, Madrak LJ, et al. Strength duration curve for left ventricular epicardial stimulation in patients undergoing cardiac resynchronization therapy. Pacing Clin Electrophysiol 2009;32(9):1146–51.
27. Scally M, Heston KJ, Rudnick AG, et al. Strength duration curve for epicardial left ventricular stimulation. Pacing Clin Electrophysiol 2007;30(5):612–5.
28. Hjortshoj S, Heath F, Haugland M, et al. Long pacing pulses reduce phrenic nerve stimulation in left ventricular pacing. J Cardiovasc Electrophysiol 2014;25(5):485–90.
29. Oh S, Kim WY, Kim HC, et al. Left ventricular pacing with long pulse duration can avoid phrenic nerve stimulation. Heart Rhythm 2011;8(10):1637–40.
30. Ellenbogen KA. Clinical cardiac pacing, defibrillation, and resynchronization therapy. 3rd edition. Philadelphia: Saunders/Elsevier; 2007.
31. Moss AJ, Schuger C, Beck CA, et al. Reduction in inappropriate therapy and mortality through ICD programming. N Engl J Med 2012;367(24):2275–83.
32. Reynolds D, Duray GZ, Omar R, et al. A leadless intracardiac transcatheter pacing system. N Engl J Med 2016;374(6):533–41.
33. Duray GZ, Ritter P, El-Chami M, et al. Long-term performance of a transcatheter pacing system: 12-month results from the Micra Transcatheter Pacing study. Heart Rhythm 2017;14(5):702–9.
34. Theuns DA, Crozier IG, Barr CS, et al. Longevity of the subcutaneous implantable defibrillator: long-term follow-up of the European Regulatory Trial Cohort. Circ Arrhythm Electrophysiol 2015;8(5):1159–63.
35. Pokorney SD, Greenfield RA, Atwater BD, et al. Novel mechanism of premature battery failure due to lithium cluster formation in implantable cardioverter-defibrillators. Heart Rhythm 2014;11(12):2190–5.
36. Aggarwal A, Sarmiento JJ, Charles DR, et al. Accelerated implantable defibrillator battery depletion secondary to lithium cluster formation: a case series. Pacing Clin Electrophysiol 2016;39(4):375–7.
37. Boriani G, Ritter P, Biffi M, et al. Battery drain in daily practice and medium-term projections on longevity of cardioverter-defibrillators: an analysis from a remote monitoring database. Europace 2016;18(9):1366–73.

Use of the Wearable Cardioverter Defibrillator as a Bridge to Implantable Cardioverter Defibrillator

Jonathan Weinstock, MD

KEYWORDS

• Sudden cardiac death • Wearable defibrillator • Cardiomyopathy • Ventricular arrhythmias

KEY POINTS

• The wearable cardioverter defibrillator has been shown to be effective in terminating ventricular arrhythmias in patients at risk for sudden cardiac death.
• There are numerous scenarios in which implant of a permanent implantable cardioverter defibrillator is temporarily contraindicated or not advisable and a wearable cardioverter defibrillator may be beneficial.
• There are no prospective randomized studies published that provide conclusive guidance toward the use of the wearable cardioverter defibrillator, and thus, patient management needs to be individualized based on the available data.

INTRODUCTION

The advent of the implantable cardioverter defibrillator (ICD) has revolutionized the primary and secondary prevention of sudden cardiac death (SCD). However, several potential situations exist in which the implantation of an ICD, either transvenous or subcutaneous, at a given point in time is not advisable or indicated for other reasons. The wearable cardioverter defibrillator (WCD) provides a potential temporary alternative to ICD implantation in such situations. This review summarizes the technical aspects of the WCD, efficacy, and potential indications for use as a bridge to an ICD.

THE WEARABLE CARDIOVERTER DEFIBRILLATOR

The WCD was approved for clinical use by the US Food and Drug Administration in 2001.[1] At the time of this writing, the device is produced by a single manufacturer (LifeVest; Zoll Medical Corporation, Chelmsford, MA, USA). Its application requires no surgical procedure, and unlike implanted ICD technology, requires significant participation from the patient. The device consists of a garment and a battery pack. The garment is customized to fit the individual patient's body habitus and contains 4 electrodes for cardiac rhythm sensing and 3 defibrillation pads arranged in a posterior to apical configuration. The battery pack functions as the monitor and defibrillator, is connected to the garment, and is carried with a shoulder strap or via a holster at the waist. The patient is provided with a battery charger and a modem. The WCD has the ability to store and transmit data remotely to a secure Internet portal, including electrocardiogram (ECG) recordings of events leading to

Disclosure: Dr J. Weinstock is the local principal investigator at Tufts Medical Center for the VEST study, sponsored by Zoll Inc.
Department of Medicine, Division of Cardiology, Tufts University School of Medicine, Cardiac Arrhythmia Center, Tufts Medical Center, 800 Washington Street, Boston, MA 02118, USA
E-mail address: Jweinstock1@tuftsmedicalcenter.org

Card Electrophysiol Clin 10 (2018) 11–16
https://doi.org/10.1016/j.ccep.2017.11.002

shocks, nonsustained arrhythmias above the rate cutoff, asystolic events, patient-initiated recordings, and patient compliance.

Rate cutoff parameters for ventricular tachycardia (VT) and ventricular fibrillation (VF) can be programmed as can the shock energy (between 75 and 150 J) for each shock. The VT zone can be programmed to between 120 and 250 bpm, up to the floor of the VF zone. The default parameters are 150 to 200 bpm for VT, greater than 200 bpm for VF, and 150 J per shock. The device can deliver a maximum of 5 shocks per episode. The garment requires replacement after an episode is treated. The WCD cannot provide any pacing.[2]

Once the WCD detects an arrhythmia above the prescribed rate cutoff, morphology analysis compares it with a template of the patient's baseline rhythm as well as other filters to attempt to exclude external interference. If the device algorithms confirm a ventricular arrhythmia, a series of patient responsiveness alerts are initiated, which include an audible alarm, vibration of elements of the garment, and a message on the monitor pack. A conscious patient has the ability to depress 2 buttons on the monitor simultaneously, which will abort the shock. If the shock is not aborted, gel is automatically applied by the device to the defibrillation pads, and a shock or shocks are delivered. Detection within the VT zone results in a synchronized shock, as opposed to the VF zone, which triggers an unsynchronized shock. The elapsed time from arrhythmia onset to shock delivery is approximately 45 to 50 seconds. That time consists of detection criteria of 5 to 10 seconds, arrhythmia confirmation of 10 seconds, and 25 seconds of the arrhythmia alarm mechanism, during which the patient can manually abort the shock.[3]

SENSING AND SHOCK EFFICACY

The sensing algorithm of the WCD has been reported to result in a high sensitivity (90%–100%) and specificity (98%–99%). The rate of inappropriate shocks in clinical studies has been low (0.5%–2% per month).[3–5] Data regarding efficacy of the WCD are comparable to implanted ICDs and are derived from induced VF and from clinical studies. Twenty-two episodes of VF induced during electrophysiology study were successfully terminated with either a 70- or a 100-J biphasic shock from a WCD in 12 patients, providing a wide safety margin up to 150 J from the device.[6] In a study of 8453 patient prescribed a WCD after myocardial infarction (MI), a total of 146 arrhythmia events occurred in 133 patients, with a successful conversion rate of 82%. The short-term survival rate in those patients who received a shock was 91%.[5] In a registry of 2000 patients prescribed a WCD, a total of 30 appropriate shocks in 22 patients were delivered, all of which were successful in terminating VT or VF. Of note, in that same registry, therapies for 90 true arrhythmic events in 22 patients were manually aborted by the patient.[4]

PATIENT COMPLIANCE

A key element in the potential efficacy of the WCD is patient adherence. Directions accompanying device use are to wear it at all times, other than during bathing. Factors limiting the use of the device most commonly relate to patient discomfort and limitation on lifestyle. In 2 large nonrandomized series of patients using a WCD, median daily use was 21.7 and 22.5 hours, respectively.[4,5] In published studies, 14% to 25% of patients stopped using the WCD prematurely mostly because of comfort issues.[5,6]

WEARABLE CARDIOVERTER DEFIBRILLATOR CLINICAL STUDIES

It is important to note that at this time there are no published randomized data to guide the use of the WCD. As such, patient care decisions are based on data from nonrandomized prospective studies or retrospective analyses of patients wearing the WCD.

The first major study to address the clinical use of the WCD was the Wearable Defibrillator Investigative Trial and Bridge to ICD in Patients at Risk of Arrhythmic Death (WEARIT/BIROAD) study.[7] The publication was the combined results of 2 separate investigations. The WEARIT study enrolled patients with a left ventricular ejection fraction (LVEF) of less than 30% and New York Heart Association (NYHA) class III to IV congestive heart failure (CHF) symptoms who were not eligible for an ICD based on indications at that time. The BIROAD study enrolled patients for 4 months with several factors deemed to be high risk, including patients who had experienced a recent MI with VT/VF within 48 hours, LVEF of less than 30% more than 3 days after an MI, or cardiac arrest more than 48 hours after the MI, but otherwise not a candidate for an ICD. Other inclusion criteria included a ventricular arrhythmia within 48 hours after coronary artery bypass graft (CABG), LVEF of less than 30% at least 3 days after CABG, cardiac arrest or syncope at least 48 hours after CABG, but not able to have an ICD implanted, ICD candidates at home who were not expected to receive an ICD for 4 months, or patients who had refused ICD implantation. A total of 289 patients were enrolled in the combined studies. There were a total of 8 attempts at WCD defibrillation in follow-up, 6 of which were successful. The 2 unsuccessful attempts were both in patients who were not wearing the device correctly: one of which was shocked successfully with an external defibrillator, and the other died suddenly. Twelve patients died during the study, none of whom were wearing the device correctly at the time of death. Six of the 12 deaths were non-sudden, and 5 patients died suddenly while not wearing the device. There were 6 inappropriate shocks in 6 patients from the WCD during follow-up. Sixty-five of 289 patients withdrew from the study before reaching an endpoint, because of comfort or lifestyle issues. This study documented the effectiveness of the WCD in preventing sudden death in compliant patients who wore the device correctly.

Data were analyzed from a manufacturer registry of 3569 patients who wore a WCD for a mean of 53 ± 70 days between 2002 and 2006.[8] Indications for WCD use were prior ICD explanation (23%), ventricular arrhythmia before planned ICD implant (16%), recent MI (16%) or CABG (16%), and recent cardiomyopathy diagnosed, with an LVEF of less than 35% (28%). Fourteen percent of patients prematurely discontinued use of the WCD, a lower rate than previously observed likely because of the lighter and smaller size of the newer generation of WCD used. Median daily use of the WCD was 21.7 hours. Eighty sustained VT/VF episodes occurred in 59 patients (1.7% of patients). Effectiveness of the first shock was 99%, and survival after successful shock was 89.5%. Importantly, non-VT/VF events, specifically asystole and pulseless electrical activity, accounted for 24.5 of cardiac arrests during WCD use. The investigators concluded that survival after VT/VF with the WCD was comparable to ICD studies, but that non-VT/VF events accounted for a significant proportion of sudden death in this setting.

In a similar retrospective analysis of 8453 patient prescribed a WCD within 3 months of an MI between 2005 and 2011, 1.6% of patients received an appropriate shock. The median time from the index event to the first appropriate shock was 9 days, and survival from the event was 93%. While wearing the WCD, 1.2% of patients received inappropriate shocks.[5]

The WEARIT-II registry prospectively enrolled 2000 patients between 2011 and 2014, with a mix of indications including ischemic and nonischemic cardiomyopathy (NICM) and congenital heart disease. Forty-one patients had sustained VT during WCD use, with a total of 120 episodes. Importantly, 90 events were manually aborted (in 22 patients). The remaining events were successfully terminated with a shock from the WCD. The inappropriate shock rate was low at 0.5%. Patients with NICM had a lower probability of receiving a shock when compared with ischemic cardiomyopathy and NICM. Three patients died during follow-up with an asystolic event recorded on the WCD. Eighty-five percent of the patients who had an appropriate shock subsequently underwent ICD implant, whereas less than half who had no therapy had an ICD implanted.[4]

Several other smaller case series and retrospective analyses studied the use of the WCD in other more specific populations, such as patients newly diagnosed with a cardiomyopathy listed for heart transplantation,[7] peripartum cardiomyopathy,[9] patients younger than 21 years old,[10] and inherited arrhythmias.[11] The larger studies discussed above as well as these smaller studies are summarized in **Table 1**.

POTENTIAL WEARABLE CARDIOVERTER DEFIBRILLATOR INDICATIONS
After Myocardial Infarction

The evidence from 2 major clinical trials has resulted in guidelines discouraging the use of an ICD within 40 days of an MI. The Immediate Risk Stratification Improves Survival (IRIS) study randomized 898 patients 5 to 31 days after an MI to medical therapy or an ICD (with medical therapy).[12] Enrollment criteria included LVEF less than 40% with a high resting heart rate on the first available ECG, nonsustained VT, or both. Overall mortality was similar in both arms with lower arrhythmic death offset by higher nonarrhythmic death. The DINAMIT (Defibrillator and Acute Myocardial Infarction Trial) study similarly randomized 674 patients with LVEF less than 35%, 6 to 40 days after MI, with cardiac autonomic dysfunction or high heart rate on monitoring to medical therapy or ICD.[13] Mirroring the results of IRIS, there was no difference in mortality in the 2 arms for similar reasons.

In the absence of randomized data, an American Heart Association/Heart Rhythm Society Science advisory in 2015 listed WCD use in this scenario as a class IIb indication with level of evidence C (may be appropriate to use WCD).[2] It is hoped that clearer guidance will be forthcoming from the VEST (Vest Prevention of Early Sudden Death Trial), which is an ongoing study randomizing patients after MI with an LVEF of 35% or less to a WCD or medical therapy.[14]

Table 1
Summary of larger clinical studies of wearable cardioverter defibrillator use

Author, Year	Number of Subjects	Population Description	Hours/ Day Worn	Shock Rate Appropriate (%)	Shock Rate Inappropriate (%)	Survival (%)
Kutyifa et al,[4] 2015	2000	Ischemic, nonischemic, congenital/inherited heart disease prescribed WCD	22.5	1.1	0.5	99.8
Epstein et al,[5] 2013	8453	Within 3 mo of MI	21.8	1.6	1.3	93
Mitrani et al,[21] 2013	134	Recent revascularization or new diagnosis of cardiomyopathy	14	0	0	98
Zishiri et al,[23] 2013	809	LVEF <35 and recent PCI or CABG	N/A	1.3	1.6	98
Kao et al,[22] 2012	82	Patient with CHF listed for transplant, on inotropic therapy or new diagnosis	20	0	0	100
Saltzberg et al,[9] 2012	159 107	NICM Peripartum cardiomyopathy	17 18	0.6 0	0 0	97 85
Rao et al,[11] 2012	119 43	Inherited arrhythmia Congenital heart disease	19 19	2.5 0	5.9 0	97 87
Chung et al,[8] 2010	3569	US Manufacturer Registry	20	1.7	1.9	99
Collins et al,[10] 2010	103 81	Age 19–21 Age <19	19 20	1.9 0	0.9 1.2	91 89
Klein et al,[3] 2010	354	Aggregate German data	21	3.1	0.8	N/A
Feldman et al,[7] 2004	289	WEARIT/BIROAD CHF or bridge to ICD	N/A	1.0	2.1	96

Abbreviations: N/A, not available; PCI, percutaneous coronary intervention.
Data from Piccini JP, Allen LA, Kudenchuk PJ, et al. Wearable cardioverter-defibrillator therapy for the prevention of sudden cardiac death: a science advisory from the American Heart Association. Circulation 2016;133(17):1715–27.

TEMPORARY IMPAIRMENT OF LEFT VENTRICULAR FUNCTION

There are several scenarios in which LV dysfunction exists but may be a temporary condition that could be improved by an active intervention. Examples of this scenario include the immediate period following coronary revascularization, or a newly diagnosed NICM initiating medical therapy.

ICD implantation has shown to not improve mortality when used in the period immediately following coronary bypass surgery.[15] There is a heightened risk of SCD in patients with an LVEF of less than 35%, but yet there is improvement in LV function in as many as half of patients undergoing CABG.[16] Because of these data, guideline statements and government payers currently mandate a waiting period of 90 days following coronary revascularization with subsequent reevaluation of LVEF, before implanting an ICD.

The Sudden Cardiac Death Heart Failure trial (SCD-HeFT) trial demonstrated the benefit of a single-chamber ICD for the primary prevention of SCD in patients with a NICM, NYHA class II to III symptoms, and LVEF less than 35%. Notably, the design of the study enrolled patients only after a minimum of 3 months from the initial diagnosis, and on optimal medical therapy.[17] When the ICD was studied in a similar population with a diagnosis of NICM within 9 months of enrollment, no mortality benefit was shown.[18] Similar to coronary revascularization, the possibility of improvement in LV function exists in NICM with medical therapy. Current practice is to wait for at least 3 months from the diagnosis of NICM and to repeat assessment of LV function before committing to an ICD.

Several other temporary or correctable scenarios with uncertain risk of SCD may be appropriate settings for use of a WCD. These conditions include peripartum cardiomyopathy, tachycardia-induced cardiomyopathy, stress cardiomyopathy, and others. The likelihood of recovery of LV dysfunction in these situations is high, and yet the risk of SCD during recovery is poorly understood.

Combined, these situations of potentially temporary periods of SCD risk, where ICD implantation is not recommended, constitute a class IIb indication with level of evidence C (may be appropriate to use WCD). It may be helpful to consider other high-risk features such as nonsustained ventricular tachycardia or a high burden of premature ventricular contractions in deciding on the use of the WCD in such patients.

After Implantable Cardioverter Defibrillator Extraction

ICD system infection often results in lead extraction and removal of the ICD generator. Depending of the extent of the infection, the duration of antibiotic therapy and delay to reimplantation can be prolonged. For short periods, and depending on other patient factors, it may be reasonable to keep a patient in a hospital until a new ICD is implanted. For longer waiting periods of antibiotic therapy, the WCD can provide a temporary measure as a means of SCD prevention. In making the decision to use the WCD in this scenario, the underlying risk of SCD could be considered. Specifically, a patient who was initially implanted for secondary prevention or had prior appropriate therapy may have a stronger indication than a similar primary prevention indication. Current guidelines indicate this set of circumstances to be reasonable (class IIa recommendation, level of evidence C).[2]

DECISION MAKING AND THE WEARABLE CARDIOVERTER DEFIBRILLATOR

As discussed earlier in this review, there are currently no published randomized data regarding the use of the WCD in any clinical situation. The lack of data limits any scientific statements/guidelines from making any class I recommendation. The last few decades have seen numerous instances of cardiovascular therapies that appear intuitively beneficial that have subsequently gone on to not impart any benefit, or even be harmful when studied in a randomized clinical trial.[13,19] Although the WCD appears effective in preventing SCD in a variety of situations, the absence of a control arm confounds any definite recommendation of widespread application of the technology. It is possible that in this vulnerable population, the stress caused to patients by its use or a sympathetic surge resulting from WCD alarms caused by telemetry noise may outweigh any benefit.[20] It is hoped that the ongoing VEST study will address these limitations in the immediate post-MI population, which represents a large proportion of the patients in which WCD could be used.

As with any medical therapy, the use of the WCD has to be individualized to a particular patient. The underlying risk of SCD in the time period of use of the WCD has to be weighed against any potential downside. Importantly, patient compliance and the ability to interact with the device have to be taken into account. For example, a patient undergoing an ICD extraction, with prior frequent appropriate shocks, in which compliance with wearing the WCD is expected to be low, alternative solutions (such as a rehabilitation facility with telemetry) may need to be favored over WCD prescription. In addition, the inability to apply the device correctly and understand the shock abort mechanism may serve as a contraindication to WCD use.

SUMMARY

The WCD is an effective tool in the prevention of SCD as a temporary bridge to ICD therapy in a variety of scenarios. The data guiding the use of the WCD are derived from prospective nonrandomized studies or retrospective analyses. Although the WCD can be considered a bridge to an ICD in these situations, it is difficult to make definite wide-ranging recommendations. As such, decisions regarding the use of the WCD have to be individualized, taking into account the temporary risk of SCD in the given time period, and the likelihood of patient compliance and ability to use the device. Results of an upcoming randomized study addressing the use of the WCD in the immediate post-MI period will be helpful, but better-designed prospective randomized studies in other scenarios are needed.

REFERENCES

1. Premarket Approval (PMA). Available at: https://www.accessdata.fda.gov/scripts/cdrh/cfdocs/cfpma/pma.cfm?id=P010030. Accessed July 6, 2017.
2. Piccini JP, Allen LA, Kudenchuk PJ, et al. Wearable cardioverter-defibrillator therapy for the prevention of sudden cardiac death: a science advisory from the American Heart Association. Circulation 2016; 133(17):1715–27.
3. Klein HU, Meltendorf U, Reek S, et al. Bridging a temporary high risk of sudden arrhythmic death. Experience with the wearable cardioverter defibrillator (WCD). Pacing Clin Electrophysiol 2010;33(3): 353–67.
4. Kutyifa V, Moss AJ, Klein H, et al. Use of the wearable cardioverter defibrillator in high-risk cardiac patients. Circulation 2015;132(17):1613–9.
5. Epstein AE, Abraham WT, Bianco NR, et al. Wearable cardioverter-defibrillator use in patients perceived to be at high risk early post-myocardial infarction. J Am Coll Cardiol 2013;62(21):2000–7.
6. Reek S, Geller JC, Meltendorf U, et al. Clinical efficacy of a wearable defibrillator in acutely terminating episodes of ventricular fibrillation using biphasic shocks. Pacing Clin Electrophysiol 2003;26(10): 2016–22.
7. Feldman AM, Klein H, Tchou P, et al. Use of a wearable defibrillator in terminating tachyarrhythmias in patients at high risk for sudden death: results of the WEARIT/BIROAD. Pacing Clin Electrophysiol 2004;27(1):4–9.
8. Chung MK, Szymkiewicz SJ, Shao M, et al. Aggregate national experience with the wearable cardioverter-defibrillator. J Am Coll Cardiol 2010;56(3): 194–203.
9. Saltzberg MT, Szymkiewicz S, Bianco NR. Characteristics and outcomes of peripartum versus nonperipartum cardiomyopathy in women using a wearable cardiac defibrillator. J Card Fail 2012;18(1):21–7.
10. Collins KK, Silva JNA, Rhee EK, et al. Use of a wearable automated defibrillator in children compared to young adults. Pacing Clin Electrophysiol 2010;33(9): 1119–24.
11. Rao M, Goldenberg I, Moss AJ, et al. Wearable defibrillator in congenital structural heart disease and inherited arrhythmias. Am J Cardiol 2011;108(11): 1632–8.
12. Steinbeck G, Andresen D, Seidl K, et al. Defibrillator implantation early after myocardial infarction. N Engl J Med 2009;361(15):1427–36.
13. Hohnloser SH, Kuck KH, Dorian P, et al. Prophylactic use of an implantable cardioverter–defibrillator after acute myocardial infarction. N Engl J Med 2004; 351(24):2481–8.
14. Vest Prevention of Early Sudden Death Trial and VEST Registry - Full Text View - ClinicalTrials.gov. Available at: https://clinicaltrials.gov/ct2/show/NCT01446965. Accessed July 22, 2017.
15. Bigger JT. Prophylactic use of implanted cardiac defibrillators in patients at high risk for ventricular arrhythmias after coronary-artery bypass graft surgery. N Engl J Med 1997;337(22):1569–75.
16. Toda K, Mackenzie K, Mehra MR, et al. Revascularization in severe ventricular dysfunction (15% < OR = LVEF < OR = 30%): a comparison of bypass grafting and percutaneous intervention. Ann Thorac Surg 2002;74(6):2082–7.
17. Bardy GH, Lee KL, Mark DB, et al. Amiodarone or an implantable cardioverter–defibrillator for congestive heart failure. N Engl J Med 2005;352(3):225–37.
18. Bänsch D, Antz M, Boczor S, et al. Primary prevention of sudden cardiac death in idiopathic dilated cardiomyopathy: the cardiomyopathy trial (CAT). Circulation 2002;105(12):1453–8.
19. Echt DS, Liebson PR, Mitchell LB, et al. Mortality and morbidity in patients receiving encainide, flecainide, or placebo. N Engl J Med 1991;324(12): 781–8.
20. Lee BK, Olgin JE. The wearable cardioverter-defibrillator. Circulation 2016;134(9):644–6.
21. Mitrani RD, Mcardle A, Slane M, et al. Wearable defibrillators in uninsured patients with newly diagnosed cardiomyopathy or recent revascularization in a community medical center. Am Heart J 2013; 165(3):386–92.
22. Kao AC, Krause SW, Handa R, et al. Wearable defibrillator use in heart failure (WIF): results of a prospective registry. BMC Cardiovasc Disord 2012; 12(1):123.
23. Zishiri ET, Williams S, Cronin EM, et al. Early risk of mortality after coronary artery revascularization in patients with left ventricular dysfunction and potential role of the wearable cardioverter defibrillator clinical perspective. Circ Arrhythmia Electrophysiol 2013;6(1).

Leadless Pacemakers
State of the Art and Future Perspectives

Domenico G. Della Rocca, MD[a], Carola Gianni, MD, PhD[a],
Luigi Di Biase, MD, PhD[a,b,c,d], Andrea Natale, MD[a,c,e,f,g,h,i],
Amin Al-Ahmad, MD[a,*]

KEYWORDS

- Cardiac pacing • Cardiac arrhythmias • Leadless pacemaker • Transvenous pacemaker
- Bradyarrhythmias • Transvenous leads • Cardiac resynchronization therapy

KEY POINTS

- Conventional cardiac pacemakers are prone to multiple potential short- and long-term complications owing to the surgical pocket and/or placement of epicardial or transvenous leads.
- Leadless pacemaker therapy is a new technology that aims at avoiding lead- and pocket-related complications of conventional transvenous and epicardial pacing.
- Two self-contained leadless pacemakers for right ventricular pacing are available clinically: the Nanostim Leadless Pacemaker System and the Micra Transcatheter Pacing System.
- A new multicomponent leadless pacemaker for endocardial left ventricular pacing (WiSE-CRT) has been proposed as an alternative for cardiac resynchronization therapy.

INTRODUCTION

Leadless pacemaker (PMK) therapy is a new technology that has been recently introduced into clinical practice. The aim of leadless pacing is to avoid lead- and pocket-related complications. Conventional cardiac PMKs are prone to multiple potential short- and long-term complications as a result of the creation of a surgical pocket and/or the placement of epicardial or transvenous leads. In this article, we sought to describe the state of the art of leadless pacing and compare the currently available devices with traditional transvenous PMKs. This article also addresses the future perspectives of leadless pacing.

Disclosures: Dr L. Di Biase is a consultant for Biosense Webster, Boston Scientific, Stereotaxis, and St. Jude Medical; and has received speaker honoraria from Medtronic, AtriCure, EPiEP, and Biotronik. Dr A. Natale has received speaker honoraria from Boston Scientific, Biosense Webster, St. Jude Medical, Biotronik, and Medtronic, and is a consultant for Biosense Webster, St. Jude Medical, and Janssen. Dr A. Al-Ahmad has received honoraria from Medtronic and St. Jude Medical. All other authors have reported that they have no relationships relevant to the contents of this paper to disclose.

[a] Texas Cardiac Arrhythmia Institute, St. David's Medical Center, 3000 North IH-35, Suite 720, Austin, TX 78705, USA; [b] Albert Einstein College of Medicine, Montefiore Hospital, Bronx, NY, USA; [c] Department of Biomedical Engineering, Cockrell School of Engineering, University of Texas, Austin, TX, USA; [d] Department of Cardiology, University of Foggia, Foggia, Italy; [e] Department of Internal Medicine, Dell Medical School, University of Texas, Austin, TX, USA; [f] Interventional Electrophysiology, Scripps Clinic, La Jolla, CA, USA; [g] Department of Cardiology, MetroHealth Medical Center, Case Western Reserve University School of Medicine, Cleveland, OH, USA; [h] Division of Cardiology, Stanford University, Stanford, CA, USA; [i] Atrial Fibrillation and Arrhythmia Center, California Pacific Medical Center, San Francisco, CA, USA
* Corresponding author.
E-mail address: aalahmadmd@gmail.com

Card Electrophysiol Clin 10 (2018) 17–29
https://doi.org/10.1016/j.ccep.2017.11.003

PACEMAKER TECHNOLOGY: HISTORICAL CONSIDERATIONS AND STATISTICS

In 1932, Albert S. Hyman reported for the first time the effect of an external cardiac PMK: a bipolar needle electrode introduced via an intercostal space was used to direct electrical impulses into the patient's right atrium at pacing rates of 30, 60, or 120 per minutes. Since the report on the successful implantation of the first epicardial pacing system by Rune Elmquist and Åke Senning and of the first transvenous temporary pacing lead in 1958, technology for conventional cardiac pacing has evolved considerably. Initially, efforts were addressed to size and battery life, in an attempt to downsize the body and prolong longevity.

In the mid 1980s, rate-responsive PMKs were developed; this feature can adapt the pacing rates according to the patient's physical activity. In the 1990s, microprocessor-driven PMKs were introduced into clinical practice; as a result of the development of several algorithms, devices became automatically capable of adapting their internal parameters to the changing needs of the patient. The idea of biventricular pacing was developed in the late 1980s and early 1990s, after the results of several animal studies that demonstrated a linear decrease in left ventricular pressure as the QRS duration increases.[1] In 1996, Cazeau and colleagues[2] demonstrated that biventricular pacing is associated with an acute and sustained hemodynamic improvement in patients with end-stage heart failure. In patients undergoing cardiac resynchronization therapy (CRT), an additional lead is generally introduced to the epicardial surface of the left ventricle (LV) via the coronary sinus, in the attempt to resynchronize contraction of the LV, thereby improving cardiac function and symptoms.

Despite remarkable advances in cardiac pacing and resynchronization therapy,[3–5] this technology is still prone to several potential acute and chronic complications.

Overall, approximately 1 million pacemakers are implanted worldwide, with 26% of the total being replacement devices.[6] Complications are mainly related to the transvenous leads and the subcutaneous generator pocket. Short-term complications often related to the procedure include pneumothorax, cardiac tamponade, lead dislodgement, and pocket hematoma. Long-term complications include insulation breaches, lead fractures, skin erosions, pocket infections, and septicemia. Transvenous leads can also cause upper extremity deep vein thrombosis, venous obstruction, tricuspid valve insufficiency, and endocarditis. The incidence of postoperative adverse events has been estimated as high as 10%.[7] Transvenous leads are the most vulnerable components of the system: in addition to insulation defects and fractures, which require reintervention, endocarditis can be a life-threatening complication with mortality rates of 12% to 31%.[8,9] Pocket-related complications occur in 0.7% to 2.4% of patients[10,11]: a clinically significant pocket hematoma is an important risk factor of infection, which is associated with a greater than 7-fold increased risk of hospitalization owing to infection within 1 year after device implantation.[11]

Leadless cardiac pacing was proposed in the 1970s[12] as an alternative solution to conventional pacing, with the aim to avoid transvenous leads and the need for a subcutaneous device pocket, thereby eliminating lead- and pocket-related complications. Additionally, a self-contained device, delivered directly to the heart, prevents any cosmetic concern by eliminating the physical signs of the device.

The leadless pacing system proposed in 1970[12] was a prototype capsule, 8 mm in diameter and 18 mm in length, designed to allow transvenous insertion in animal models. The intracardiac system was powered by a mercury battery and had a radially directed spiral barb system that showed stable thresholds. The system was implanted in a dog and showed stable pacing rates even during severe exercise. The further development of these technologies have led to the introduction of 2 different leadless pacing systems.

To date, 2 self-contained leadless pacemakers are clinically available: the Nanostim Leadless Pacemaker System (LPS; St. Jude Medical, Sylmar, CA) and the Micra Transcatheter Pacing System (TPS; Medtronic, Minneapolis, MN).

TECHNOLOGICAL FEATURES OF CURRENTLY AVAILABLE SINGLE-COMPONENT LEADLESS PACEMAKERS
Technological Aspects

The Nanostim LPS (St. Jude Medical) was the world's first commercially available leadless pacing system: it received the CE mark in October 2013, but is still awaiting US Food and Drug Administration approval. The Micra TPS (Medtronic) received the CE mark in April 2015 and US Food and Drug Administration approval in April 2016. A comparison of the characteristics of the 2 pacing systems is reported in **Table 1**. The Nanostim LPS measures 41.4 × 5.99 mm and has a volume of 1 cm^3. The Micra TPS is a 25.9 × 6.7-mm device, which displaces a volume of 0.8 cm^3. The 2 currently available leadless pacing systems share a few similarities: (a) they are delivered

Table 1
Characteristics of the leadless pacing systems

Specifications	Nanostim Leadless Cardiac Pacemaker	Micra Transcatheter Pacing System
Dimensions (mm)	41.4 × 5.99	25.9 × 6.7
Volume (cm^3)	1.0	0.8
Weight (g)	2	2
Primary fixation system	Helix (screw-in)	Nitinol tines
Secondary fixation system	Nylon tines	—
Pacing mode	VVI (R)	VVI (R)
Rate response sensor	Temperature	3-axis accelerometer
Battery	Lithium carbon-monofluoride (integrated)	Lithium silver vanadium oxide/carbon monofluoride (integrated)
Battery longevity (y)	8.5–9.8	4.7–9.6
Retrieval option	Yes	Yes
Sheath size (French)	18	23
Communication	Conductive	Rediofrequency
MRI compatibility	Full body MRI conditionally safe	Full body MRI conditionally safe

through the femoral vein via a deflectable catheter, (b) pacing features are similar to a conventional single chamber ventricular (VVI) PMK, (c) both units incorporate a motion sensor and a rate-response algorithm, (d) both include steroid-eluting tips, which reduce inflammation and maintain low stimulation thresholds, and (e) the proximal end of the devices has been designed to recapture the system if repositioning is necessary or if the device needs to be retrieved.

The main differences between the 2 systems are (a) fixation, (b) programming systems, and (c) motion sensor function. The Nanostim LPS fixation system is a screw-in helix; a secondary fixation mechanism is provided by 4 nylon tines. A steroid-eluting disc located at the center of the helix acts as the cathode, whereas the anode is the uncoated ring of the titanium case. The Micra TPS attaches to the apical septum through the use of 4 flexible, electrically inactive, nitinol tines. The cathode is a steroid-eluting tip, which is spaced 18 mm from a titanium nitride ring acting as the anode.

Interrogation and programming of the devices are achieved via 2 different communication systems. The Nanostim LPS uses conductive communication via a dedicated programmer, which uses skin leads to apply subliminal 250 kHz pulses for signal transmission and programming. The Micra TPS uses a conventional radiofrequency communication via the same programmer used for conventional Medtronic pacemakers; threshold measurements are performed automatically by the device on a daily basis. As mentioned, both units incorporate a motion sensor and a rate-response algorithm. However, the Nanostim LPS uses a temperature-based sensor, whereas the Micra TPS a 3-axis accelerometer to provide rate-response.

Battery longevity, based on fixed programming at the ISO International Organization for Standardization (ISO 14708) standard guidelines (2.5 V, 0.4 ms, 600 Ω, 60 beats/min, and 100% pacing), has been estimated to be 9.8 years for the Nanostim LCP and 4.7 years for the Micra TPS. However, owing to the innovative design, which optimizes energy consumption and the electrode/tissue interface, the estimated longevity is approximately 10 years for both devices. These longevities are comparable with those of a standard PMK.

As reported recently, the combination of a leadless system and a subcutaneous implantable cardioverter-defibrillator (ICD) seems to be feasible, without interference in pacing and sensing.[13]

From this perspective, Boston Scientific has developed a modular system, based on the combined implant of an antitachycardia pacing–enabled leadless cardiac PMK and a subcutaneous ICD. A key feature of the device is unidirectional device–device communication (subcutaneous ICD to leadless PMK) and antitachycardia pacing delivery by the leadless system. In a preclinical study in an ovine model, appropriate PMK functionality, as well as successful ICD to leadless system communication and antitachycardia pacing delivery by the device, were observed.[14]

Implantation Technique

Both devices can be implanted in the electrophysiology or interventional suite under local anesthesia and fluoroscopic guidance (**Figs. 1** and **2**). The devices are advanced into the right ventricle (RV) through the femoral vein via dedicated deflectable sheaths, which measure 18-F (inner diameter)/21-F (outer diameter) for the Nanostim LPS, and 23-F (inner diameter)/27-F (outer diameter) for the Micra TPS. Once the device is advanced into the RV, contrast medium is injected through the sheath to visualize the appropriate apical septal position. Fixation is achieved by rotating the screw-in helix of the Nanostim LPS with 1.25 turns or by retracting the outer sheath of the delivery system to deploy the tines of the Micra TPS. The screw-in helix of the Nanostim can penetrate in the myocardium for a maximum depth of 1.3 mm.

After the PMK is deployed to the myocardium, electrical parameter measurements are acquired.

Device stability is then evaluated via a gentle tug test. With appropriate electrical parameters and stability of the device, the system is released from the sheath by unlocking the tethering.

SAFETY AND EFFICACY OF SINGLE-COMPONENT LEADLESS PACEMAKERS
Clinical Data for the Nanostim Leadless Pacemaker System

The LEADLESS trial[15] (NCT01700244) was a prospective, nonrandomized, single-arm multicentre study that tested the safety and clinical performance of the Nanostim LPS. The study enrolled 33 patients (mean age, 77 ± 8 years; 67% males) who underwent device implantation between December 2012 and April 2013 in 3 different participating centers. The indications for cardiac pacing were permanent atrial fibrillation with atrioventricular (AV) block (n = 22/33; 67%), second- or third-degree AV block in patients with a low level of physical activity or short expected lifespan (n = 6/33; 18%), sinus bradycardia with

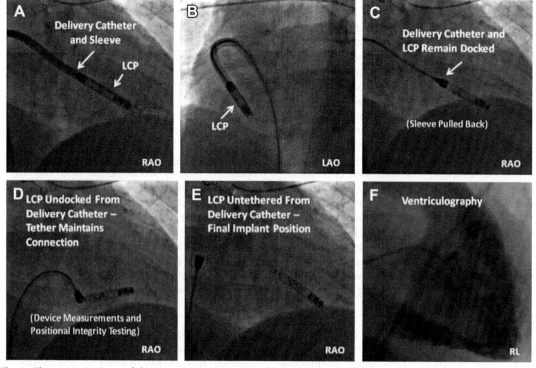

Fig. 1. Fluoroscopic views of the Nanostim LCP implantation procedure. (*A, B*) The delivery catheter and LCP positioning in the RV apex in RAO and LAO views, respectively. (*C*) Withdrawal of the delivery sleeve and maintenance of the connection between the LCP and the delivery catheter. (*D*) Demonstration of positional integrity testing with downward and upward traction applied to the LCP, while the device remains tethered to the delivery catheter. (*E*) Final implant position of the LCP once the delivery catheter has been undocked from the LCP. (*F*) Ventriculogram of the final implant position at the RV apex. LAO, left anterior oblique; LCP, leadless cardiac pacemaker; RAO, right anterior oblique; RL, right lateral; RV, right ventricular. (*From* Reddy VY, Knops RE, Sperzel J, et al. Permanent leadless cardiac pacing: Results of the LEADLESS trial. Circulation 2014;129(14):1466–71; with permission.)

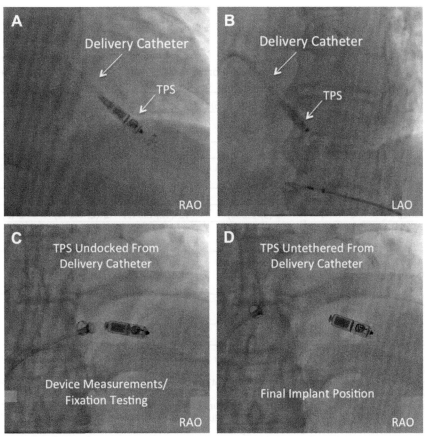

Fig. 2. Fluoroscopic views of the Micra TPS implantation procedure. (*A, B*) The delivery catheter and the TPS positioning in the RV in the RAO and LAO views, respectively. (*C*) Withdrawal of the delivery sleeve and maintenance of the connection between the TPS and the delivery catheter. (*D*) Final implant position of the TPS once the delivery catheter has been undocked from the TPS. LAO, left anterior oblique; RAO, right anterior oblique; RV, right ventricle; TPS, transcatheter pacing system.

infrequent pauses or unexplained syncope with electrophysiologic findings (n = 5/33; 15%). The primary safety endpoint was freedom from serious adverse device events at 90 days; the second safety point was implant success rate. PMK performance characteristics were also evaluated, including R-wave amplitude, pacing threshold, pacing impedance, pacing percentage, and cell charge. The device was successfully implanted in 32 patients (97%), with an average procedural time of 28 ± 17 minutes (**Table 2**). In 23 of 32 patients, the device was implanted without the need of further repositioning or the use of more than 1 system during the procedure. Five patients required more than 1 LCP during the procedure: 1 patient had an inadvertent placement of the device into the LV through a patent foramen ovale (the device was retrieved and another system was positioned in the RV during the same procedure); 4 patients experience problems with the delivery system or the device (malfunction of the release knob [n = 1], dysfunction of the deflection mechanism [n = 1], damage of the catheter secondary to

tortuosity of the venous system [n = 1], damage to the LCP helix during insertion [n = 1]). The overall complication-free rate was 94% (n = 31/33) and 1 serious adverse device effect was reported (see **Table 2**). Over the 3-month follow-up period, electrical parameters significantly improved and no adverse events requiring a revision of the system were needed. The 1-year follow-up results of the LEADLESS trial[15,16] showed no PMK-related adverse events and stable electrical performance.

The LEADLESS II trial[17] was a prospective, nonrandomized, multicenter clinical study that enrolled a total cohort of 526 patients (mean age, 75.8 ± 12.1 years; 61.8% males) with indication for permanent VVI pacing between February 2014 and June 2015 in 56 different participating centers in 3 countries. The primary efficacy endpoint was both an acceptable pacing threshold and R-wave amplitude; the primary safety endpoint was freedom from device-related serious adverse events at 6 months of follow-up. Non–device-related serious adverse events were also

Table 2
Device-related major complications

	Leadless I[15] (n = 33)	Leadless II,[17] Primary Cohort (n = 300)	Leadless II,[17] Total Cohort (n = 526)	Micra TPS Study[18] (n = 725)	Micra TPS Registry[20] (n = 795)
Success rate, % (n/N)	97 (32/33)	95.8 (504/526)		99.2 (719/725)	99.6 (792/795)
Procedure duration (min)	28 ± 17	29 ± 18		35 ± 24	—
Adverse events,[a] number of events (patients, %)					
Total major complications	1 (1, 3.0%)	22 (20, 6.7%)	40 (34, 6.5%)	28 (25, 3.4%)	13 (12, 1.5%)
Cardiac injury[b]	1 (1, 3.0%)	4 (4, 1.3%)	8 (8, 1.5%)	11 (11, 1.5%)	1 (1, 0.1%)
Pacing issues[c]	0	9 (9, 3.0%)	12 (12, 2.3%)	2 (2, 0.3%)	2 (2, 0.2%)
Event at groin puncture site[d]	0	4 (4, 1.3%)	6 (6, 1.1%)	5 (5, 0.7%)	6 (6, 0.8)
Arrhythmia during device implantation[e]	0[h]	2 (2, 0.7%)	4 (4, 0.8%)	0	0
Embolism and thrombosis[f]	0	1 (1, 0.3%)	2 (2, 0.4%)	2 (2, 0.3%)	1 (1, 0.1%)
Other[g]	0	2 (2, 0.7%)	8 (8, 1.5%)	8 (8, 1.1%)	3 (3, 0.4)

[a] See the Clinical Data for the Nanostim Leadless Pacemaker System and Clinical Data for the Micra Transcatheter Pacing System sections for definitions of serious adverse events.
[b] Cardiac injury includes cardiac tamponade with intervention, cardiac perforation with intervention, and pericardial effusion with no intervention.
[c] Pacing issues are device dislodgment, device migration during implantation, and pacing threshold elevation.
[d] Event at groin puncture site is an arteriovenous fistula, failure of vascular closure, hematoma, incision site hemorrhage, persistent lymphatic fistula, or vascular pseudoaneurysm.
[e] Arrhythmia during device implantation is asystole, ventricular tachycardia or ventricular fibrillation, or cardiac arrest.
[f] Embolism and thrombosis include pulmonary embolism, deep vein thrombosis, and ischemic stroke.
[g] Other includes acute myocardial infarction, angina pectoris, chest pain, cardiac failure, contrast induced nephropathy, hemothorax, metabolic acidosis, neurologic symptoms (aphasia, confusion, dysarthria, lethargy), orthstatic hypotension, pacemaker syndrome, pericarditis, presyncope, pulmonary oedema, sepsis, and syncope.
[h] An 86-year-old patient was admitted 2 days after discharge owing to recurrent syncope. Inpatient cardiac monitoring documented monomorphic ventricular tachycardia at 260 bpm, accompanied by syncope. The system was removed 5 days after following the implant and replaced by a single-chamber transvenous implantable cardioverter-defibrillator system.

evaluated. The device was implanted successfully in 504 of the 526 patients (96%), with an average procedural time of 29 ± 18 minutes (see **Table 2**). The primary safety endpoint among the primary cohort of 300 patients who completed the 6-month follow-up was 93.3% (n = 280). Twenty-two device-related serious adverse events were observed among 20 patients (6.7%), and included cardiac perforation (1.3%), device dislodgement (1.7%), elevated pacing thresholds requiring retrieval and replacement (1.3%), and vascular complications (1.3%; see **Table 2**). A similar rate of device-related serious adverse events (6.5%) was reported in the total cohort of 526 patients (cardiac perforation, 1.5%; device dislodgement, 1.1%; device retrieval, 0.8%). Six dislodgements were observed (4 into the pulmonary artery; 2 into the right femoral vein), which occurred after an average of 8.0 ± 6.4 days after device implantation and were

successfully treated percutaneously (see **Table 2**). Among the 28 deaths (5.3%) during follow-up, none was classified as device related and 2 (0.4%) were considered to be procedure related. The primary efficacy endpoint was reached by 270 of the 300 patients in the primary cohort; device implantation was unsuccessful in 11 patients and another 19 patients with successful implantation did not reach the primary efficacy endpoint owing to inadequate pacing capture (n = 4), inadequate sensed R-wave amplitudes (n = 16), or both (n = 1). Overall, electrical parameters significantly improved during follow-up.

Clinical Data for the Micra Transcatheter Pacing System

The Micra Transcatheter Pacing Study[18,19] was a prospective, nonrandomized, single study group, multicenter trial that evaluated the safety and efficacy of the Micra TPS. Overall, 725 patients (mean age, 75.9 ± 10.9 years; 58.8% males) with class I or II guideline-based indications for permanent VVI pacing were enrolled at 56 centers in 19 countries. The indications for cardiac pacing were persistent or permanent atrial tachyarrhythmia and bradycardia (64%), sinus node dysfunction (17.5%), AV block (14.8%), or others (3.7%). The primary efficacy endpoint was an acceptable pacing threshold at 6 months of follow-up; the primary safety endpoint was freedom from device- and procedure-related serious adverse events. Among the 725 patients who underwent an implantation attempt, the device was successfully placed in 719 patients (99.2%; see **Table 2**). The procedure was unsuccessful in 6 patients owing to a major complication (n = 4; 3 cardiac perforations and 1 pericardial effusion), tortuous venous anatomy (n = 1), and unsatisfactory pacing capture threshold (n = 1). There were no dislodgments or infections during follow-up. Overall, 28 major complications were reported in 25 patients (11 cardiac injuries, 5 groin puncture site complications, 2 episodes of thromboembolism, 2 pacing issues, and 8 other complications resulting in hospitalization or prolongation of hospitalization; see **Table 2**). One patient with end-stage renal failure who underwent both AV nodal ablation and Micra TPS implantation died as a result of metabolic acidosis attributable to a prolonged procedure time. In 3 cases, a system revision was required; in 1 case the system was retrieved owing to intermittent loss of capture without radiographic evidence of dislodgment and in 2 patients the system was turned off but not retrieved owing to an elevated pacing capture threshold (n = 1) and the development of a PMK syndrome (n = 1). The primary efficacy endpoint was reached by 292 of the 297 patients (98.3%) who reached the 6-month follow-up. Overall, electrical parameters improved during follow-up.

The Micra Transcatheter Pacing System Post-Approval Registry[20] was a prospective, nonrandomized, multicenter registry aiming to assess the safety and effectiveness of the Micra system in a postapproval setting. The study is still on-going and has a projected total enrollment of 1830 patients. An interim analysis on the first 795 patients (mean age, 75.1 ± 14.2 years; 62.3% males) implanted between July 2015 and January 2017 has been recently published. The aim of the preliminary report is to assess device- and procedure-related serious adverse events during a follow-up period of 30 days after implantation. The indications for cardiac pacing were persistent or permanent atrial tachyarrhythmia and bradycardia (57.7%), AV block (14.7%), syncope (14.1%), sinus node dysfunction (8%), and other or not specified indications (5.5%). One hundred fourteen patients had a previously implanted cardiac device. Among the 795 patients who underwent an implantation attempt, the device was successfully placed in 792 patients (99.6%; see **Table 2**). A total of 13 serious adverse events were reported in 12 patients during the 30-day follow-up (see **Table 2**): 6 groin puncture site complications (in one resulting in arteriovenous fistula), hematoma (n = 2), site haemorrhage (n = 1), persistent lymphatic fistula (n = 1), pseudoaneurysm (n = 1), dislodgment without embolization of the device, which was successfully repositioned 50 days after implantation (n = 1), pericardial effusion/perforation, which was treated with pericardiocentesis on the same day of the procedure (n = 1), deep vein thrombosis (n = 1), others (n = 4); chest pain (n = 1), pulmonary edema (n = 1), sepsis (n = 1), and a device pacing issue (n = 1). Overall, 5 cardiac effusions or perforations were observed, but only 1 case met the criteria for major complication (event resulting in death, prolonged hospitalization ≥48 hours, rehospitalization, system revision, or permanent loss of device function). Twenty-two patients died during the study, but none of the deaths was attributable to the Micra system.

Patients with Limited Upper Venous Access or/and Contraindications for Traditional Pacing

Leadless pacing has been proposed as an alternative and effective solution in patients with limited venous anatomy or contraindications against traditional transvenous pacing. Among them, superior vena cava occlusion, bilateral subclavian thrombosis, recurrent infections at the implant site, and chronic kidney disease with limited venous access, may contraindicate transvenous PMK implantation in the pectoral region and have required a surgical epicardial approach as the only alternative so far.

Venous thrombosis and stenosis are common complications of transvenous implantable cardiac devices and occur more frequently in patients with multiple transvenous leads and without antiplatelet or anticoagulant therapy.[21] The prevalence of venous obstruction or occlusion has been reported to be as high as 12%, but it is even higher in patients with infections, probably as the result of the infection itself.[21] Although venous occlusion is generally symptomless, implantation of new leads, as well as the revision or extraction of previously implanted leads, can be difficult or impossible. Leadless cardiac pacing can be a valid alternative in patients with end-stage kidney disease and limited venous access. In this subset of patients, a high risk of morbidity and mortality, as well as device-related infections, has been reported.[22] Several factors may promote infections, such as immunosuppression, anemia, a higher incidence of pocket hematoma after implantation, catheter-related bacteraemia, the presence of long-term dialysis catheters, advanced age, and related comorbidities. Additionally, the incidence of venous stenosis is significantly higher (32%) among patients on dialysis,[23] who frequently have central catheters, which exclude the use of transvenous cardiac leads.

Device infections are serious complications that imply the need for complete device removal and long-term antibiotic treatment before implanting a new device. From this perspective, leadless technology may bypass these contraindications and prevent the need for an epicardial approach. Limited data are still available[24–28]: in the Micra Transcatheter Pacing System Post-Approval Registry,[20] 166 of 795 patients (20.9%) were allocated to a leadless cardiac system owing to at least 1 condition contraindicating a transvenous approach. Among them, the majority was on dialysis (n = 38), had compromised venous access (n = 72), or a history of or risk for infection (n = 70).

Recently, Da Costa and colleague[24] reported their experience with the Micra system in a cohort of patients with traditional PMK contraindication or limited venous access. Among the 14 patients enrolled in the analysis, bilateral subclavian occlusion was present in 4 patients, total vena cava occlusion in 3, bilaterally infected pectoral tissue in 3, and end-stage renal disease with dialysis and device infection or presence of long-term dialysis catheter in 8. The leadless system was successfully implanted in all the patients and no device-related serious adverse events were observed. Transcatheter leadless cardiac pacing could represent a valuable alternative also in case of congenital venous abnormalities,[26] as well as in patients with severe and recurrent infections with or without bilateral device infection.[27,28]

Complications and the Impact of Operator Experience

Comparison between leadless systems

Complication rates of the 2 commercially available leadless PMK systems are reported in **Table 2**. Overall, both systems demonstrated a high implant success rate and low serious adverse event rate. Additionally, the vast majority of patients who had a successful device implantation met the prespecified primary efficacy endpoint. Further improvement in the mean sensing and pacing threshold values was reported during follow-up, compared with those observed at the time of PMK implantation. In a recent subanalysis of the Micra Transcatheter Pacing Study,[18] patients with a pacing threshold of less than 2 V at implant showed a pacing threshold of 1 V or less during a 12-month follow-up in the vast majority of cases, whereas those with a pacing threshold of greater than 2 V had a significantly higher risk of persistently elevated values at follow-up.[29]

The choice of a leadless pacing system prevents any complication related to the creation of a surgical pocket and/or the placement of epicardial or transvenous leads. Of note, the Micra Transcatheter Pacing Study[18] showed a 51% decrease in the risk of complications compared with traditional PMKs during the first 6 months of follow-up, as well as a lower risk of infections. However, the implantation technique carries a certain risk of femoral vascular complications, which is exclusive to leadless devices as a result of the delivery system. In the 3 larger trials published to date,[17,18,20] the incidence of adverse events at the groin puncture site, such as arteriovenous fistula, failure of vascular closure, hematoma, incision site hemorrhage, persistent lymphatic fistula, and vascular pseudoaneurysm, ranged from 0.7% to 1.3% and was comparable between the 2 systems. It has been hypothesized that leadless pacing might be associated with a higher risk of arrhythmias as a result of the greater area of endocardial contact and fibrosis; however, data from clinical trials have not supported this hypothesis.

Other possible complications are device dislodgment and cardiac injury, such as cardiac tamponade, cardiac perforation, or pericardial effusion. Among Nanostim LPS-implanted patients, device dislodgment was not observed in any of the 33 patients enrolled in the LEADLESS trial[15] and occurred in 6 of the 526 patients in the LEADLESS II trial (1.1%).[17,30] Dislodged devices were identified 8.0 ± 6.4 days after implantation and all were successfully retrieved percutaneously from the pulmonary artery (n = 4) or the right femoral vein (n = 2). Among Micra TPS-implanted patients, no dislodgments were described among the 725 patients of the Micra Transcatheter Pacing Study[18] (in 1 patient, the system was retrieved 17 days after implantation owing to intermittent pacing without radiographic evidence of dislodgment). Device dislodgment without embolization occurred in 1 of the 795 patients (0.1%) enrolled in the Micra Transcatheter Pacing System Post-Approval Registry[20]; dislodgment was noted 2 days after implantation and the device was successfully repositioned 50 days after the procedure without other pacing issues. The significantly different incidence of device dislodgment reported in the main leadless pacing trials[15,17,18,20] (6 cases among 559 patients with the Nanostim system [1.1%] versus 1 case among 1520 patients with the Micra system [0.1%]) might be the result of the different fixation mechanisms, such as a screw-in helix in the first case or a passive fixation mechanism (4 nitilon tines) in the second case.

The incidence of cardiac injury (resulting in cardiac tamponade, cardiac perforation, or pericardial effusion) reported in the LEADLESS II trial[17] was similar to that in the Micra Transcatheter Pacing Study[18] (1.5% in both). However, real-world studies reported different results. In The Micra Transcatheter Pacing System Post-Approval Registry,[20] 5 of 795 patients (0.6%) had cardiac effusion or perforation: among them, only 1 met the major complication criterion of prolonged hospitalization, 3 required no intervention, and 1 was treated via pericardial drainage. In contrast, in the ongoing European LEADLESS Observational Study (NCT02051972), investigators reported 6 instances of pericardial effusion or perforation among the first 147 patients implanted with the Nanostim system (4.1%); in 2 cases, perforation led to patient death.[31]

The higher incidence of cardiac injury among Nanostim patients implanted in a real-world setting can be explained in this way. Effective fixation of the Nanostim system can be achieved via an adequate myocardial penetration, which reduces the risk of dislodgment (owing to insufficient penetration) without increasing the risk of cardiac perforation (owing to excessive penetration). Achieving stable active fixation has been demonstrated to be experience related. In the LEADLESS II trial,[17] the risk of device-related serious adverse events decreased after the first 10 implants per operator (6.8% vs 3.6%; $P = .56$). Similar findings were observed in the ongoing European LEADLESS Observational Study (NCT02051972): the study was voluntarily paused for evaluation of safety after 2 deaths caused by myocardial perforation.[31] Several corrective actions were applied, which resulted in a decrease in the overall perforation rate in the period after the study was paused. Specifically, the incidence of pericardial effusion or perforation decreased from 4.1% to 2.2% as well as the risk of device dislodgment (from 1.4% to 0.0%).

In a subanalysis of the Micra Study,[18,32] the rate of serious adverse events remained low, regardless of the operator experience. The risk of pericardial effusion after Micra was higher in patients with older age, lower body mass index, female sex, prior myocardial infarction, chronic obstructive pulmonary disease, and chronic lung disease,[32] as well as after any additional device repositioning during the index procedure, which was associated with a 1.35 higher odds of effusion.[29]

Recently, the Nanostim cardiac PMK has been taken off the market owing to battery malfunction occurring between 29 and 37 months after implantation. The malfunction was observed in 7 of 1423 patients (0.5%) implanted with the leadless system, which experienced abrupt battery depletion with consequent loss of pacing and communication.

Comparison between leadless and transvenous systems

A recent review compared short-term ($\leq$2 months) and long-term (>2 months) complication rates between leadless versus traditional VVI pacing.[33] Data from 10 different studies, enrolling a total of 14,330 patients with a VVI device (historic VVI cohort), were compared with those of the 3 leadless pacing trials (leadless cohort; n = 1284 patients). The short-term complication rate of leadless PMKs is slightly higher (4.8%) compared with that of the traditional cohort (4.1%). Cardiac perforation and pacing threshold elevation requiring intervention are more frequent in leadless recipients compared with traditional VVI patients (1.5% vs 0.1% for cardiac perforation; 0.5% vs 0.0% for pacing threshold elevation), whereas acute lead or device dislocation rates were similar between the 2 groups (0.5% vs 0.4%). As mentioned, some complications, such as those related to the femoral vascular access site, are exclusively attributable to the leadless PMK implantation procedure, as well as others (eg, pneumothorax, lead- and pocket-related complications) are solely attributable to the traditional implant procedure. A comparison between Nanostim-implanted patients and a propensity-matched cohort of VVI PMK recipients[34] reported a 71% reduction in complications in the leadless cohort, during both short-term ($\leq$1 month after implantation) and mid-term (1–24 months after implantation) follow-up. Compared with standard PMK patients, patients implanted with a Micra system[35] showed a 48% reduction in the 1-year complication rate, with 47% fewer hospitalizations and an 82% decrease in PMK system revision procedures.

Acute and Chronic Retrievability

The proximal end of the leadless devices has been designed to recapture the system if repositioning is necessary or if the device needs to be retrieved. Repositioning can be achieved easily during implantation and before unlocking the tethering, in case of unsatisfactory electrical parameters or device stability. As observed in histologic sections, it takes approximately 6 weeks to develop a fibrous capsule around a traditional steroid-eluting lead.[36] On the basis of these observations, retrieval is classified as acute when performed within 6 weeks after implantation or chronic if the implant was performed more than 6 weeks before retrieval.

Nanostim system retrieval

The Nanostim retrieval catheter has a deflectable tip and is introduced via the femoral vein. The deflectable tip of the catheter has either a single-loop or a triple-loop snare, and is integrated in a protective sleeve. An 18-F sheath is required for the system. Once coaxial alignment of the snare with the docking system is confirmed with fluoroscopy, the snare can be locked to dock the device. The system is then unscrewed via counterclockwise rotation of the snare control handle (2 full rotations of the PMK) and fully covered with the sleeve for retrieval from the body as a single unit.

Histologic changes owing to Nanostim system implantation were first assessed in an in vivo ovine model[37]: 11 animals underwent leadless device implantation and were humanley killed 3 months after the procedure. Mild degrees of fibrotic thickening of the endocardium were observed at the area of the helix and of the RV wall facing the device. Some degrees of myocardial calcification and adipose tissue formation were observed, as a normal dystrophic reaction to a foreign body. Overall, the mean pacing thresholds improved overtime in both groups.

In the LEADLESS II trial,[17] device retrieval was achieved successfully in 7 patients after 160 ± 180 days after implantation (range, 1–413) without complications.

A recent multicenter study sought to assess safety and effectiveness of acute (<6 weeks after implantation) and chronic (≥6 weeks after implantation) retrieval of the Nanostim system.[38] In the acute retrieval cohort, the procedure success rate was 100% (5/5 patients). Among the 11 patients in the chronic retrieval group the success rate was 91% (10/11 patients); two-thirds of the patients had been implanted for more than 6 months with a mean time from implant to retrieval of 346 days. None of the patients experienced any adverse events at 30 days after retrieval.

Micra system retrieval

Micra system retrieval can be achieved using a percutaneous gooseneck snare. In the Micra Transcatheter Pacing Study,[18] there were 3 system revisions: in 2 cases, the device was turned off and remained in the RV; in one patient the system was successfully and safely retrieved 17 days after implantation and another leadless system was positioned.

In the Micra Transcatheter Pacing System Post-Approval Registry,[20] a device dislodgment was noted and the same system successfully repositioned 50 days after the implant.

Thirteen system revisions have been reported[39]: the device was successfully removed in 8 of 10 patients and turned off and left in situ in 3 plus the 2 patients in which retrieval was unsuccessful. The mean time from implant to successful retrieval was 25 days (range: 1–61 days); in one case, the system was surgically removed during mitral valve repair. The mean time from implant to unsuccessful retrieval was 244 days (range: 229–259 days). Of note, postmortem histopathological examination of some Micra devices demonstrated significant encapsulation of the device at different time-points.[40–42] If we consider the limited volume of the system, it seems reasonable to turn-off the device and abandon it in the RV. As previously demonstrated, multiple leadless implants in a swine model did not seem to have a negative impact on cardiac function,[43] as the RV could accommodate multiple Micra devices.[44]

SAFETY AND EFFICACY OF MULTICOMPONENT LEADLESS PACEMAKERS

LV pacing site is one of the major determinants of response in patients receiving a transvenous lead for CRT via the tributaries of the coronary sinus (epicardial pacing). Among CRT recipients, the rate of patients who do not benefit from this technology is approximately 30%. Endocardial LV pacing has been proposed as an alternative solution to overcome any limitation related to CS venous anatomy and lead stability, thereby increasing response to CRT. Endocarial LV pacing can by achieved by placing a lead in the LV via a transseptal approach.[45]

The wireless cardiac stimulation (WiCS)-LV system is a new approach for LV pacing based on a multicomponent, leadless ultrasound-based endocardial PMK for CRT. The system is based on a pulse generator (transmitter) and a receiver-electrode (electrode). The transmitter is surgically implanted subcutaneously at the level of the left lateral thorax and delivers acoustic energy (ultrasounds) to the electrode. The receiver is implanted into the endocardium of the LV via a retrograde transaortic catheter approach. The receiver is able to convert the energy at ultrasonic frequencies to an electrical pacing impulse, which is delivered to the LV. The WiCS-LV system is compatible with any PMK, ICD or CRT device and is able to discriminate right atrial pacing (if present) from RV pacing. As a result, only RV signals sensed by the system can trigger LV stimulation (3 ms of delay). In the first report,[46] the system was successfully implanted in 3 patients: an ICD patient, a patient with a CRT system with loss of capture of the LV lead, and a patient classified as non-responder to CRT. Functional New York Heart Association (NYHA) class and LV ejection fraction significantly improved at 6 months of follow-up. The Wireless Stimulation Endocardially for CRT (WiSE-CRT) study was a multicentre, prospective study, which intended to enroll 100 patients who met the criteria for conventional CRT.[47] However, only 17 patients were enrolled in the trial prior to suspension owing to safety issues. Among them, 13 patients were successfully implanted with a WiCS-LV system. Three other patients (18%) had severe pericardial effusion leading to hemodynamic instability and death in one case and one patient did not have a sufficient implant site. During follow-up, one patient had rapid battery depletion, and 2 others had loss of LV pacing, which required electrode revision. After 6 months after implantation, two-thirds of the patients experienced at least one NYHA functional class change; LV ejection fraction significantly improved by 6 points ($P<.01$).

As a result of electrode-related major adverse events, the receiver was redesigned to avoid any implant-related complication. Safety and effectiveness of the new system has been recently evaluated in the Safety and Performance of Electrodes Implanted in the Left Ventricle (SELECT-LV) study. This multicentre, prospective study enrolled 35 patients who were classified as non-responder to CRT and received a WiSE-CRT system. The device was successfully implanted in 34 (97.1%) patients. The procedure was unsuccessful in one patient who developed ventricular arrhythmia during the procedure. At 6 months of follow-up, the clinical composite score improved in 84.8% of patients and 21 (66%) showed a significant echocardiographic response with ≥5% increase in LV ejection fraction. Although further study on safety and effectiveness of this device are needed, preliminary results demonstrated that the system may provide significant benefits to patients who did not respond to CRT.

SUMMARY

Leadless pacing is a new innovative approach, which was recently introduced into clinical practice as an alternative to conventional transvenous systems. Leadless devices have been designed to overcome lead- and pocket-related complications. Although these devices are still limited to patients with an indication for single-chamber pacing, multicomponent, wireless communicating leadless systems will open up their application for dual-chamber pacing and CRT. Further randomized controlled trials comparing leadless and transvenous systems are required to assess safety, retrievability and long-term performance.

REFERENCES

1. Burkhoff D, Oikawa RY, Sagawa K. Influence of pacing site on canine left ventricular contraction. Am J Physiol 1986;251(2 Pt 2):H428–35. Available at: http://www.ncbi.nlm.nih.gov/pubmed/3740295.
2. Cazeau S, Ritter P, Lazarus A, et al. Multisite pacing for end-stage heart failure: early experience. Pacing Clin Electrophysiol 1996;19(11):1748–57.
3. Forleo GB, Della Rocca DG, Papavasileiou LP, et al. Left ventricular pacing with a new quadripolar transvenous lead for CRT: early results of a prospective comparison with conventional implant outcomes. Heart Rhythm 2011;8(1):31–7.
4. Della Rocca DG, Forleo GB, Santini L, et al. Without a quadripolar left ventricular lead you don't succeed: a challenging case of phrenic nerve stimulation. Int J Cardiol 2012;155(2):e37–8.
5. Zanon F, Baracca E, Pastore G, et al. Multipoint pacing by a left ventricular quadripolar lead improves the acute hemodynamic response to CRT compared with conventional biventricular pacing at any site. Heart Rhythm 2015;12(5):975–81.
6. Mond HG, Proclemer A. The 11th world survey of cardiac pacing and implantable cardioverter-defibrillators: calendar year 2009-A world society of Arrhythmia's project. Pacing Clin Electrophysiol 2011;34(8):1013–27.
7. Kirkfeldt RE, Johansen JB, Nohr EA, et al. Complications after cardiac implantable electronic device implantations: an analysis of a complete, nationwide cohort in Denmark. Eur Heart J 2014;35(18):1186–94.
8. Tarakji KG, Wazni OM, Harb S, et al. Risk factors for 1-year mortality among patients with cardiac implantable electronic device infection undergoing transvenous lead extraction: the impact of the infection type and the presence of vegetation on survival. Europace 2014;16(10):1490–5.
9. Brunner MP, Cronin EM, Wazni O, et al. Outcomes of patients requiring emergent surgical or endovascular intervention for catastrophic complications during transvenous lead extraction. Heart Rhythm 2014;11(3):419–25.
10. Klug D, Balde M, Pavin D, et al. Risk factors related to infections of implanted pacemakers and

cardioverter-defibrillators: results of a large prospective study. Circulation 2007;116(12):1349–55.

11. Essebag V, Verma A, Healey JS, et al. Clinically significant pocket hematoma increases long-term risk of device infection: BRUISE CONTROL INFECTION study. J Am Coll Cardiol 2016;67(11):1300–8.

12. Spickler JW, Rasor NS, Kezdi P, et al. Totally self-contained intracardiac pacemaker. J Electrocardiol 1970;3(3–4):325–31.

13. Tjong FVY, Brouwer TF, Smeding L, et al. Combined leadless pacemaker and subcutaneous implantable defibrillator therapy: feasibility, safety, and performance. Europace 2016;18(11):1740–7.

14. Tjong FVY, Brouwer TF, Kooiman KM, et al. Communicating antitachycardia pacing-enabled leadless pacemaker and subcutaneous implantable defibrillator. J Am Coll Cardiol 2016;67(15):1865–6.

15. Reddy VY, Knops RE, Sperzel J, et al. Permanent leadless cardiac pacing: results of the LEADLESS trial. Circulation 2014;129(14):1466–71.

16. Knops RE, Tjong FVY, Neuzil P, et al. Chronic performance of a leadless cardiac pacemaker: 1-year follow-up of the LEADLESS trial. J Am Coll Cardiol 2015;65(15):1497–504.

17. Reddy VY, Exner DV, Cantillon DJ, et al. Percutaneous implantation of an entirely intracardiac leadless pacemaker. N Engl J Med 2015;373(12): 1125–35.

18. Reynolds D, Duray GZ, Omar R, et al. A leadless intracardiac transcatheter pacing system. N Engl J Med 2015;374(6):533–41.

19. Ritter P, Duray GZ, Zhang S, et al. The rationale and design of the Micra Transcatheter Pacing Study: safety and efficacy of a novel miniaturized pacemaker. Europace 2015;17(5):807–13.

20. Roberts PR, Clementy N, Al Samadi F, et al. A leadless pacemaker in the real-world setting: the micra transcatheter pacing system post-approval registry. Heart Rhythm 2017. https://doi.org/10.1016/j.hrthm.2017.05.017.

21. Li X, Ze F, Wang L, et al. Prevalence of venous occlusion in patients referred for lead extraction: implications for tool selection. Europace 2014;16(12): 1795–9.

22. Bloom H, Heeke B, Leon A, et al. Renal insufficiency and the risk of infection from pacemaker or defibrillator surgery. Pacing Clin Electrophysiol 2006;29(2): 142–5.

23. Drew DA, Meyer KB, Weiner DE. Transvenous cardiac device wires and vascular access in hemodialysis patients. Am J Kidney Dis 2011;58(3):494–6.

24. Da Costa A, Axiotis A, Romeyer-Bouchard C, et al. Transcatheter leadless cardiac pacing. Int J Cardiol 2017;227:122–6.

25. Lau CP, Lee KLF. Transcatheter leadless cardiac pacing in renal failure with limited venous access. Pacing Clin Electrophysiol 2016;39(11):1281–4.

26. Garweg C, Ector J, Willems R. Leadless cardiac pacemaker as alternative in case of congenital vascular abnormality and pocket infection. Europace 2016;18(10):1564.

27. Tjong FVY, Kooiman KM, de Groot JR, et al. A leadless solution. Europace 2015;17(5):800.

28. Kypta A, Blessberger H, Kammler J, et al. Leadless cardiac pacemaker implantation after lead extraction in patients with severe device infection. J Cardiovasc Electrophysiol 2016; 27(9):1067–71.

29. Piccini JP, Stromberg K, Jackson KP, et al. Long-term outcomes in leadless micra transcatheter pacemakers with elevated thresholds at implantation: results from the micra transcatheter pacing system global clinical trial. Heart Rhythm 2017; 14(5):685–91.

30. Sundaram S, Choe W. The one that got away: a leadless pacemaker embolizes to the lungs. Heart Rhythm 2016;13(12):2316.

31. Nanostim Leadless Pacemaker System. Executive Summary for the Circulatory System Devices Panel of the Medical Devices Advisory Committee Meeting date: February 18, 2016. Version 01/20/2016. Available at: http://www.fda.gov/downloads/AdvisoryCommittees/CommitteesMeetingMaterials/MedicalDevices/MedicalDevicesAdvisoryCommittee/CirculatorySystemDevicesPanel/UCM485095.pdf. Accessed May 22, 2017.

32. El Chami M, Kowal RC. Impact of operator experience and training strategy on procedural outcomes with leadless pacing: insights from the Micra Transcatheter pacing study. Pacing Clin Electrophysiol 2017. https://doi.org/10.1111/pace.13094.This.

33. Tjong FVY, Reddy VY. Permanent leadless cardiac pacemaker therapy: a comprehensive review. Circulation 2017;135(15):1458–70.

34. Reddy V, Cantillon D, Ip J. A comparative study of acute and mid-term complications of leadless vs transvenous pacemakers. In: Abstract Presented at Heart Rhythm Society Annual Meeting 2016 as LBCT02-04, San Francisco, CA, USA. 2016. Available at: http://www.hrssessions.org/Program-Events/Program-Highlights/Late-Breaking-Clinical-Trials%5Cnhttp://www.medpagetoday.com/meeting coverage/hrs/57810.

35. Ritter P, Duray GZ, Yalagudri S, et al. Long-term performance of a transcatheter pacing system: 12 month results from the Micra Global Clinical Trial. In: European Society of Cardiology Congress 2016. 2016. Available at: http://www.medtronic.com/us-en/healthcare-professionals/products/cardiac-rhythm/pacemakers/micra-pacing-system.html.

36. Dvorak P, Novak M, Kamaryt P, et al. Histological findings around electrodes in pacemaker and implantable cardioverter-defibrillator patients: comparison of steroid-eluting and non-steroid-eluting electrodes. Europace 2012;14(1):117–23.

37. Koruth JS, Rippy MK, Khairkhahan A, et al. Feasibility and efficacy of percutaneously delivered leadless cardiac pacing in an in vivo ovine model. J Cardiovasc Electrophysiol 2015;26(3):322–8.

38. Reddy VY, Miller MA, Knops RE, et al. Retrieval of the leadless cardiac pacemaker: a multicenter experience. Circ Arrhythm Electrophysiol 2016; 9(12). https://doi.org/10.1161/CIRCEP.116.004626.

39. Micra Transcatheter Pacing System (TPS). FDA Panel pack for Circulatory Systems Devices Panel, meeting date February 18, 2016. Available at: http://www.fda. gov/downloads/AdvisoryCommittees/Committees MeetingMaterials/%0DMedicalDevices/MedicalDevices Advisory%0DCommittee/CirculatorySystemDevices Panel/UCM485094.pdf. Accessed May 24, 2017.

40. Tjong FVY, Stam OCG, Van Der Wal AC, et al. Postmortem histopathological examination of a leadless pacemaker shows partial encapsulation after 19 months. Circ Arrhythm Electrophysiol 2015;8(5): 1293–5.

41. Kypta A, Blessberger H, Lichtenauer M, et al. Complete encapsulation of a leadless cardiac pacemaker. Clin Res Cardiol 2016;105(1):94.

42. Kypta A, Blessberger H, Kammler J, et al. First autopsy description of changes 1 year after implantation of a leadless cardiac pacemaker: unexpected ingrowth and severe chronic inflammation. Can J Cardiol 2017;32(12):1578.e1–2.

43. Chen K, Zheng X, Dai Y, et al. Multiple leadless pacemakers implanted in the right ventricle of swine. Europace 2016;18(11):1748–52.

44. Omdahl P, Eggen MD, Bonner MD, et al. Right ventricular anatomy can accommodate multiple micra transcatheter pacemakers. Pacing Clin Electrophysiol 2016;39(4):393–7.

45. Jaïs P, Takahashi A, Garrigue S, et al. Mid-term follow-up of endocardial biventricular pacing. Pacing Clin Electrophysiol 2000;23(11P2):1744–7.

46. Auricchio A, Delnoy PP, Regoli F, et al. First-in-man implantation of leadless ultrasound-based cardiac stimulation pacing system: novel endocardial left ventricular resynchronization therapy in heart failure patients. Europace 2013;15(8):1191–7.

47. Auricchio A, Delnoy PP, Butter C, et al. Feasibility, safety, and short-term outcome of leadless ultrasound-based endocardial left ventricular resynchronization in heart failure patients: results of the Wireless Stimulation Endocardially for CRT (WiSE-CRT) study. Europace 2014;16(5):681–8.

Right Ventricular Pacing and Cardiac Resynchronization Devices

Tharian S. Cherian, MD[a], Gaurav A. Upadhyay, MD[b],*

KEYWORDS

- Right ventricular pacing • CRT • Pacemaker-induced cardiomyopathy

KEY POINTS

- Cardiac resynchronization is associated with benefit for patients with pacing-induced cardiomyopathy and clinical heart failure.
- There is insufficient evidence to recommend cardiac resynchronization therapy to all patients undergoing right ventricular pacemaker implantation, particularly in patients with normal left ventricular function.
- There is a low risk for pacing-induced cardiomyopathy in a majority of patients with low degree of right ventricular pacing.
- Risk factors for developing pacing-induced cardiomyopathy include burden of right ventricular pacing, with 40% identified as a threshold for development of cardiomyopathy in large randomized trials.

INTRODUCTION

The incidence and prevalence of cardiac conduction disease has been increasing worldwide owing to the aging population. There has been a concomitant increase in the number of patients receiving pacemakers. Between 1993 and 2009, approximately 3 million patients in the United States received pacemakers, during which time overall rate of implantation increased by 56%.[1] Worsening congestive heart failure (CHF) attributed to chronic right ventricular pacing (RVP) has now been recognized in patients receiving high-degree of RVP for both sinus node dysfunction and atrioventricular (AV) block.[2–5] As such, pacing-induced cardiomyopathy (PICM) has been a concern for clinicians recommending and implanting pacemakers.[6,7] With the advent of cardiac resynchronization therapy (CRT), several trials (notably Biventricular versus Right Ventricular Pacing in Heart Failure Patients with Atrioventricular Block [BLOCK HF][8]) have shown that more physiologic pacing afforded by this device may mitigate the risk of patients developing PICM. This raises the question of whether all patients expected to be RVP should receive a CRT device *a priori*. This topic is explored through a series of questions in this review.

WHAT IS THE SEQUENCE OF NORMAL EXCITATION OF THE HUMAN HEART?

Physiologic ventricular contraction is a coordinated process mediated by rapid and homogenous

Disclosures: T.S. Cherian has no disclosures. G.A. Upadhyay receives research support from Medtronic and Biotronik.
[a] Section of Cardiology, The University of Chicago Medicine, Pritzker School of Medicine, 5841 South Maryland Avenue, Chicago, IL 60637, USA; [b] Section of Cardiology, Center for Arrhythmia Care, Heart and Vascular Center, The University of Chicago Medicine, Pritzker School of Medicine, 5841 South Maryland Avenue, MC 9024, Chicago, IL 60637, USA
* Corresponding author.
E-mail address: gupadhyay@medicine.bsd.uchicago.edu

Card Electrophysiol Clin 10 (2018) 31–42
https://doi.org/10.1016/j.ccep.2017.11.004
1877-9182/18/© 2017 Elsevier Inc. All rights reserved.

myocardial activation orchestrated by the His-Purkinje system. Normal electrical activation of the left ventricle (LV) commences synchronously in 3 endocardial areas near the interventricular septum—high anterior paraseptal wall, central left surface of interventricular septum, and the posterior paraseptal wall. Within the first 30 ms, electrical activation progresses to the apex, anterior LV, and parts of the right ventricular (RV) septal and free walls. The wavefront then propagates through the anterior and inferior walls of the LV, ending in the posterobasal region approximately 50 ms after the initiation of the LV potential.[9] This coordinated progression of electrical activity leads to synchronous mechanical activation and efficient ventricular contraction.

HOW IS VENTRICULAR CONDUCTION DERANGED IN RIGHT VENTRICULAR PACING?

In pure RVP in the absence of fusion (or anodal stimulation), electrical depolarization is cathodal—beginning at the lead tip—with an electrical wavefront that depolarizes myocyte to myocyte from the RV to the LV.[10] This leads to a functional left bundle branch block (LBBB). Depending on the proximity to the native His-Purkinje system, there may or may not be any engagement of specialized conduction fibers; therefore, activation is delayed and inscribes a wide QRS. This slower progression of ventricular activation results in reduced efficiency of contraction, particularly from the apical RV lead position.[4,11–13] At a cellular level, abnormal electrical activation leads to disturbances in shortening of myocardial fibers, mechanical work, blood flow, and oxygen consumption.[12,14,15]

WHAT ARE THE CLINICAL SEQUELAE OF CHRONIC RIGHT VENTRICULAR PACING?

PICM refers to the development and manifestation of significant LV dysfunction attributable to the adverse physiologic changes arising from chronic RVP. The diagnosis is made in the absence of other identifiable causes of cardiomyopathy. In clinical studies, PICM definitions have ranged from LV ejection fraction (LVEF) less than 45%, decline in LVEF greater than 10%, or decline in LVEF necessitating CRT upgrade.[7,16,17] The pathophysiologic changes contributing to the development of PICM happens almost immediately after the initiation of RVP. Nahlawi and colleagues[18] studied echocardiographic changes from RVP in 12 patients with a dual-chamber pacemaker and normal LV function who were atrial paced (control) and near 100% RVP over periods of 2 hours and 1 week. They found that there was a significant decline in LVEF after just 2 hours of pacing (decrease in LVEF from 66% to 60%), which worsened after 1 week of pacing (decrease in LVEF from 66% to 53%). Although LVEF recovered after pacing termination, it took 32 hours for LVEF to recover to baseline.

Despite the dramatic echocardiographic changes noted, only a subset of RVP patients develop clinical manifestations of PICM. Implantation of CRT device in all patients requiring RVP would be reasonable if a significant proportion of RVP patients developed PICM. Studies of RVP have shown that prevalence of PICM ranges from 3% to 50%, over a wide range of follow-up durations (**Fig. 1**, **Tables 1** and **2**). This suggests that there are several patient-related and pacing-related parameters that influence the development of PICM. Thus, selecting patients who are at high

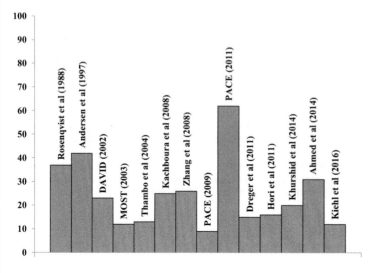

Fig. 1. Varying incidences of LV dysfunction and clinical HF in RVP patients in clinical studies.

Table 1
Incidence of heart failure and pacing-induced cardiomyopathy in studies of right ventricular pacing

Clinical Trial or Study	Number of Patients	Follow-up (Mean)	Pacing Mode	Permanent Pacemaker Implantation Indication	Clinical Heart Failure/ Pacing-induced Cardiomyopathy	Left Ventricular Dysfunction
Rosenqvist et al,[48] 1988	168	4 y	AAI vs VVI	SND	15% vs 37%	—
Andersen et al,[49] 1997	225	8 y	AAI vs VVI	SND	23 vs 42% (NYHA III-IV)	—
DAVID,[26] (2002)	506	8 mo	DDD vs VVI	—	23% vs 13% (HF + death)	—
MOST,[28] (2003)	2010	2.8 y	DDD vs VVI	SND	12% vs 10%	—
Thambo et al,[3] 2004	23	9.7 y	DDD	Congenital AVB	13% (NYHA II-III)	13%
Kachboura et al,[50] 2008	43	18 mo	DDD and VVI	AVB	25%	25%
Zhang et al,[34] 2008	304	7.8 y	DDD and VVI	AVB	26%	—
PACE,[40] (2009); PACE,[51] (2011)	163 / 163	1 y / 2 y	DDD vs CRT / DDD vs CRT	SND and AVB / SND and AVB	—	9% vs 1% (LVEF <45%) / 62% vs 20% (>5% decline in LVEF)
Dreger et al,[16] 2011	26	25 y	DDD	AVB	—	15% (mean LVEF 41%)
Hori et al,[52] 2011	367	113 mo	DDD and VVI	SND and AVB	16%	Baseline mean LVEF 56% in HF group compared with 65% in non-HF group
Khurshid et al,[17] 2014	277	3.3 y	RVP	SND and AVB	20%	Decline in mean LVEF: 62% to 36%
Ahmed et al,[53] 2014	91	28 mo	DDD and VVI	AVB	31%	Decline in mean LVEF 60% to 49%
Kiehl et al,[7] 2016	823	4.3 y	DDD, VVI, AAI + MVP, DDI	AVB	12%	Mean LVEF 34% in PICM vs 58% without PICM

Abbreviations: AVB, AV node block; PPM, permanent pacemaker implantation; SND, sinus node dysfunction.
Studies of ventricular pacing showing a wide range of incidence of LV dysfunction and clinical HF with RVP.

Table 2
Randomized controlled trials evaluating right ventricular pacing versus of cardiac resynchronization therapy

Clinical Trial or Study	Patient Population	QRS Duration (Mean)	Left Ventricular Ejection Fraction (Mean)	Summary of Study Findings
HOBIPACE,[54] (2006)	AV block and LV dysfunction	174 ms	26%	Significantly lower LVEDV, LVESV, NT-proBNP, improved exercise capacity and quality life with BiV pacing
PACE,[40] (2009)	SND, advanced AV block	107 ms	62%	Significantly lower LVEF and significantly higher LVESV in RVP group. No difference in clinical outcome.
COMBAT,[55] (2010)	AV block and LV dysfunction	148 ms (RVP) 154 ms (CRT)	30%	Significant improvement in QOL, FC, LVEF, LVESV with BiVP, increased mortality in RVP
PREVENT-HF,[41] (2011)	Expected VP >80%	124 ms	55%	No significant difference in LVEDV at 1 y
BLOCK-HF,[8] (2013)	Expected high degree of RVP	125 ms	43%	Significant reduction in composite of mortality, HF requiring intravenous diuretic, or ≥15% increase in LVESVI (56% vs 45%)
BioPace (2014)[a],[38]	Expected high degree of RVP	118 ms	55%	No significant reduction in composite of mortality and HF hospitalization

Abbreviations: FC, functional class; LVEDV, LV end-diastolic volume; LVESV, LV end-systolic volume; LVESVI, LV end-systolic volume index; NT-proBNP, N terminal pro B-type Natriuretic Peptide; QOL, quality of life; SND, sinus node dysfunction; VP, ventricular pacing.

   CRT seems associated with grater clinical benefit relative to RVP in patients in trials with significant LV dysfunction at baseline, but not in trials with normal or preserved LVEF at baseline.

   [a] Based on preliminary reported results.

risk of developing PICM with RVP for CRT implantation would ensure that any incremental risks of CRT relative to traditional RVP are minimized.

HOW DOES VENTRICULAR ACTIVATION IN CARDIAC RESYNCHRONIZATION THERAPY RESTORE PHYSIOLOGIC ACTIVATION OF THE LEFT VENTRICLE?

In contrast RVP, CRT represents the fusion of at least 2 wavefronts: 1 from the epicardial LV lead and another from the RV lead or with fusion from activation of the native His-Purkinje system (as in LV-only pacing). During biventricular (BiV) pacing, an epicardial LV wavefront fuses with an RV wavefront, along with possible participation of native His-Purkinje activation from the AV node as well. Together, the goal of pacing from the LV lead is to restore earlier activation of the LV. Although LV activation direction is nonphysiologic (epicardial to endocardial) from the LV lead, the overall activation time is shorter and, in CRT responders, the

cardiac output increases due to better coordination of the RV and LV.

DO ALL PATIENTS RECEIVING CARDIAC RESYNCHRONIZATION THERAPY FOR PACING-INDUCED CARDIOMYOPATHY RETURN TO NORMAL LEFT VENTRICULAR FUNCTION?

Echocardiographic parameters of LV function often improve after BiV upgrade for RVP patients who develop PICM (**Fig. 2**). Shimano and colleagues[19] evaluated a cohort of 18 patients who developed heart failure (HF) after chronic near complete RVP for AV block. One year after CRT upgrade, New York Heart Association (NYHA) classification significantly increased and number of hospitalizations significantly decreased. They noted, however, that CRT response (assessed by LV end-diastolic dimension) was greater in patients who had been paced for a shorter duration (<5 years). Fröhlich and colleagues[20] reported a

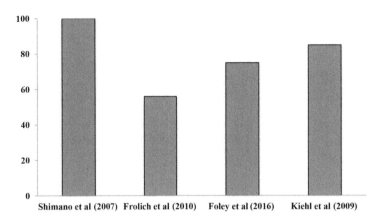

Fig. 2. Rates of improvement in LV function in patients with PICM from retrospective studies.

56% response rate to CRT upgrade in patients with PICM, defined as absolute increase in LVEF greater than 10%. In this study, there was a mean 11% absolute increase in LVEF, significant decrease in LV end-diastolic diameter-index, and a significant decrease in LV end-systolic diameter. Kiehl and colleagues[7] reported that among 30% of PICM patients in their cohort who received CRT device, the response rate was substantial, at 85% (defined as increase in LVEF ≥10% and decrease in LVESV ≥15%). Similarly, Foley and colleagues[21] reported a 75% response rate with CRT upgrade, defined as improvement greater than or equal to 1 NYHA class or greater than or equal to 25% increase in 6-minute walking distance and freedom from HF hospitalization for 1 year. As with the studies discussed previously, there were significant favorable improvements in echocardiographic parameters with CRT upgrade, including reduction in LVESV and improvement in LVEF. A significant limitation of these studies is their retrospective nature and potentially significant confounders with respect to selection bias.

IS THERE A THRESHOLD OF RIGHT VENTRICULAR PACING BURDEN THAT PREDICTS DEVELOPMENT OF PACING-INDUCED CARDIOMYOPATHY?

Intuitively, greater time with RVP—and, therefore, increased time in dyssynchrony—leads to higher likelihood of developing PICM. Accordingly, randomized controlled trials and subgroup analyses have demonstrated that high burden of RVP, rather than pacing mode, is an independent predictor of LV dysfunction (**Table 3**). Smit and colleagues[22] studied patients who received an implantable cardioverter-defibrillator (ICD) without symptomatic HF and in a multivariate analysis

found that new HF, hospitalization for HF, or death due to HF was significantly higher in patients who were paced more than 50% of the time and baseline LVEF less than 26%.

Nielsen and colleagues[23] randomized patients receiving pacemaker for sick sinus syndrome into 3 groups: AAIR and DDDR with a short rate-adaptive AV delay (DDDR-S) and DDDR with a fixed long AV delay (DDDR-I). RVP burden was 90% in the DDDR-S group and 17% in the DDDR-I group. Left atrial diameter increased significantly in both DDDR groups, but LV fractional shortening significantly decreased in DDDR-S group and not in the DDDR-I group. The implication of this finding was that normalizing the P–R interval and mandating RVP has a detrimental impact on the LV and has no significant benefit with respect to atrial dimension.

A retrospective analysis of the Multicenter Automatic Defibrillator Implantation Trial (MADIT) II evaluated the effect of RVP on clinical outcomes in postmyocardial infarction patients with reduced LVEF who had ICD therapy. There was a bimodal distribution of cumulative pacing noted—1 group with median pacing of 96% and other with median pacing of 0.2%. The group with frequent pacing had significantly higher risk of new or worsened HF and ventricular tachycardia (VT)/ventricular fibrillation (VF) requiring ICD therapy.[24] An 8-year follow-up of the same 2 groups showed attenuation of device efficacy and significant increase in mortality in the group with high RVP burden.[25]

A few studies have identified a pacing burden of 40% as the threshold where the risk of developing PICM increases substantially. The Dual Chamber and VVI Implantable Defibrillator (DAVID) trial randomly assigned patients with LV dysfunction receiving ICDs to VVI pacing mode at 40 beats per minute or DDDR pacing mode

Table 3
Predictors of right ventricular pacing-induced cardiomyopathy

Clinical Variable	Clinical Trial or Study	Observed Thresholds Predictive of Cardiomyopathy/ Heart Failure
Higher RVP burden	Nielsen et al,[23] 2003	Significant LVEF decline in patients with pacing burden 90% vs 17%
	MOST,[28] (2003)	>40% RVP associated with 3× increase in HF hospitalization; 20% increase in HF hospitalization with 10% increase in RVP
	MADIT II,[24] (2005)	Higher risk of new or worsened HF and VT/VF in patients with pacing burden 96% vs 0.2%
	DAVID,[26] (2005)	>40% RVP associated with increased death or CHF hospitalization
	Kiehl et al,[7] 2016	≥20% RVP associated with PICM (CRT upgrade/post-PPM LVEF ≤40%)
Longer paced QRS duration	MOST,[56] (2003)	10 ms increase in QRS duration associated with 18% increase in HF in patients with normal LVEF
Lower baseline LVEF	MADIT II,[24] (2002)	Baseline LVEF <30%, at 1 y, 93% increased risk of new or worsened HF with RVP
	DAVID,[26] (2005)	Baseline LVEF <40%, at 1 y, 61% increased risk for mortality and HF hospitalization with RVP
	PACE,[40] (2009)	Baseline LVEF 62%, at 1 y mean LVEF in RVP 55%, no difference in HF hospitalization
	Kiehl et al,[7] 2016	1% lower LVEF associated with 5% increased risk PICM (CRT upgrade/post-PPM ejection fraction ≤40%)

Abbreviations: LVESV, LV end-systolic; PPM, permanent pacemaker implantation.
Overall greater degree of RVP, longer paced QRS duration, and lower baseline LVEF predict PICM.

at 70 beats per minute. In the DDDR group, 60% of ventricular beats were paced whereas 1% ventricular beats were paced in the VVI group. Higher burden of RVP in the DDDR group was associated with increased risk of primary endpoint of death or CHF hospitalization.[26] A subsequent analysis of the DAVID trial showed that RVP burden greater than 40% was predictive of the primary endpoint in patients in the DDDR group with less than or equal to 40% pacing burden had similar or better outcomes compared with the VVI group.[27]

The Mode Selection Trial (MOST) randomized patients with sick sinus syndrome and intact AV node function to DDDR and VVIR pacing. A majority of patients in this study had normal LVEF and approximately 20% had reported CHF, 90% of whom had NYHA class I or II symptoms. Cumulative ventricular pacing was greater in the DDDR group compared with the VVIR group (90% vs 58%). In the DDDR group, ventricular pacing greater than 40% was associated with an approximately 3-fold increase in HF hospitalizations compared with less than 40% pacing burden. There was an incremental 20% increase in HF hospitalization with 10% increase in RVP. In the VVIR group, ventricular pacing greater than 80% was associated with a

2.6-fold increase in HF hospitalization. There was a linear increase in risk of atrial fibrillation (AF) with cumulative pacing burden in both groups.[28] These data and those from the DAVID trial serve as the foundation for the current device guideline recommendations to consider CRT in patients who will receive at least 40% RVP at the time of implant or generator change (class IIa, level of evidence C).[29]

There is some evidence that an even lower RVP burden may increase risk of developing PICM. A retrospective study of 823 patients by Kiehl and colleagues,[7] for instance, showed that an RVP burden greater than 20% was associated with 6-fold increase in likelihood of developing PICM (defined as drop in LVEF to <40% post–pacemaker implantation or requiring upgrade to CRT device). In a more recent study of 991 patients with normal (>55%) or mildly reduced LVEF (41%–55%) by Ebert and colleagues,[30] however, there was no significant correlation between percentage of RVP and clinical outcome. Therefore, although some studies have indicated that degree of RVP burden is a strong risk factor for development of PICM, further research needs to address the relative contribution of pacing burden and the threshold where risk of PICM becomes substantial.

IF HIGH PACING BURDEN IS ASSOCIATED WITH PACING-INDUCED CARDIOMYOPATHY, SHOULD ALL PATIENTS UNDERGOING ATRIOVENTRICULAR NODAL ABLATION FOR ATRIAL FIBRILLATION RECEIVE A CARDIAC RESYNCHRONIZATION THERAPY DEVICE?

Given the association of RVP burden with PICM, it seems reasonable that patients expected to be paced 100% due to AV node ablation would benefit from CRT therapy. There are several studies from the CRT literature that have suggested that AV junction ablation guarantees BiV capture and improves CRT outcomes.[31,32] Only a single randomized trial, however, has explored the distinct question of whether RVP or BiV pacing should be performed after AV node ablation for the treatment of rapid AF. The Post AV Nodal Ablation Evaluation (PAVE) study[33] randomized 184 patients undergoing AV nodal ablation for AF with rapid ventricular rates to receive BiV device or RVP. At 6 months of follow-up, patients who received CRT had a significantly improved 6-minute walk distance and significantly higher LVEF. The patients in this trial were older (mean age 69) and had baseline clinical HF symptoms (NYHA II or III) and also demonstrated baseline abnormal LVEF (mean LVEF 47%).[33] Whether the benefits of CRT extend to younger patients without HF undergoing AV node ablation is not clear.

WHAT FACTORS IN ADDITION TO RIGHT VENTRICULAR PACING BURDEN CONTRIBUTE TO DEVELOPMENT OF PACING-INDUCED CARDIOMYOPATHY?

Retrospective studies have demonstrated that not all patients with RVP develop HF, and there are factors in addition to high burden of RVP that are predictive of poor outcomes in patients who develop HF. Longer duration of RVP, wider QRS morphology, and lower baseline LV function have been demonstrated to be predictors of PICM (see **Table 3**). A retrospective study of 304 patients without prior history of HF receiving RVP for AV block (all of whom were paced close to 100% of the time) demonstrated that only 26% of the patients developed HF at a median follow-up of 8 years. Multivariate analysis identified older age at implantation, a wider paced QRS duration, and coronary artery disease were independent predictors of HF.[34] New-onset HF and older age at implantation were independent predictors of mortality.[34] Similarly, a retrospective study by Khurshid and colleagues[17] reported a wider QRS duration to be independently associated with PICM (defined as decrease in LVEF >10%)—a

3% increased risk for PICM with a 1-ms increase in QRS width.

WHAT IS THE BENEFIT OF CARDIAC RESYNCHRONIZATION THERAPY DEVICES IN PATIENTS WITH LEFT VENTRICULAR DYSFUNCTION?

The benefits of CRT in patients with reduced LVEF, prolonged QRS duration, and HF symptoms despite guideline-directed medical therapy have been demonstrated in several large randomized controlled trials.[35–37] CRT now enjoys an established role in the armamentarium of device-based therapy for clinical HF, particularly in patients with LBBB greater than 150 ms, where it is a class I indication. The 2012 American College of Cardiology Foundation/American Heart Association/Heart Rhythm Society (HRS) focused update for device-based therapy for cardiac rhythm abnormalities practice guideline document recommends CRT implantation in patients with NYHA II–IV symptoms, with LVEF less than or equal to 35%, with strongest recommendations in patients with QRS duration greater than or equal to 150 ms.[29]

DO CARDIAC RESYNCHRONIZATION THERAPY DEVICES BENEFIT PATIENTS WITH LEFT VENTRICULAR DYSFUNCTION AND A NORMAL QRS DURATION?

Given the benefit of CRT devices in patients with LV dysfunction, several trials have evaluated whether these benefits extend to patients without LBBB or a widened QRS. The BLOCK HF trial randomized 691 patients with LVEF less than or equal to 50% and NYHA class I–III HF and indications for pacing for AV block to CRT or RVP. Baseline LVEF and QRS durations in the trial patients were approximately 40% and 125 ms, respectively. All patients, however, were required to demonstrate evidence that they would require a high percentage of ventricular pacing, either because of documented third-degree AV block, advanced second-degree block, or first-degree block with P–R interval greater than or equal to 300 ms when paced at 100 beats per minute. This led to an average pacing percentage of 97% or greater in all 3 groups. At 37 months' follow-up, CRT significantly reduced composite outcomes of LV end-systolic volume index, urgent care visit for HF that required intravenous therapy, or death. There was no statistically significant improvement in mortality.[8]

A more recent, large randomized trial examining the role of CRT versus RVP was the

Biventricular Pacing for Atrioventricular Block to Prevent Cardiac Desynchronization (BioPace) trial. Preliminary data were reported in 2014, with the final results not yet published. This was a large study of 1810 patients who were randomized to RV versus BiV pacing and followed for a mean duration of 5.6 years. Inclusion criteria were similar to those for BLOCK HF but with a lower observed rate of RVP (86%), higher baseline LVEF (55% overall), and lower mean QRS duration (118 ms). LBBB was present in 17% of patients overall and AF in 25%. Although there was a trend toward a reduction in mortality and HF hospitalization among those assigned to BiV pacing overall, this did not reach significance (hazard ratio [HR] 0.87; 95% 0.75–1.01; $P = .08$). This trend was less clear in patients with LV dysfunction (571 patients: mean LVEF $41.2 \pm 8.8\%$; HR 0.92; 95% CI, 0.73–1.16; $P = .48$).[38] Criticisms of BioPace have included suboptimal rates of BiV pacing (90% at 1 month) and lack of rigorous criteria for LV lead positioning. In addition, there was a high rate of initial implant failure (14.8%) to those assigned to the BiV group, which limits interpretability of findings. With that noted, the overall results of BioPace raise caution for *a priori* use of BiV pacing in patients with underlying normal QRS width.

Perhaps the most significant study evaluating the role of CRT in patients with LV dysfunction and narrow QRS was Echocardiography Guided Cardiac Resynchronization Therapy (EchoCRT), which raises the specter of possible harm with BiV pacing in patients who do not need it. This study randomized 809 patients with NYHA III or IV HF, LVEF less than 35%, QRS duration less than 130 ms, and echocardiographic evidence of dyssynchrony to receive CRT therapy or no pacing. EchoCRT was stopped early due to futility, and at a follow-up of 19 months, mortality was significantly higher in the CRT group.[39]

DOES CARDIAC RESYNCHRONIZATION THERAPY BENEFIT PATIENTS WITH PRESERVED LEFT VENTRICULAR FUNCTION AND A HIGH PACING BURDEN?

There have been 2 published randomized controlled trials that have evaluated the effects of RVP compared with BiV pacing in patients with preserved LV function. Both studies show changes in echocardiographic parameters of LV function with RVP relative to BiV, including greater decline in LVEF and increased enlargement in chamber size. Neither study, however, showed significant differences in mortality, hospitalization for HF, or quality of life.

The Pacing to Avoid Cardiac Enlargement (PACE) trial was a prospective, double-blind, multicenter study, which randomized 177 patients with sinus node dysfunction or bradycardia due to high-grade AV block and preserved LV function (baseline ejection fraction 62%) to BiV pacing or apical RVP. At 12 months of follow-up, mean LVEF was significantly lower in the RVP group compared with the BiV pacing group, with an absolute difference of 7% points (55% vs 62%); 8 patients in the RVP group and 1 patient in the BiV pacing group had LVEF less than 45%. LV end-systolic volume was significantly higher in the RVP group. There was no significant difference noted, however, in deaths, hospitalizations for HF, or quality of life as assessed by the 36-Item Short Form Health Survey score between the 2 groups.[40]

The Preventing Ventricular Dysfunction in Pacemaker Patients Without Advanced Heart Failure (PREVENT-HF) randomized 108 patients with normal LVEF who met indications for pacing to RV apical or CRT. Baseline LVEF was 55% in RVP group and 58% in the BiV pacing group. At 12 months, there was no significant difference in the primary outcome of LV end-diastolic volume. Furthermore, there were no significant differences in the secondary endpoints of LVEF and LV end-systolic volume.[41]

As discussed previously, the largest trial examining the role of upfront BiV versus RVP is the BioPace trial, which is yet to be formally published. In BioPace, 1239 patients demonstrated LVEF greater than 50% at baseline (mean $61.9\% \pm 7.0\%$). At 96 months' follow-up, there was no significant difference in the combined endpoint of mortality and HF hospitalization in the preserved LVEF group (HR 0.88; 95% CI, 0.72–1.07; $P = .18$).[38]

WHAT ADDITIONAL PROCEDURAL RISKS ARE INVOLVED WITH IMPLANTATION OF A CARDIAC RESYNCHRONIZATION THERAPY DEVICE?

Compared with implantation of an RV pacemaker, there are additional technical challenges to implantation and maintenance of a BiV pacemaker. There are complications unique to a CRT implantation, such as a coronary sinus (CS) dissection and failure to implant a CS lead or a CS lead dislodgement. In the BLOCK HF trial, successful implantation rate was approximately 94% and LV lead-related complications occurred in approximately 6% of patients.[8] A meta-analysis by

Adabag and colleagues[42] demonstrated that compared with ICD implantation, *de novo* CRT implantation was associated with significantly higher rates of adverse events, including failure to implant (6.6% vs <0.1%), pneumothorax (1.5% vs 0.8%), pocket hematoma (2.5% vs 1.8%), and infection (1.7% vs 1.3%). van Rees and colleagues[43] reported a 2% CS lead complications in patients undergoing CRT and a higher lead dislodgment rate (6% vs 2%) compared with ICD implantation. In addition, data from the REPLACE registry showed that complication rates were approximately 4-fold in patients undergoing addition of a transvenous lead. In particular, upgrade to a CRT device was associated with a 19% rate of complications.[44] Similarly, the 2012 European Heart Rhythm Association/HRS expert consensus statement on CRT therapy in HF reported a 5% to 9% implantation failure and CS lead dislodgement rate of 3% to 7%.[45]

FUTURE DIRECTIONS

His bundle pacing (HBP) is emerging as a viable and attractive alternative to RVP. This technique harnesses the intact native conduction of the heart to provide a physiologic pacing alternative that minimizes dyssynchrony. Sharma and colleagues[46] reported a series of patients requiring RVP who underwent routine attempt at HBP at 1 center and RVP at another. HBP success rate was 80% and fluoroscopy time was similar between the 2 groups. In patients who required greater than 40% pacing, HF hospitalization was significantly lower in the HBP group, and

no difference in mortality was noted between the 2 groups. Randomized controlled trials are ongoing to evaluate the safety and efficacy of these devices compared with the traditional CRT devices.[47] The authors view HBP as an attractive option particularly for those patients who are expected to undergo a high degree of pacing with only modest LV dysfunction at baseline (**Table 4**).

A SIMPLIFIED APPROACH

The authors' approach to selection of CRT in all patients who are expected to be RVP is summarized in **Table 4**. It evaluates whether the patient in consideration demonstrates 1 or both high-risk features for development of PICM: (1) Is the patient expected to receive greater than 40% RVP and (2) Does the patient have significant LV dysfunction? If the answer is no to both questions, the authors proceed with RVP. If the answer is yes to both questions, then the authors strongly consider CRT implantation, particularly if a patient has HF and a prolonged QRS. If the answer is yes to 1 of the questions, the authors proceed with RV or His pacing, with close monitoring for the development of PICM in follow-up. The authors also carefully monitor the RVP devices to maximize native conduction and therefore minimize dyssynchrony and mitigate the risk of PICM. The authors' approach is rooted in the principle of first, do no harm, believing that the risks associated with CRT implantation outweigh the benefits in patients who are not at risk for developing PICM. More research into reliable predictors of PICM is needed

Table 4
Approach to decision making regarding cardiac resynchronization therapy in patients expected to receive right ventricular pacing

	Patients with Severe Left Ventricular Dysfunction (Left Ventricular Ejection Fraction ≤35%)	Patients with Modest Left Ventricular Dysfunction (Left Ventricular Ejection Fraction 36%–49%)	Patients with Preserved Left Ventricular Function (Left Ventricular Ejection Fraction ≥50%)
Low pacing burden (RVP <40%)	ICD placement with programming parameters adjusted to minimize ventricular pacing	RV (or His) pacemaker with parameters adjusted to minimize degree of ventricular pacing	Traditional pacemaker (RVP or His) CRT device should not be implanted *a priori*
High pacing burden (RVP ≥40%)	CRT device with goal BiV pacing >95%	Consideration for upfront His lead in patients with clinical HF in whom narrow QRS and acceptable threshold can be achieved	Traditional pacemaker reasonable (RVP or His) with close attention to development of PICM in follow-up

to refine this approach moving forward, because it would aid in patient selection for CRT up front.

SUMMARY

Long-term RVP may lead to development of PICM in a subset of patients. Patients with a high degree of pacing burden and reduced LV function prior to pacemaker implantation are at the greatest risk for developing PICM. One therapy for PICM is upgrade to a CRT device, which can help restore electrical and mechanical synchrony and improve LV function in a majority of patients. Implantation of CRT devices carry additional upfront procedural risks, and robust quality clinical data are not yet available to support the use of *a priori* CRT in patients without LV dysfunction and who are expected to require a high degree of RVP. Among patients with LV dysfunction, degree of RVP and QRS width seems associated with higher risk of PICM, and these patients should be followed closely. Further research is needed to identify patient characteristics that portend higher risk of developing PICM in patients with normal LVEF at baseline.

REFERENCES

1. Greenspon AJ, Patel JD, Lau E, et al. Trends in permanent pacemaker implantation in the United States from 1993 to 2009: increasing complexity of patients and procedures. J Am Coll Cardiol 2012;60(16): 1540–5.
2. Nielsen JC, Andersen HR, Thomsen PE, et al. Heart failure and echocardiographic changes during long-term follow-up of patients with sick sinus syndrome randomized to single-chamber atrial or ventricular pacing. Circulation 1998;97(10):987–95.
3. Thambo JB, Bordachar P, Garrigue S, et al. Detrimental ventricular remodeling in patients with congenital complete heart block and chronic right ventricular apical pacing. Circulation 2004;110(25): 3766–72.
4. Tse HF, Yu C, Wong KK, et al. Functional abnormalities in patients with permanent right ventricular pacing: the effect of sites of electrical stimulation. J Am Coll Cardiol 2002;40(8):1451–8.
5. O'Keefe JH Jr, Abuissa H, Jones PG, et al. Effect of chronic right ventricular apical pacing on left ventricular function. Am J Cardiol 2005;95(6):771–3.
6. Ferrari AD, Borges AP, Albuquerque LC, et al. Cardiomyopathy induced by artificial cardiac pacing: myth or reality sustained by evidence? Rev Bras Cir Cardiovasc 2014;29(3):402–13.
7. Kiehl EL, Makki T, Kumar R, et al. Incidence and predictors of right ventricular pacing-induced cardiomyopathy in patients with complete atrioventricular

8. Curtis AB, Worley SJ, Adamson PB, et al. Biventricular pacing for atrioventricular block and systolic dysfunction. N Engl J Med 2013;368(17):1585–93.
9. Durrer D, van Dam RT, Freud GE, et al. Total excitation of the isolated human heart. Circulation 1970; 41(6):899–912.
10. Wiggers CJ. The muscular reactions of the mammalian ventricles to artificial surface stimuli. American Journal of Physiology–Legacy Content 1925;73(2): 346–78.
11. Prinzen FW, Augustijn CH, Arts T, et al. Redistribution of myocardial fiber strain and blood flow by asynchronous activation. Am J Physiol 1990;259(2 Pt 2):H300–8.
12. Lee MA, Dae MW, Langberg JJ, et al. Effects of long-term right ventricular apical pacing on left ventricular perfusion, innervation, function and histology. J Am Coll Cardiol 1994;24(1):225–32.
13. Prinzen FW, Peschar M. Relation between the pacing induced sequence of activation and left ventricular pump function in animals. Pacing Clin Electrophysiol 2002;25(4 Pt 1):484–98.
14. Delhaas T, Arts T, Prinzen FW, et al. Regional fibre stress-fibre strain area as an estimate of regional blood flow and oxygen demand in the canine heart. J Physiol 1994;477(3):481–96.
15. van Oosterhout MF, Arts T, Bassingthwaighte JB, et al. Relation between local myocardial growth and blood flow during chronic ventricular pacing. Cardiovasc Res 2002;53(4):831–40.
16. Dreger H, Maethner K, Bondke H, et al. Pacing-induced cardiomyopathy in patients with right ventricular stimulation for>15 years. Europace 2011; 14(2):238–42.
17. Khurshid S, Epstein AE, Verdino RJ, et al. Incidence and predictors of right ventricular pacing-induced cardiomyopathy. Heart Rhythm 2014;11(9):1619–25.
18. Nahlawi M, Waligora M, Spies SM, et al. Left ventricular function during and after right ventricular pacing. J Am Coll Cardiol 2004;44(9):1883–8.
19. Shimano M, Tsuji Y, Yoshida Y, et al. Acute and chronic effects of cardiac resynchronization in patients developing heart failure with long-term pacemaker therapy for acquired complete atrioventricular block. Europace 2007;9(10):869–74.
20. Fröhlich G, Steffel J, Hurlimann D, et al. Upgrading to resynchronization therapy after chronic right ventricular pacing improves left ventricular remodelling. Eur Heart J 2010;31(12):1477–85.
21. Foley PW, Muhyaldeen SA, Chalil S, et al. Long-term effects of upgrading from right ventricular pacing to cardiac resynchronization therapy in patients with heart failure. Europace 2009;11(4):495–501.
22. Smit MD, Van Dessel PF, Nieuwland W, et al. Right ventricular pacing and the risk of heart failure in

implantable cardioverter-defibrillator patients. Heart Rhythm 2006;3(12):1397–403.

23. Nielsen JC, Kristensen L, Andersen HR, et al. A randomized comparison ofatrial and dual-chamber pacing in177 consecutive patients with sick sinus syndrome: echocardiographic and clinical outcome. J Am Coll Cardiol 2003;42(4):614–23.

24. Steinberg JS, Fischer A, Wang P, et al. The clinical implications of cumulative right ventricular pacing in the multicenter automatic defibrillator trial II. J Cardiovasc Electrophysiol 2005;16(4):359–65.

25. Barsheshet A, Moss AJ, McNitt S, et al. Long-term implications of cumulative right ventricular pacing among patients with an implantable cardioverter-defibrillator. Heart Rhythm 2011;8(2):212–8.

26. Wilkoff BL, Cook JR, Epstein AE, et al. Dual-chamber pacing or ventricular backup pacing in patients with an implantable defibrillator: the Dual Chamber and VVI Implantable Defibrillator (DAVID) Trial. JAMA 2002;288(24):3115–23.

27. Sharma AD, Rizo-Patron C, Hallstrom AP, et al. Percent right ventricular pacing predicts outcomes in the DAVID trial. Heart Rhythm 2005; 2(8):830–4.

28. Sweeney MO, Hellkamp AS, Ellenbogen KA, et al. Adverse effect of ventricular pacing on heart failure and atrial fibrillation among patients with normal baseline QRS duration in a clinical trial of pacemaker therapy for sinus node dysfunction. Circulation 2003;107(23):2932–7.

29. Epstein AE, DiMarco JP, Ellenbogen KA, et al. 2012 ACCF/AHA/HRS focused update incorporated into the ACCF/AHA/HRS 2008 guidelines for device-based therapy of cardiac rhythm abnormalities: a report of the American College of Cardiology Foundation/American Heart Association Task Force on Practice Guidelines and the Heart Rhythm Society. J Am Coll Cardiol 2013;61(3):e6–75.

30. Ebert M, Jander N, Minners J, et al. Long-term impact of right ventricular pacing on left ventricular systolic function in pacemaker recipients with preserved ejection fraction: results from a large single-center registry. J Am Heart Assoc 2016;5(7) [pii:e003485].

31. Ganesan AN, Brooks AG, Roberts-Thomson KC, et al. Role of AV nodal ablation in cardiac resynchronization in patients with coexistent atrial fibrillation and heart failure a systematic review. J Am Coll Cardiol 2012;59(8):719–26.

32. Upadhyay GA, Choudhry NK, Auricchio A, et al. Cardiac resynchronization in patients with atrial fibrillation: a meta-analysis of prospective cohort studies. J Am Coll Cardiol 2008;52(15):1239–46.

33. Doshi RN, Daoud EG, Fellows C, et al. Left ventricular-based cardiac stimulation post AV nodal ablation evaluation (the PAVE study). J Cardiovasc Electrophysiol 2005;16(11):1160–5.

34. Zhang XH, Chen H, Siu CW, et al. New-onset heart failure after permanent right ventricular apical pacing in patients with acquired high-grade atrioventricular block and normal left ventricular function. J Cardiovasc Electrophysiol 2008;19(2): 136–41.

35. Al-Majed NS, McAlister FA, Bakal JA, et al. Meta-analysis: cardiac resynchronization therapy for patients with less symptomatic heart failure. Ann Intern Med 2011;154(6):401–12.

36. Woods B, Hawkins N, Mealing S, et al. Individual patient data network meta-analysis of mortality effects of implantable cardiac devices. Heart 2015; 101(22):1800–6.

37. Rickard J, Michtalik H, Sharma R, et al. Use of cardiac resynchronization therapy in the medicare population. Rockville (MD): Agency for Healthcare Research and Quality; 2015.

38. Coordinators BTIa. BioPace Trial Preliminary Results. 2014. Available at: http://clinicaltrialresults. org/Slides/TCT2014/Blanc_Biopace.pdf. Accessed July 16, 2017.

39. Ruschitzka F, Abraham WT, Singh JP, et al. Cardiac-resynchronization therapy in heart failure with a narrow QRS complex. N Engl J Med 2013;369(15): 1395–405.

40. Yu CM, Chan JY, Zhang Q, et al. Biventricular pacing in patients with bradycardia and normal ejection fraction. N Engl J Med 2009;361(22):2123–34.

41. Stockburger M, Gomez-Doblas JJ, Lamas G, et al. Preventing ventricular dysfunction in pacemaker patients without advanced heart failure: results from a multicentre international randomized trial (PREVENT-HF). Eur J Heart Fail 2011;13(6):633–41.

42. Adabag S, Roukoz H, Anand IS, et al. Cardiac resynchronization therapy in patients with minimal heart failure: a systematic review and meta-analysis. J Am Coll Cardiol 2011;58(9):935–41.

43. van Rees JB, de Bie MK, Thijssen J, et al. Implantation-related complications of implantable cardioverter-defibrillators and cardiac resynchronization therapy devices: a systematic review of randomized clinical trials. J Am Coll Cardiol 2011;58(10):995–1000.

44. Poole JE, Gleva MJ, Mela T, et al. Complication rates associated with pacemaker or implantable cardioverter-defibrillator generator replacements and upgrade procedures: results from the REPLACE registry. Circulation 2010;122(16):1553–61.

45. European Heart Rhythm Association, European Society of Cardiology, Heart Rhythm Society, et al. 2012 EHRA/HRS expert consensus statement on cardiac resynchronization therapy in heart failure: implant and follow-up recommendations and management. Heart Rhythm 2012;9(9):1524–76.

46. Sharma PS, Dandamudi G, Naperkowski A, et al. Permanent His-bundle pacing is feasible, safe,

and superior to right ventricular pacing in routine clinical practice. Heart Rhythm 2015;12(2):305–12.

47. His bundle pacing versus coronary sinus pacing for cardiac resynchronization therapy (His-SYNC). 2017. Available at: https://clinicaltrials.gov/ct2/show/NCT02700425. Accessed July 20, 2017.

48. Rosenqvist M, Brandt J, Schuller H. Long-term pacing in sinus node disease: effects of stimulation mode on cardiovascular morbidity and mortality. Am Heart J 1988;116(1 Pt 1):16–22.

49. Andersen HR, Nielsen JC, Thomsen PE, et al. Long-term follow-up of patients from a randomised trial of atrial versus ventricular pacing for sick-sinus syndrome. Lancet 1997;350(9086):1210–6.

50. Kachboura S, Ben Halima A, Fersi I, et al. Assessment of heart failure and left ventricular systolic dysfunction after cardiac pacing in patients with preserved left ventricular systolic function. Ann Cardiol Angeiol (Paris) 2008;57(1):29–36.

51. Chan JY, Fang F, Zhang Q, et al. Biventricular pacing is superior to right ventricular pacing in bradycardia patients with preserved systolic function: 2-year results of the PACE trial. Eur Heart J 2011; 32(20):2533–40.

52. Hori Y, Tada H, Nakamura K, et al. Presence of structural heart disease and left ventricular dysfunction predict hospitalizations for new-onset heart failure after right ventricular apical pacing. Europace 2011;13(2):230–6.

53. Ahmed M, Gorcsan J 3rd, Marek J, et al. Right ventricular apical pacing-induced left ventricular dyssynchrony is associated with a subsequent decline in ejection fraction. Heart Rhythm 2014; 11(4):602–8.

54. Kindermann M, Hennen B, Jung J, et al. Biventricular versus conventional right ventricular stimulation for patients with standard pacing indication and left ventricular dysfunction: the Homburg Biventricular Pacing Evaluation (HOBIPACE). J Am Coll Cardiol 2006;47(10):1927–37.

55. Martinelli Filho M, de Siqueira SF, Costa R, et al. Conventional versus biventricular pacing in heart failure and bradyarrhythmia: the COMBAT study. J Card Fail 2010;16(4):293–300.

56. Shukla HH, Hellkamp AS, James EA, et al. Heart failure hospitalization is more common in pacemaker patients with sinus node dysfunction and a prolonged paced QRS duration. Heart Rhythm 2005; 2(3):245–51.

Remote Monitoring for Chronic Disease Management
Atrial Fibrillation and Heart Failure

Maki Ono, MD, PhD[a,b], Niraj Varma, MD, PhD[b],*

KEYWORDS

- Remote monitoring • Heart failure • Atrial fibrillation • Cardiac implantable electronic devices
- Pacemaker • Implantable cardioverter defibrillator • Cardiac resynchronization therapy

KEY POINTS

- Remote monitoring for cardiac implantable electronic devices is a class I recommendation.
- Device-detected atrial fibrillation increases the risk of stroke and remote monitoring is useful for early detection and intervention for atrial fibrillation.
- Definitive data for merits of early anticoagulation to reduce the risk of stroke are awaited, but current evidence does not support discontinuation of anticoagulation based on remote monitoring.
- Multiparameter monitoring with automatic transmission is useful for heart failure management including mortality benefit.
- Thoracic impedance alone lacks the evidence to support its usefulness for clinical outcome for heart failure.

INTRODUCTION

More than 10 years have passed since the introduction of automatic remote monitoring (RM) of cardiac implantable electronic devices (CIEDs) and strong evidence has been built for its usefulness for the early detection of ventricular arrhythmias and the evaluation of system performance, such as lead failure and battery depletion.[1–5] Now we enter a new growth era to effectively use RM for chronic heart disease management, specifically for atrial fibrillation and heart failure.

In developed countries, atrial fibrillation and heart failure pose a significant medical burden. Atrial fibrillation, apart from triggering inappropriate shocks in implantable cardioverter-defibrillators (ICDs), affects patients in 2 major ways: (1) increased thromboembolic risk such as stroke and (2) precipitation of heart failure owing to the loss of atrial contraction and biventricular pacing, variation in ventricular cycle duration, or higher ventricular response rate. For the former, prompt anticoagulation decisions based on RM alerts and patient's profile such as embolic risk score (eg, CHADS2 or CHA2DS2-VASc2) and bleeding risk score (eg, HAS-BLED score) is ideal. For the latter, RM may prevent heart failure deterioration, with or without atrial fibrillation. Central to these aims is the early detection ability provided by RM.

Disclosure: No funding was received for this article. M. Ono reports no conflict of interest. N. Varma has served as a consultant/speaker for remote monitoring for Medtronic, Biotronik, Sorin, and Abbott.
[a] Department of Cardiology, Kameda General Hospital, 929 Higashi-cho, Kamogawa City, Chiba 296-8602, Japan; [b] Cardiac Pacing and Electrophysiology, Heart and Vascular Institute, Cleveland Clinic, J2-2, 9500 Euclid Avenue, Cleveland, OH 44195, USA
* Corresponding author.
E-mail address: varman@ccf.org

Card Electrophysiol Clin 10 (2018) 43–58
https://doi.org/10.1016/j.ccep.2017.11.005

In this article, we provide an overview on the latest evidence of RM in terms of atrial fibrillation and heart failure management, update the current technology relating to the method, and discuss the future of RM.

REMOTE MONITORING AND ATRIAL FIBRILLATION
Current Evidence About Device-Detected Atrial Fibrillation

Prior studies have shown that the detection of device-based rapid atrial rate correlated well with electrocardiographic documentation of atrial fibrillation[6–8] and that either a high burden of atrial fibrillation or arrhythmia episodes are independent predictors for stroke and mortality.[9–13] Implanted devices provide a more sensitive and accurate measure of atrial fibrillation than symptoms.[14–16] The ASymptomatic atrial fibrillation and stroke Evaluation in pacemaker patients and the atrial fibrillation reduction atrial pacing trial (ASSERT) Investigators documented that device-detected atrial tachyarrhythmias, even asymptomatic subclinical atrial fibrillation, were associated with a significant increase of ischemic stroke or systemic embolism.[17–19]

The relationship between atrial fibrillation and stroke was, however, not as simple and direct as anticipated. This link was shown by the time lag between atrial fibrillation and thromboembolic event.[20] A subanalysis of the ASSERT trial clarified that, although subclinical atrial fibrillation was associated with an increased risk of stroke and embolism, very few patients had subclinical atrial fibrillation in the month before their event.[21] In another observational study, Shanmugam and colleagues[22] demonstrated that the majority of patients (73%) did not show a temporal association with the detected atrial episode and their adverse event, with a mean lag period of 46.7 ± 71.9 days before the thromboembolic complication. Thus, the link between atrial fibrillation and stroke seems to be more complex than previously appreciated, and subclinical atrial fibrillation may simply be a risk marker for stroke or may cause stroke via an indirect mechanism. Atrial fibrillation burden may play a role. Shanmugam and colleagues[22] demonstrated that patients with device-detected atrial high rate of greater than 3.8 hours over a day were 9 times more likely to develop thromboembolic events compared with patients without atrial high rate episodes (P<.006). A recent subanalysis of the ASSERT trial demonstrated a relationship of duration of subclinical atrial fibrillation and embolism. Patients with a duration of atrial fibrillation of greater than 24 hours had a significantly increased risk of subsequent stroke or systemic embolism (adjusted hazard ratio, 3.24; 95% confidence interval [CI], 1.51–6.95; P = .003).[23] The other end of the spectrum, short (<30-s) atrial fibrillation duration was not associated with increased risk.[24] Thus, although the causal relationship between atrial fibrillation and stroke remains unclear, current data indicate that a longer duration of atrial fibrillation (ie, >24 hours) is associated with a higher risk of stroke.

Current Evidence About Remote Monitoring and Atrial Fibrillation

The automatic intervention algorithm to suppress atrial fibrillation (eg, AF Suppression, continuous atrial overdrive pacing) was not only ineffective but also poorly tolerated for the management of new-onset atrial fibrillation, and it accelerated battery depletion.[25] Therefore, medical intervention by medical professionals, such as optimization of medication including anticoagulation with or without invasive methods such as cardioversion or ablation, should be considered. The next clinical question is whether we can reduce embolism and heart failure precipitated by atrial fibrillation by RM or not,[26] and if we can, what is the most efficient way of intervening.

The reliability of RM for atrial arrhythmia detection, quantification, and early notification has been well-established.[27] The percentage of inappropriate atrial fibrillation detection (owing to far-field R wave oversensing, T wave oversensing, repetitive nonreentrant V-A synchrony, or noise) is reduced using RM that permits visualization of intracardiac electrograms.[7,28] The HomeGuide Registry clarified that automatic RM had a high sensitivity and positive predictive value for major cardiovascular events, including atrial fibrillation.[29] Among the true positive events, 36% were atrial tachyarrhythmias and 93% of the atrial events were detected by RM. This technology allowed early detection of atrial fibrillation in CIED patients and appropriate reaction to optimize medical treatment on average 148 days earlier.[30] Computer modeling suggested that automatic daily monitoring of patients potentially reduced the stroke risk by 9% to 18% with an absolute reduction of 0.2% to 0.6% compared with standard follow-up with intervals of 6 to 12 months.[31] These observational studies and registry promised a potential paradigm shift for the care of patients with atrial fibrillation. However, data from randomized, controlled trials have not been so definitive.

In the Cardiovascular Outcomes for People Using Anticoagulation Strategies (COMPAS) trial[32] hospitalizations for atrial arrhythmias (6 vs 18) and strokes (2 vs 8) were fewer (P<.05) in RM group than in the control group. However, the IMPACT trial showed a neutral result about improvement of clinical outcome (stroke, systemic embolism, or major bleeding) by the early initiation of anticoagulation based on RM.[33] This is again possibly owing to temporal dissociation between atrial fibrillation and stroke, and stroke mechanisms not linked to atrial fibrillation. This study also did have a limitation in that more than 90% of patients with stroke were not under anticoagulation or had suboptimal International Normalized Ratio values. Furthermore, subanalysis of the IMPACT study indicated the suboptimal anticoagulation (mean TTR [time in therapeutic range] of 0.536 ± 0.23) overall.[34] A subanalysis of the HomeGuide study, however, showed the potential benefit of RM; the incidence of thromboembolic events was less than one-half the estimations based on the CHA2DS2-VASc risk profile, which could be due to appropriate medical intervention (85% of events that necessitate intervention were detected by RM with a short reaction time of 1 day [range, 0–6]).[35]

Hence, in summary, the current status is that (1) device-detected atrial fibrillation is associated with increased stroke risk, (2) RM is useful for early detection and quantification,[36] but (3) early anticoagulation based on RM has not been shown to reduce stroke risk, and there are no data to support the safety of the discontinuation of anticoagulation based on the absence of device-detected atrial fibrillation for a certain period. The latter may be guided by results of Tailored Anticoagulation for Noncontinuous AF (TACTIC-AF), a multicenter, randomized, controlled pilot study of RM to evaluate the intermittent use of anticoagulation in patients with established but infrequent atrial fibrillation. In this study, anticoagulation is initiated or discontinued based on the atrial fibrillation burden detected by RM transmitted twice a week. In the future, to better classify the clinical relevance and importance of alerts for atrial fibrillation, an automatic system that integrates alert information and the patient data extracted from the electronic health record may guide appropriate and effective anticoagulation decisions.[37–39]

Fig. 1 shows the assessment of RM and atrial fibrillation. Recent registries and randomized, controlled trials are grouped and discussed in **Table 1**. Ongoing studies of RM related to atrial fibrillation are listed in **Table 2**, as registered on ClinicalTrials.gov as of May 2017.

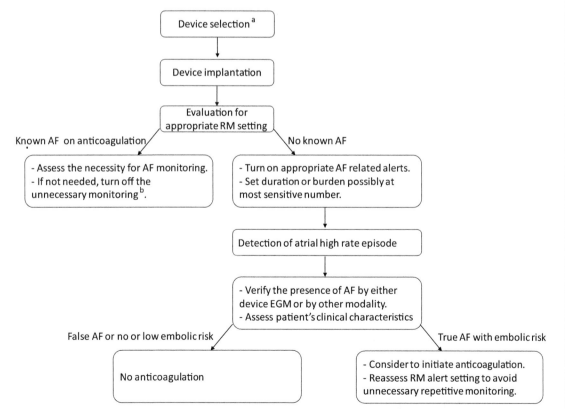

Fig. 1. Management of atrial fibrillation with remote monitoring. [a] Content of remote monitoring (RM) can be one of the selection criteria. [b] Area needed to be studied for the appropriate alert setting for patients with known atrial fibrillation (AF). EGM, electrogram.

Table 1
Clinical evidence of RM about atrial fibrillation

Study Name	Year	Type	n	Inclusion Criteria	Endpoints	Definition of AF	Results	Statistical Values	Findings
Randomized trials									
IMPACT	2015	Randomized, prospective, multicenter	2718	ICD/CRTD, Biotronik HM, CHADS2 ≥1	First occurrence of stroke, systemic embolism, or major bleeding	Duration depends on the risk (any duration to >48 h)	2.4 per 100 patient-years in HM vs 2.3 per 100 patient-years in control	P = .732	No difference in stroke or all-cause mortality between RM and control
SETAM	2017	Randomized, prospective, multicenter	595	PM, Biotronik HM, CHA2DS2VASc ≥2 No known prior AF	Time between implantation and the first treated atrial arrhythmia	Duration >6 h or burden >10%/d	114 d in HM vs 224 d in control	P = .01	Patients with RM were diagnosed and treated earlier.
Registries, observational cohort studies									
HomeGuide Registry	2013	Nonrandomized, prospective, observational	1650	PM/ICD/CRTD, Biotronik HM	All major CV event	AF burden >10% for ≥5 d, AF burden = 100% for 2 d	Events found in 51% of patients (82% in HM, 18% in-person visit)	Sensitivity 84.3%; PPV 97.4%	RM was effective in detecting and managing clinical events in CIED patients

Abbreviations: AF, atrial fibrillation; CIED, cardiac implantable electronic device; CRTD, cardiac resynchronization therapy defibrillator; CV, cardiovascular; HM, home monitoring; ICD, implantable cardioverter defibrillator; PM, pacemaker; PPV, positive predictive value; RM, remote monitoring.

Table 2
Ongoing studies of remote monitoring related to atrial fibrillation as of May 2017

Study	NCT Identifier	Sponsor	Design	Outcomes	Locations	Status
TACTIC AF	NCT01650298	St. Jude Medical	Randomized, parallel assignment, open label	All-cause heart failure, cardiovascular, and stroke hospitalizations and death over 1 year	United States	Estimated primary completion date in February 2017
RACE V	NCT02726698	Maastricht University Medical Center	Observational, prospective cohort	Progression of atrial fibrillation burden over 2.5 y	The Netherlands	Recruiting
SILENT	NCT02004509	InCor Heart Institute	Randomized, parallel assignment, open label	Stroke or systemic embolism	Brazil	Estimated primary completion date in Oct 2020

From https://clinicaltrials.gov. Accessed May 31, 2017.

It is important to note that devices from different manufacturers may categorize and notify atrial fibrillation[40] differently, and this factor should be considered when selecting devices. **Table 3** shows the technical aspects of current RM platforms. Some offer automatic continuous monitoring, yet others do not have alert mechanisms. Each manufacturer has its own definition of an atrial high rate, and detection depends on its setting (eg, cutoff rate) and atrial sensitivity. Some detect duration, and others monitor burden (whether these atrial fibrillation patterns influence stroke risk is unknown[41]). Some parameters are set to "on" as the initial setting, and others have to be turned on manually.

Remote Monitoring for Atrial Fibrillation: Beyond Anticoagulation Decisions

Management of atrial fibrillation using RM promotes cost effectiveness[42] and reduces manpower utilization[29,43] compared with conventional ambulatory control. In the HomeGuide model with a nurse-centered organizational system, expert nurses reviewed 70% of all transmissions. Only 15% were submitted to physicians for clinical evaluation, which showed the effectiveness and time savings of the management of data.

Atrial fibrillation is one of the major cause of the unnecessary ICD therapies.[44] Prompt management of atrial fibrillation by RM may reduce the inappropriate therapies by ICDs, which will prevent harm to heart. Atrial fibrillation may precipitate heart failure.

REMOTE MONITORING AND HEART FAILURE
Current Evidence About Remote Monitoring and Heart Failure

Two large nationwide mega cohort analyses (Aliskiren Trial in Type 2 Diabetes Using Cardiorenal Endpoints [ALTITUDE][45] and MERLIN[46]) demonstrated a large survival benefit associated with the use of RM. The level of adherence to RM had shown to be related to the survival. The limitations of cohort studies were that each cohort was restricted to devices from a single manufacturer and lacked clinical details.

The Patient Related Determinants of ICD Remote Monitoring (PREDICT RM) study,[47,48] based on ALTITUDE, added patient demographics and confirmed that RM patients (hazard ratio, 0.67; 95% CI, 0.64–0.71; $P<.0001$) compared with conventionally managed patients (hazard ratio, 0.82; 95% CI, 0.80–0.84; $P<.0001$) had a lower risk of mortality and hospitalization.

Nonrandomized studies show benefit of RM. Smaller studies inclusive of differing RM technologies (eg, the prospective clinical efficacy in the management of heart failure [EFFECT] trial[49] and the retrospective analysis by Portugal and colleagues[50]) suggested that RM improved clinical outcomes of death and cardiovascular hospitalizations. Also, a matched cohort study based on Contemporary Modalities In Treatment of Heart Failure Registry (COMMIT-HF; an ongoing prospective observational registry) showed that RM of ICD/cardiac resynchronization therapy

Table 3
Technical aspects of current RM platforms about AF

Brand Name of RM Manufacture	MyCareLink (Medtronic)	Merlin.net (Abbott, St. Jude Medical)	Latitude NXT (Boston Scientific)	Home Monitoring (Biotronik)	SMARTVIEW (LivaNova, Sorin)
Parameters transmitted via alert (range of the alert)					
Pacemaker	(Alert not available)	AT/AF duration (0.5–24 h)[a] AT/AF burden (0.5–48 h/d or week)[a] Average V rate during AT/AF (90–200 bpm/1–12 h)[a]	A arrhythmia burden (0–24 h/24 h)	AHR episode (1–50/d)[a] AT/AF burden (0%–75%/d)[a] MS (20–50/d)[a] MS duration (10%–75%/d) average V rate during MS (110–150 bpm/5%–30%)[a]	(Alert not available)
ICD/CRTD	AT/AF duration (0.5–24 h) average V rate during AT/AF (90–150 bpm/0.5–24 h)	AT/AF duration (0.5–24 h)[a] AT/AF burden (0.5–48 h/d or week)[a] Average V rate during AT/AF (90–200 bpm/1–12 h)[a]	A arrhythmia burden (0–24 h/24 h)	AT/AF burden (0%–75%) average V rate during AT/AF (110–150 bpm/5%–30%) detection of AT/AF (every time, 3/wk), long A arrhythmia episode (6–12 h)[a]	AT/AF burden (0.5–24 h/24 h)[a] Average V rate during AT/AF (80–120 bpm/0.5–24 h)[a]

Abbreviations: A, atrial; AF, atrial fibrillation; AHR, atrial high rate; AT, atrial tachyarrhythmia; CRT, cardiac resynchronization therapy; ICD, implantable cardioverter-defibrillator; MS, mode switch; RM, remote monitoring; V, ventricular.

[a] Initial setting of the alert is OFF.

defibrillator significantly reduced long-term mortality in a real-world clinical condition.[51] This registry includes patients with heart failure with CIED not limited to a single manufacturer. The latest nationwide cohort study[52] with a large number of patients (n = 92,566) with implanted devices from any manufacturer, demonstrated that patients using RM had a lower adjusted risk of all-cause hospitalization, at a hazard ratio of 0.82 (95% CI, 0.80–0.84; $P<.001$), and a shorter mean duration of hospitalization (5.3 days vs 8.1 days; $P<.001$) during follow-up. This cohort proved that RM had the power to reduce the hospitalization associated with heart failure, no matter which manufacturer and device were selected. The REmote SUpervision to Decrease HospitaLization RaTe (RESULT) study[53] is an ongoing randomized study including 3 brands (St. Jude Medical, Biotronik, and Medtronic) to assess the composite outcome of death for any reason or hospitalization owing to cardiovascular reasons. With the result of RESULT, we will know whether the benefit of RM is system specific or not.

Current large, prospective, randomized controlled trials, however, have shown mixed results. The landmark Implant-Based Multiparameter Telemonitoring of Patients With Heart Failure (IN-TIME) trial[54] showed the survival benefit of RM with daily automatic multiparameter data transmission (excluding thoracic impedance) in Biotronik devices (but hospitalization was unchanged). Evaluation of fluid status based in Medtronic devices in prospective randomized trials have not shown benefit with RM of thoracic impedance.[55–58] The recent OptiLink HF trial[56] did not show a significant difference of a composite of all-cause death and cardiovascular hospitalization (45.0% in RM arm and 48.1% in the control arm at 1.9 years; $P = .13$). The MOnitoring Resynchronization dEvices and CARdiac patiEnts (MORE-CARE) trial[57] showed no difference about a composite of death or cardiovascular- and device-related hospitalization (29.7% in RM arm and 28.7% in the control arm at 2 years; $P = .89$). The Remote Management of Heart Failure Using Implantable Electronic Devices (REM-HF) trial[58] showed no additive impact of weekly RM with thoracic impedance in outcome during a median follow-up period of 2.8 years (primary composite outcome in 42.4% of the weekly RM group and in 40.8% of the control group; $P = .87$). These studies are listed in detail in **Table 4**.

The neutral results of recent randomized controlled trials with thoracic impedance are considered to be due to several limitations in demographics of patients and design of the studies.

Compared with IN-TIME,[54] REM-HF[58] enrolled less severe patients with fewer New York Heart Association functional class III or IV, MORE-CARE[57] had a lower mortality rate in its control group and high comorbidity rate, and OptiLink[56] had fewer successful data transmission, and a low intervention rate. All of them would have mitigated the impact of RM on heart failure management. Also, REM-HF[58] showed the addition of weekly RM to patients who already had well-controlled symptoms possibly with satisfactory adherence to any heart failure treatment was no better than standard care. In the real world, however, adherence to heart failure treatment is challenging, and for those patients who are nonadherent, RM may play an important role in the early detection of disease deterioration.

Recent metaanalyses yield differing results. In one,[59] assessing 11 randomized controlled studies up to 2015 showed RM was associated with a reduction in total number of visits (relative risk, 0.56; 95% CI ,0.43–0.73; $P<.001$), but not on cardiac hospitalization or total and cardiac mortality. Parthiban and colleagues[60] included 7 randomized controlled RM trials and showed that overall, clinical outcomes were comparable to conventional follow-up in terms of all-cause mortality (odds ratio [OR], 0.83; $P = .285$), cardiovascular mortality (OR, 0.66; $P = .103$), and hospitalization (OR, 0.83; $P = .196$). However, a survival benefit (OR, 0.65; $P = .021$) was noted in the 3 trials only featuring RM with daily automatic multiparameter data transmission (Biotronik, Home Monitoring) characterized by high reliability of daily transmission.[61] This finding was confirmed by the latest metaanalysis of 3 trials (Lumos-T Safely Reduces Routine Office Device Follow-up [TRUST], ECOST, and IN-TIME) using Home Monitoring.[62] This analysis demonstrated that home monitoring reduced all-cause death ($P = .037$) and the composite endpoints of worsening heart failure hospitalization and all-cause or worsening heart failure death ($P = .007$).

On balance, the data indicate the following. (1) Thoracic impedance alone lacks any evidence to support its usefulness for clinical outcome. (2) Multiparameter monitoring (without thoracic impedance) with daily transmission is useful for heart failure management including mortality benefit. Operational characteristics (eg, automaticity, frequency of transmission, and its reliability) may provide the level of connectivity necessary to observe these effects.[61]

Several studies are ongoing for the further evidence of RM about heart failure and are shown in **Table 5**, as registered on ClinicalTrials.gov as of May 2017.

Table 4
Clinical evidence of RM about heart failure

Study Name or Author, Year	Study Type	No. of Patients	Inclusion Criteria	Endpoints	Results	Statistical Values	Findings
Randomized trials							
TRUST, 2010	Randomized, prospective, multicenter	1339	ICDs, Biotronik HM, no PM dependent	Total in-hospital device evaluations	2.1 per patient-year in the RM arm vs 3.8 per patient-year in the control arm.	P<.001	RM was safe in supplanting 'routine' in-office visits allowing an early event detection in ICD recipients.
				Overall adverse event rate	10.4% in both groups at 12 mo	P = .005	
				Time from event onset to physician evaluation	RM reduced event detection by >30 d	Noninferiority P<.001	
IN-TIME, 2014	Randomized, prospective, multicenter	716	ICDs/CRTDs, Biotronik HM, NYHA functional class II/III, LVEF ≤35%	Primary outcome: composite clinical score combining all-cause death, overnight hospital admission for HF, change in NYHA functional class, and change in patient global self-assessment	18.9% patients in HM group vs 27.2% in control group worsened at 1 y	P = .013	The first RCT that showed RM reduced all-cause mortality
				Secondary outcome: all-cause mortality and hospital admission heart failure admissions	1-y all-cause mortality in the HM group was 3.4% vs 8.7% in control group RM did not affect HF admissions	P = .004 P = .38	

Study, year	Design	Number	Device	Endpoint	Result	P value	Conclusion
OptiLink, 2016	Randomized, prospective, multicenter	1002	ICDs/CRTDs, Medtronic CareLink, NYHA functional II/III, LVEF ≤35%	A composite of all-cause death and CV hospitalization	45.0% in RM arm and 48.1% in the control arm at 1.9 y	$P = .13$	RM of fluid status did not significantly improve clinical outcome. Adherence was found to be a challenge
REM-HF, presented in 2016	Randomized, prospective, multicenter	1650	ICDs/CRTs, Medtronic, SJM, or Boston, NYHA functional class II–IV	A composite of time to first event of all-cause death or unplanned CV hospitalization	Occurred in 42.4% of the weekly RM group and in 40.8% of the control group at 2.8 y	$P = .87$	Adding weekly RM to well-controlled patients is no better than standard HF care with standard RM
MORE-CARE, 2016	Randomized, prospective, multicenter	865	CRTDs, Medtronic CareLink	A composite of death and CV and device-related hospitalization	29.7% in RM arm and 28.7% in the control arm at 2 y	$P = .89$	RM of CRTDs did not reduce mortality or CV and device-related hospitalization
Registries, observational cohort studies							
ALTITUDE, 2010	Nonrandomized, prospective, networked patients	185,778	ICDs/CRTDs, Boston Latitude	Patient survival	1- and 5-y survival rates were higher in RM patients	$P<.0001$ 50% reduction	RM improves survival
MERLIN, 2015	Nonrandomized, networked patients	Consecutive 269,471	PMs/ICDs/CRTs, SJM Merlin.net	Survival according to level of adherence to RM and device type	>75% adherence to RM promoted best survival. PM patients gained similar survival advantage with >75% adherence to RM	$P<.001$ $P<.001$	RM mediated survival depends on degree of adherence, but not on device type

(continued on next page)

Table 4
(continued)

Study Name or Author, Year	Study Type	No. of Patients	Inclusion Criteria	Endpoints	Results	Statistical Values	Findings
EFFECT, 2015	Nonrandomized, prospective, observational	987	ICDs/CRTDs, Medtronic, SJM, Boston, or Biotronik	A composite of all-cause death and CV hospitalization	0.15 events/year in RM arm and 0.27 events/year in standard arm at 1 y	P<.001	RM reduced mortality and CV hospitalization
Piccini et al,[52] 2016	Retrospective, observational	92,566	PMs/ICDs/CRTs, any manufacturer	All-cause hospitalization	0.39 per patient-year in RM arm vs 0.49 per patient-year in no RM arm	P<.001	RM reduced hospitalization and cost
				Health care costs	$8720 mean cost per patient-year in RM arm vs $12,423 mean cost per patient-year in no RM arm	P<.001	
Metaanalyses							
Parthiban et al,[60] 2015	Metaanalysis of RCTs	4932 from 7 RCTs for mortality	ICDs	All-cause mortality	RM demonstrated mortality comparable with office follow-up	P = .285	Survival benefit was noted in only Biotronik HM
Klersy et al,[59] 2016	Metaanalysis of RCTs	5702 from 11 RCTs	PMs/ICDs/CRTs	Total number of CV hospitalization	Similar between RM and standard care	P = .60	RM was not associated with reduction of hospitalization
				Total number of hospital visits	RM was associated with a reduction in visits	P<.001	

Abbreviations: CRT, cardiac resynchronization therapy; CRTD, cardiac resynchronization therapy defibrillator; CV, cardiovascular; HF, heart failure; HM, Home Monitoring; ICD, implantable cardioverter defibrillator; LVEF, left ventricular ejection fraction; NYHA, New York Heart Association; PM, pacemaker; RCT, randomized controlled trials; RM, remote monitoring; SJM, St. Jude Medical.

Table 5
Ongoing studies of remote monitoring about heart failure as of May 2017

Study	NCT Identifier	Sponsor	Design	Outcomes	Locations	Status
RESULT	NCT02409225	Silesian Centre for Heart Diseases	Randomized, parallel assignment, open label	Death for any reason or hospitalization owing to cardiovascular reasons	Poland	Active, not recruiting
REMOTE-CIED	NCT01691586	UMC Utrecht	Observational, prospective cohort	Patient-reported health status and device acceptance	The Netherland	Active, not recruiting
ECOST-CRT	NCT03012490	University Hospital, Lille	Randomized, parallel assignment, open label	All-cause mortality or worsening heart failure hospitalization	France	Not yet open for recruiting
BioDetectHFIV	NCT01836510	Biotronik	Observational, prospective cohort	First hospitalization for worsening heart failure	Italy	Active, not recruiting
IMPLANTED	NCT03061747	Azienda Ospedaliera Cardinale G. Panico	Observational, retrospective cohort	Death for any cause	Italy	Recruiting
COR-HF	NCT01482598	St. Jude Medical	Randomized, parallel assignment, open label	Combined endpoint on patient clinical outcome	Italy	Active, not recruiting

From https://clinicaltrials.gov. Accessed May 31, 2017.

Table 6
Technical aspects of current RM platforms about heart

Brand Name of RM Manufacture	MyCareLink (Medtronic)	Merlin.net (Abbott, St. Jude Medical)	Latitude NXT (Boston Scientific)	Home Monitoring (Biotronik)	SMARTVIEW (LivaNova, Sorin)
1. Parameters transmitted via alert (range of the alert)	(Alert not available)	RV pacing (0%–95%, 1–90 d) CorVue (8–18 d beyond threshold) BiV pacing (60%–100%/1–90 d)	RV pacing (10%–50%) Body weight (1–10 lb, 1–7 d) CRT pacing (50%–95%)	RV pacing (10%–90%) Average V rate (70–140 bpm) Average V rate at rest (70–140 bpm) Average PVC (10–250 beats/h) BiV pacing (50%–95%) CRT pacing (50%–95%)	CRT pacing (50%–95%)
2. Parameters not transmitted via alert (evaluated on the website)	RV pacing (%) Average V rate (bpm) Patient activity (h/d) Thoracic impedance (ohm) HRV (ms) OptiVol 2.0[a]	Activity (h) Heart rate (bpm)	Blood pressure (mm Hg) Activity level (%) Heart rate (bpm) Respiratory rate (/min) AP scan (/h) HRV footprint (%) SDANN (ms) Autonomic balance monitor	HRV (ms) Activity (%/d) Thoracic impedance (ohm)	(Not available)

Abbreviations: AP, atrial pacing; BiV, biventricular pacing; CRT, cardiac resynchronization therapy; HRV, heart rate variability; PVC, premature ventricular contraction; RM, remote monitoring; RV, right ventricle; SDANN, standard deviation of averaged normal-to-normal intervals; V, ventricular.
[a] Can be transmitted via alert in other than the U.S.

Important Aspects When Evaluating Heart Failure and Remote Monitoring

Several important points should be considered, regarding the use of RM for heart failure. First, cost effectiveness is highly important issue in modern medicine. The nationwide cohort study mentioned[52] showed that RM was associated with a $3703 reduction in hospitalization cost per patient-year (P<.001) including all device types, and a $7358 reduction in ICD patients (43% lower; P<.001). The latest subanalysis of EFFECT trial recently confirmed the reduction in direct health care costs of RM for patients with heart failure with ICDs, particularly CRT-D, compared with standard monitoring.[63] Hence, RM is highly advocated to improve the economics of health care use among patients with CIEDs. Reimbursement should be strengthened based on these recent positive data.

Second, we have to keep in mind that the parameters and setting of RM for heart failure is highly variable among different proprietary systems (far more than for atrial fibrillation; compare **Table 3** with **Table 6**). **Table 6** shows the parameters related to heart failure. No direct comparison among each manufacturer or evidence for the optimal setting for with maximized sensitivity and specificity exist currently.

Third, the burden associated with handling RM for heart failure is far from negligible. Because the parameter varies and we do not know the optimal setting, activating alerts with low specificity will increase the workload. The standardization of technology[64] and algorithms to alert[65,66] will be required.

CURRENT GUIDELINES

The Heart Rhythm Society's (HRS) Expert Consensus Statement on RM (2015)[67] advocates a class I recommendation (level of evidence A) for the use of this technology in patients receiving all forms of CIEDs. The 2013 European Society of Cardiology guideline stated RM as a class IIa recommendation (level of evidence A).[68]

Specifically, for atrial fibrillation, the recommendation is class I (level of evidence A) in the HRS Expert Consensus, stating its usefulness for the early detection and quantification, but not for driving anticoagulation decisions. The 2016 European Society of Cardiology guideline for atrial fibrillation[69] and the Third Atrial Fibrillation Competence NETwork/European Heart Rhythm Association consensus conference[70] comment on device-detected atrial fibrillation and provide an algorithm for its management, but without comment on the usefulness of RM. The management of atrial fibrillation should be guided by the 2014 American Heart Association/American College of Cardiology/HRS guideline[71] (which also does not comment on RM).

For heart failure management, the 2015 HRS Expert Consensus statement[67] recommends class IIb (level of evidence C), stating that the effectiveness of the technique for thoracic impedance alone, or combined with other diagnostics, to manage congestive heart failure is currently uncertain. The 2013 ACCF/American Heart Association guideline for heart failure[72] or focused update in 2017[73] contained no comment on RM. The latest (2016) European guideline for heart failure[74] assigned a class IIb recommendation to RM, indicating that multiparameter monitoring based on devices (the IN-TIME approach) may be considered in symptomatic patients with heart failure with reduced ejection fraction (left ventricular ejection fraction ≤35%) to improve clinical outcomes. This support is strengthened by the recent patient-level metaanalysis of trials specifically using home monitoring technology.

With these recommendations, however, the recent deployment rate of RM among ICD patients remains less than 50% according to a nationwide cohort study.[52]

FUTURE DIRECTIONS

According to current evidence and guidelines, RM of patients receiving CIEDs is highly recommended for atrial fibrillation and should be considered for heart failure. Problems that need to be overcome are (1) clarification of optimal alert setting of CIEDs and cutoff for anticoagulation for atrial fibrillation to prevent thromboembolic events that can be used for any manufacturer, (2) the establishment of possible safety standards for the discontinuation of anticoagulation based on RM, if any, (3) construction of an automatic system that integrates the alert information and the patient data extracted from the electronic health record to prevent thromboembolic events, (4) technical advancements such as user-friendly automatic transmission with portability to improve adherence to RM of patients with heart failure, and (5) construction of a monitoring algorithm for heart failure with standardized operation for preemptive intervention.

REFERENCES

1. Varma N, Epstein AE, Irimpen A, et al. Efficacy and safety of automatic remote monitoring for implantable cardioverter-defibrillator follow-up: the Lumos-T

Safely Reduces Routine Office Device Follow-up (TRUST) trial. Circulation 2010;122:325–32.

2. Guedon-Moreau L, Chevalier P, Marquie C, et al. Contributions of remote monitoring to the follow-up of implantable cardioverter-defibrillator leads under advisory. Eur Heart J 2010;31:2246–52.

3. Guedon-Moreau L, Kouakam C, Klug D, et al. Decreased delivery of inappropriate shocks achieved by remote monitoring of ICD: a substudy of the ECOST trial. J Cardiovasc Electrophysiol 2014;25:763–70.

4. Spencker S, Coban N, Koch L, et al. Potential role of home monitoring to reduce inappropriate shocks in implantable cardioverter-defibrillator patients due to lead failure. Europace 2009;11:483–8.

5. Varma N, Michalski J, Epstein AE, et al. Automatic remote monitoring of implantable cardioverter-defibrillator lead and generator performance: the Lumos-T Safely RedUceS RouTine Office Device Follow-Up (TRUST) trial. Circ Arrhythm Electrophysiol 2010;3:428–36.

6. Pollak WM, Simmons JD, Interian A Jr, et al. Clinical utility of intraatrial pacemaker stored electrograms to diagnose atrial fibrillation and flutter. Pacing Clin Electrophysiol 2001;24:424–9.

7. Seidl K, Meisel E, VanAgt E, et al. Is the atrial high rate episode diagnostic feature reliable in detecting paroxysmal episodes of atrial tachyarrhythmias? Pacing Clin Electrophysiol 1998;21:694–700.

8. Purerfellner H, Gillis AM, Holbrook R, et al. Accuracy of atrial tachyarrhythmia detection in implantable devices with arrhythmia therapies. Pacing Clin Electrophysiol 2004;27:983–92.

9. Glotzer TV, Hellkamp AS, Zimmerman J, et al. Atrial high rate episodes detected by pacemaker diagnostics predict death and stroke: report of the Atrial Diagnostics Ancillary Study of the MOde Selection Trial (MOST). Circulation 2003;107:1614–9.

10. Glotzer TV, Daoud EG, Wyse DG, et al. The relationship between daily atrial tachyarrhythmia burden from implantable device diagnostics and stroke risk: the TRENDS study. Circ Arrhythm Electrophysiol 2009;2:474–80.

11. Capucci A, Santini M, Padeletti L, et al. Monitored atrial fibrillation duration predicts arterial embolic events in patients suffering from bradycardia and atrial fibrillation implanted with antitachycardia pacemakers. J Am Coll Cardiol 2005;46:1913–20.

12. Santini M, Gasparini M, Landolina M, et al. Device-detected atrial tachyarrhythmias predict adverse outcome in real-world patients with implantable biventricular defibrillators. J Am Coll Cardiol 2011; 57:167–72.

13. Gonzalez M, Keating RJ, Markowitz SM, et al. Newly detected atrial high rate episodes predict long-term mortality outcomes in patients with permanent pacemakers. Heart Rhythm 2014;11:2214–21.

14. Israel CW, Gronefeld G, Ehrlich JR, et al. Long-term risk of recurrent atrial fibrillation as documented by an implantable monitoring device: implications for optimal patient care. J Am Coll Cardiol 2004;43: 47–52.

15. Orlov MV, Ghali JK, Araghi-Niknam M, et al. Asymptomatic atrial fibrillation in pacemaker recipients: incidence, progression, and determinants based on the atrial high rate trial. Pacing Clin Electrophysiol 2007;30:404–11.

16. Defaye P, Dournaux F, Mouton E. Prevalence of supraventricular arrhythmias from the automated analysis of data stored in the DDD pacemakers of 617 patients: the AIDA study. The AIDA Multicenter Study Group. Automatic interpretation for diagnosis assistance. Pacing Clin Electrophysiol 1998;21: 250–5.

17. Healey JS, Connolly SJ, Gold MR, et al. Subclinical atrial fibrillation and the risk of stroke. N Engl J Med 2012;366:120–9.

18. Subclinical atrial fibrillation and the risk of stroke. N Engl J Med 2016;374:998.

19. Hohnloser SH, Capucci A, Fain E, et al. ASymptomatic atrial fibrillation and stroke Evaluation in pacemaker patients and the atrial fibrillation reduction atrial pacing trial (ASSERT). Am Heart J 2006;152:442–7.

20. Daoud EG, Glotzer TV, Wyse DG, et al. Temporal relationship of atrial tachyarrhythmias, cerebrovascular events, and systemic emboli based on stored device data: a subgroup analysis of TRENDS. Heart Rhythm 2011;8:1416–23.

21. Brambatti M, Connolly SJ, Gold MR, et al. Temporal relationship between subclinical atrial fibrillation and embolic events. Circulation 2014;129:2094–9.

22. Shanmugam N, Boerdlein A, Proff J, et al. Detection of atrial high-rate events by continuous home monitoring: clinical significance in the heart failure-cardiac resynchronization therapy population. Europace 2012;14:230–7.

23. Van Gelder IC, Healey JS, Crijns HJ, et al. Duration of device-detected subclinical atrial fibrillation and occurrence of stroke in ASSERT. Eur Heart J 2017; 38(17):1339–44.

24. Swiryn S, Orlov MV, Benditt DG, et al. Clinical implications of brief device-detected atrial tachyarrhythmias in a cardiac rhythm management device population: results from the Registry of Atrial Tachycardia and Atrial Fibrillation Episodes. Circulation 2016;134:1130–40.

25. Hohnloser SH, Healey JS, Gold MR, et al. Atrial overdrive pacing to prevent atrial fibrillation: insights from ASSERT. Heart Rhythm 2012;9:1667–73.

26. Ricci RP, Morichelli L, Santini M. Home monitoring remote control of pacemaker and implantable cardioverter defibrillator patients in clinical practice: impact on medical management and health-care resource utilization. Europace 2008;10:164–70.

27. Varma N, Stambler B, Chun S. Detection of atrial fibrillation by implanted devices with wireless data transmission capability. Pacing Clin Electrophysiol 2005;28(Suppl 1):S133–6.

28. Nagele H, Lipoldova J, Oswald H, et al. Home monitoring of implantable cardioverter-defibrillators: interpretation reliability of the second-generation "IEGM Online" system. Europace 2015;17:584–90.

29. Ricci RP, Morichelli L, D'Onofrio A, et al. Effectiveness of remote monitoring of CIEDs in detection and treatment of clinical and device-related cardiovascular events in daily practice: the HomeGuide registry. Europace 2013;15:970–7.

30. Ricci RP, Morichelli L, Santini M. Remote control of implanted devices through home monitoring technology improves detection and clinical management of atrial fibrillation. Europace 2009;11:54–61.

31. Ricci RP, Morichelli L, Gargaro A, et al. Home monitoring in patients with implantable cardiac devices: is there a potential reduction of stroke risk? Results from a computer model tested through Monte Carlo simulations. J Cardiovasc Electrophysiol 2009;20: 1244–51.

32. Mabo P, Victor F, Bazin P, et al. A randomized trial of long-term remote monitoring of pacemaker recipients (the COMPAS trial). Eur Heart J 2012;33:1105–11.

33. Healey JS, Lopes RD, Connolly SJ. The detection and treatment of subclinical atrial fibrillation: evaluating the IMPACT of a comprehensive strategy based on remote arrhythmia monitoring. Eur Heart J 2015;36:1640–2.

34. Lip GY, Waldo AL, Ip J, et al. Determinants of time in therapeutic range in patients receiving oral anticoagulants (a substudy of IMPACT). Am J Cardiol 2016;118:1680–4.

35. Ricci RP, Vaccari D, Morichelli L, et al. Stroke incidence in patients with cardiac implantable electronic devices remotely controlled with automatic alerts of atrial fibrillation. A sub-analysis of the HomeGuide study. Int J Cardiol 2016;219:251–6.

36. Amara W, Montagnier C, Cheggour S, et al. Early detection and treatment of atrial arrhythmias alleviates the arrhythmic burden in paced patients: the SETAM study. Pacing Clin Electrophysiol 2017; 40(5):527–36.

37. Rosier A, Mabo P, Temal L, et al. Remote monitoring of cardiac implantable devices: ontology driven classification of the alerts. Stud Health Technol Inform 2016;221:59–63.

38. Zoppo F, Facchin D, Molon G, et al. Improving atrial fibrillation detection in patients with implantable cardiac devices by means of a remote monitoring and management application. Pacing Clin Electrophysiol 2014;37:1610–8.

39. Rosier A, Mabo P, Temal L, et al. Personalized and automated remote monitoring of atrial fibrillation. Europace 2016;18:347–52.

40. Ploux S, Varma N, Strik M, et al. Optimizing implantable cardioverter-defibrillator remote monitoring. JACC Clin Electrophysiol 2017;3:315–28.

41. Turakhia MP, Ziegler PD, Schmitt SK, et al. Atrial fibrillation burden and short-term risk of stroke: case-crossover analysis of continuously recorded heart rhythm from cardiac electronic implanted devices. Circ Arrhythm Electrophysiol 2015;8:1040–7.

42. Lorenzoni G, Folino F, Soriani N, et al. Cost-effectiveness of early detection of atrial fibrillation via remote control of implanted devices. J Eval Clin Pract 2014; 20:570–7.

43. Ricci RP, Morichelli L, D'Onofrio A, et al. Manpower and outpatient clinic workload for remote monitoring of patients with cardiac implantable electronic devices: data from the HomeGuide Registry. J Cardiovasc Electrophysiol 2014;25:1216–23.

44. Shah H, Mezu U, Patel D, et al. Mechanisms of inappropriate defibrillator therapy in a modern cohort of remotely monitored patients. Pacing Clin Electrophysiol 2013;36:547–52.

45. Saxon LA, Hayes DL, Gilliam FR, et al. Long-term outcome after ICD and CRT implantation and influence of remote device follow-up: the ALTITUDE survival study. Circulation 2010;122:2359–67.

46. Varma N, Piccini JP, Snell J, et al. The relationship between level of adherence to automatic wireless remote monitoring and survival in pacemaker and defibrillator patients. J Am Coll Cardiol 2015;65: 2601–10.

47. Akar JG, Bao H, Jones P, et al. Use of remote monitoring of newly implanted cardioverter-defibrillators: insights from the Patient Related Determinants of ICD Remote Monitoring (PREDICT RM) study. Circulation 2013;128:2372–83.

48. Akar JG, Bao H, Jones PW, et al. Use of remote monitoring is associated with lower risk of adverse outcomes among patients with implanted cardiac defibrillators. Circ Arrhythm Electrophysiol 2015;8: 1173–80.

49. De Simone A, Leoni L, Luzi M, et al. Remote monitoring improves outcome after ICD implantation: the Clinical Efficacy in the Management of Heart Failure (EFFECT) study. Europace 2015;17:1267–75.

50. Portugal G, Cunha P, Valente B, et al. Influence of remote monitoring on long-term cardiovascular outcomes after cardioverter-defibrillator implantation. Int J Cardiol 2016;222:764–8.

51. Kurek A, Tajstra M, Gadula-Gacek E, et al. Impact of remote monitoring on long-term prognosis in heart failure patients in a real-world cohort: results from all-comers COMMIT-HF trial. J Cardiovasc Electrophysiol 2017;28:425–31.

52. Piccini JP, Mittal S, Snell J, et al. Impact of remote monitoring on clinical events and associated health care utilization: a nationwide assessment. Heart Rhythm 2016;13:2279–86.

53. Tajstra M, Sokal A, Gwozdz A, et al. REmote SUpervision to Decrease HospitaLization RaTe. Unified and integrated platform for data collected from devices manufactured by different companies: design and rationale of the RESULT study. Ann Noninvasive Electrocardiol 2017;22:e12418–12424.

54. Hindricks G, Taborsky M, Glikson M, et al. Implant-based multiparameter telemonitoring of patients with heart failure (IN-TIME): a randomised controlled trial. Lancet 2014;384:583–90.

55. Luthje L, Vollmann D, Seegers J, et al. A randomized study of remote monitoring and fluid monitoring for the management of patients with implanted cardiac arrhythmia devices. Europace 2015;17:1276–81.

56. Bohm M, Drexler H, Oswald H, et al. Fluid status telemedicine alerts for heart failure: a randomized controlled trial. Eur Heart J 2016;37(41):3154–63.

57. Boriani G, Da Costa A, Quesada A, et al. Effects of remote monitoring on clinical outcomes and use of healthcare resources in heart failure patients with biventricular defibrillators: results of the MORE-CARE multicentre randomized controlled trial. Eur J Heart Fail 2016;19(3):416–25.

58. Morgan JM, Dimitrov BD, Gill J, et al. Rationale and study design of the REM-HF study: remote management of heart failure using implanted devices and formalized follow-up procedures. Eur J Heart Fail 2014;16:1039–45.

59. Klersy C, Boriani G, De Silvestri A, et al. Effect of telemonitoring of cardiac implantable electronic devices on healthcare utilization: a meta-analysis of randomized controlled trials in patients with heart failure. Eur J Heart Fail 2016;18:195–204.

60. Parthiban N, Esterman A, Mahajan R, et al. Remote monitoring of implantable cardioverter-defibrillators: a systematic review and meta-analysis of clinical outcomes. J Am Coll Cardiol 2015;65:2591–600.

61. Varma N, Love CJ, Schweikert R, et al. Automatic remote monitoring utilizing daily transmissions: transmission reliability and implantable cardioverter defibrillator battery longevity in the TRUST trial. Europace 2017. [Epub ahead of print].

62. Hindricks G, Varma N, Kacet S, et al. Daily remote monitoring of implantable cardioverter-defibrillators: insights from the pooled patient-level data from three randomized controlled trials (IN-TIME, ECOST, TRUST). Eur Heart J 2017.

63. Capucci A, De Simone A, Luzi M, et al. Economic impact of remote monitoring after implantable defibrillators implantation in heart failure patients: an analysis from the EFFECT study. Europace 2017; 19(9):1493–9.

64. de Ruvo E, Sciarra L, Martino AM, et al. A prospective comparison of remote monitoring systems in implantable cardiac defibrillators: potential effects of frequency of transmissions. J Interv Card Electrophysiol 2016;45:81–90.

65. Bertini M, Marcantoni L, Toselli T, et al. Remote monitoring of implantable devices: should we continue to ignore it? Int J Cardiol 2016;202:368–77.

66. Arya A, Block M, Kautzner J, et al. Influence of home monitoring on the clinical status of heart failure patients: design and rationale of the IN-TIME study. Eur J Heart Fail 2008;10:1143–8.

67. Slotwiner D, Varma N, Akar JG, et al. HRS expert consensus statement on remote interrogation and monitoring for cardiovascular implantable electronic devices. Heart Rhythm 2015;12:e69–100.

68. Brignole M, Auricchio A, Baron-Esquivias G, et al. 2013 ESC Guidelines on cardiac pacing and cardiac resynchronization therapy: the Task Force on Cardiac Pacing and Resynchronization Therapy of the European Society of Cardiology (ESC). Developed in collaboration with the European Heart Rhythm Association (EHRA). Eur Heart J 2013;34:2281–329.

69. Kirchhof P, Benussi S, Kotecha D, et al. 2016 ESC guidelines for the management of atrial fibrillation developed in collaboration with EACTS. Eur Heart J 2016;37:2893–962.

70. Kirchhof P, Lip GY, Van Gelder IC, et al. Comprehensive risk reduction in patients with atrial fibrillation: emerging diagnostic and therapeutic options–a report from the 3rd Atrial Fibrillation Competence NETwork/European Heart Rhythm Association consensus conference. Europace 2012;14:8–27.

71. January CT, Wann LS, Alpert JS, et al. 2014 AHA/ACC/HRS guideline for the management of patients with atrial fibrillation: executive summary. J Am Coll Cardiol 2014;64:2246–80.

72. Writing Committee M, Yancy CW, Jessup M, et al. 2013 ACCF/AHA guideline for the management of heart failure: a report of the American College of Cardiology Foundation/American Heart Association Task Force on Practice Guidelines. Circulation 2013;128:e240–327.

73. Yancy CW, Jessup M, Bozkurt B, et al. 2017 ACC/AHA/HFSA focused update of the 2013 ACCF/AHA guideline for the management of heart failure: a report of the American College of Cardiology/American Heart Association Task Force on Clinical Practice Guidelines and the Heart Failure Society of America. Circulation 2017;136(6):e137–61.

74. Ponikowski P, Voors AA, Anker SD, et al. 2016 ESC Guidelines for the diagnosis and treatment of acute and chronic heart failure: the task Force for the diagnosis and treatment of acute and chronic heart failure of the European Society of Cardiology (ESC) developed with the special contribution of the Heart Failure Association (HFA) of the ESC. Eur Heart J 2016;37:2129–200.

Should Single-Coil Implantable Cardioverter Defibrillator Leads Be Used in all Patients?

Fahad Almehmadi, MBBS, FRCPC,
Jaimie Manlucu, MD, FRCPC*

KEYWORDS

- Single-coil • Dual-coil • Defibrillation threshold • Lead extraction • Mortality

KEY POINTS

- Dual coil implantable cardioverter defibrillator leads were originally designed to compensate for elevated defibrillation thresholds encountered with old device technology.
- The high safety margins generated by contemporary devices have rendered the modest difference in defibrillation threshold between single- and dual-coil leads clinically insignificant.
- Dual-coil leads are associated with a higher all-cause mortality, and a greater risk of major complication and/or death with transvenous lead extraction.
- Single-coil leads in conjunction with active left-pectoral generators are clinically effective, and a reasonable first choice in de novo implants and/or younger patients with longer life expectancies.

INTRODUCTION

Implantable cardioverter defibrillator (ICD) remains the mainstay therapy for patients at risk of malignant arrhythmias and sudden cardiac death (SCD).[1,2] This is achieved by the delivery of high voltage energy to the myocardium. The initial ICD platforms consisted of a large abdominal pulse generators and epicardial lead patches.[3,4] Unfortunately, implantation of these epicardial systems required a thoracotomy, which carried a reasonable risk of perioperative mortality, and a high rate of lead malfunction.[5–7] Over the past 2 decades, considerable advances in generator and lead technology have led to substantial improvements in the delivery and reliability of ICD therapy. The development of active pectoral pulse generators, biphasic waveforms, and transvenous leads

simplified the implant procedure, and dramatically improved defibrillation efficacy and safety margins. To accommodate the transition from the abdomen to an active left pectoral implant site, there came a necessary reduction in pulse generator size.[8] To compensate for the smaller generator, additional shocking coils were evaluated in an attempt to increase the defibrillation surface area. These coils were tested in multiple locations within the superior vena cava,[9,10] inferior vena cava,[11] right atrium, and coronary sinus.[12] Independent of these unipolar lead configurations, a more complex single-pass lead design was developed containing 2 separate defibrillator coils, one in the right ventricle (RV) and one in the superior vena cava (SVC).[9]

For years, dual-coil leads were preferred over ICD leads with a single coil in the RV. Used in

Disclosure Statement: J. Manlucu: Consulting for Medtronic Inc, F. Almehmadi: None.
Division of Cardiology, Department of Medicine, Western University, PO Box 5339, 339 Windermere Road, Room B6-127, London, Ontario N6A 5A5, Canada
* Corresponding author.
E-mail address: Jaimie.Manlucu@lhsc.on.ca

Card Electrophysiol Clin 10 (2018) 59–66
https://doi.org/10.1016/j.ccep.2017.11.010
1877-9182/18/© 2017 Elsevier Inc. All rights reserved.

conjunction with an active pulse generator, this 3-electrode (triad) configuration became common practice. In a large US cohort of 129,520 ICD patients, 85.2% of patients received a dual-coil lead between 2004 and 2014.[13] This practice was driven by a presumption of superior shock efficacy mainly based on early data suggesting that SVC coils may lower DFTs compared with a single coil in the RV alone.[8,10] However, the veracity of the evidence and its clinical value in light of the large safety margins achieved with contemporary high output pectoral generators are uncertain. A signal toward higher mortality rate and higher risk of lead extraction with dual-coil leads has also brought the utility of an SVC coil into question.[13,14] This article summarizes the current literature and re-evaluates the incremental benefits of a dual-coil over single-coil ICD leads.

EFFICACY
Differences in Defibrillation Threshold

The differences in defibrillation threshold between single- and dual-coil leads have been studied in several randomized and nonrandomized studies[8–10,14–24] (Table 1). Many early studies reported a statistically significant reduction in DFT with dual-coil systems.[8,10,11,18,19,23,25] However, subsequent studies showed conflicting results, with differences observed in some cohorts,[17,21–23,25] but not in others.[13,16] Two meta-analyses published earlier this year summarized the cumulative data comparing outcomes between the 2 ICD lead designs.[14,24] In a pooled analysis of 15 cohort studies and 2975 patients, a meta-analysis by Sunderland and colleagues showed that DFTs were lower in dual-coil leads compared single-coil leads. However, the absolute difference was small, with a mean difference of only 0.83 J (95% confidence interval [CI]: −1.39–0.27; $P = .004$). When the 2 randomized controlled trials were included in the analysis, no difference in DFT or first shock efficacy was observed between the 2 groups. Similar results were reported by Kumar and colleagues, where data pooled from 14 studies showed a mean DFT difference of 0.81 J (95% CI: 0.31–1.30 J; $P = .0014$) in favor of dual-coil leads with no difference in first-shock efficacy. Therefore, there appears to a real but fairly modest difference in DFT between the 2 lead models, with no difference in first-shock efficacy. With the high safety margin of contemporary biphasic, high-voltage, active pectoral pulse generators, this small difference may have limited clinical importance. Most ICDs can usually achieve a DFT that is 10 to 20J less than its maximum output with a 90% chance that

the first shock will successfully terminate the clinical arrhythmia.[26,27] Routine DFT testing has also gradually fallen out of favor. With reliable ICD technology rendering routine DFTs unnecessary,[28] and data suggesting that they are potentially harmful[29] and not predictive of shock failure[30] or death,[31] peri-implant DFT testing has become antiquated.[13]

Right-Sided Pulse Generators

Among the most instrumental innovations that led to a reduction in defibrillation thresholds was the development of an active pulse generator, where the titanium outer shell functions as a cathode. In this configuration, the anatomic location of the pulse generator becomes an important determinant of DFT and shock efficacy. Although a unipolar defibrillation system with a single coil in the RV and an active left-sided pectoral generator has proven to be a clinically reliable platform,[32,33] data on right-sided pulse generators are lacking. The few data that exist suggest that DFTs may be higher when the generator is on the right chest.[31,33–37] This observation may be due to a less favorable shock vector in this configuration. When an active pectoral generator is on the right, shock current is directed away from the left ventricle and toward the right shoulder. Because a coil in the SVC would shunt the current in a similar rightward direction, there should be no significant advantage of a dual-coil lead when partnered with a right-sided generator. This was confirmed in 2 cohort studies where, despite a lower shock impedance with dual-coil leads, no difference in DFT was observed between the 2 lead designs.[34,38] One study found that when shocking between 2 coils without an active pulse generator, the optimal position for the second coil was in the left subclavian, which directs current more toward the left ventricle compared with placing the coil in the SVC.[39] However, there was no incremental benefit to the second coil's position when an active left pectoral can was part of the shocking circuit.[18] This suggests that an SVC coil may be redundant if an active left pectoral generator is part of the circuit.

RISK
Transvenous Lead Extraction Outcomes

Much of the movement away from dual-coil leads has been fueled by data suggesting that extraction of dual-coil ICD leads are more complex and higher risk compared with single-coil leads.[40–42] Technical challenges, longer procedural times, and greater risk of serious vascular complications

Table 1
Summary of literature on DFTs in single versus dual-coil leads

Study	Study Type	N	Lead Coil Design		Efficacy Data	Safety Data
			Single	Dual		
Kumar et al,[24] 2017	Meta-Analysis	137,295	15.9%	84.1%	DC: lower DFT (mean difference 0.81 J), P<.01 No difference in first shock efficacy SC: lower overall mortality (HR = 0.91, P<.03)	
Sunderland et al,[14] 2017	Meta-analysis	138,124	16.1%	83.9%	DC: lower DFT (mean difference 0.83 J) No difference in first shock efficacy SC: lower overall mortality (HR = 0.91, P<.05)	
Lesham et al,[29] 2016	Israeli ICD Registry (2010–2015)	6343	32%	68%		No difference in all-cause mortality, heart failure hospitalization and ICD shocks
Larsen et al,[16] 2016	Danish Device Registry (2007–2011)	4769	38.9%	61.1%	DC: lower DFT (mean difference 1.1 J)	SC: lower mortality (HR 0.85, P<.05)
Hsu at al,[13] 2015	ALTITUDE database (2004–2014)	129,520	14.8%	85.2%	No difference in first shock efficacy	SC: lower mortality (HR 0.91, P<.05)
Baccillieri et al,[15] 2015	Multicenter Italian cohort	469	66%	34%	No difference in first shock efficacy (92.5%)	
Kutyifa et al,[17] 2013	MADIT-CRT substudy	1783	9.1%	90.9%	DC: lower DFT (mean difference 1.8 J) No difference in first shock efficacy (>90%)	No difference in all-cause mortality, short- (<30 d) and long-term complications
Aoukar et al,[53] 2013	SCD-HeFT substudy	811	27.9%	72.1%	No difference in mean DFT or 1st shock efficacy	No difference in overall mortality
Ellis et al,[54] 2012	St. Jude Medical ACT-ICD Registry	5424	5.4%	94.6%	No difference in 1st shock efficacy	
Verma et al,[34] 2008	Prospective single center cross-over study (order of DFT testing randomized)	42 (right-sided)	100% (SVC coil off)	100% (SVC coil on)	The only study on DFT solely right sided implants No difference in DFT with addition of SVC coil in shock configuration	

(continued on next page)

Table 1
(continued)

Study	Study Type	N	Lead Coil Design		Efficacy Data	Safety Data
			Single	**Dual**		
Lubinski et al,[25] 2005	Single center cohort study	138	55%	45%	DC: lower DFT (mean difference 1.6 J) DC: more patients with DFT <15 J (93% vs 81%)	
Rub et al,[55] 2004	Prospective single center cross-over study (order of DFT testing randomized)	11	100% (SVC coil off)	100% (SVC coil on)	No difference in DFT	
Rinaldi et al,[22] 2003	Multicentre RCT	76	50%	50%	No difference in DFT	
Schulte et al,[21] 2001	Multicentre RCT	80	50%	50%	No difference in DFT	
Libero et al,[23] 2001	Single center prospective cohort study	44	100% (SVC coil off)	100% (SVC coil on)	DC: lower DFT (mean difference 2.3 J)	
Gold et al,[18] 2000	Prospective single center cross-over study (order of DFT testing randomized)	27	100% (SVC coil off)	100% (SVC coil on)	DC: lower stored energy at peak DFT (mean difference 2.3 J) DC: more patients with DFT≤15J (96% vs 81%)	
Manolis et al,[20] 2000	Prospective study	94	34%	66%	No difference in DFT	
Gold et al,[10] 1998	Prospective single center cross-over study (order of DFT testing randomized)	50	100%	100%	DC: lower DFT (mean difference 1.4 J), lower shock impedance, and higher peak current DC: more DFT≤15 (98% vs 88%)	
Gold et al,[8] 1997	Prospective single center cross-over study (order of DFT testing randomized)	21	100% (SVC coil off)	100% (SVC coil on)	DC: lower DFT (mean difference 3.4 J) DFT ≤15 J in all patients with dual coil + active can	
Bardy et al,[9] 1994	Prospective single center cross-over study (order of DFT testing randomized)	15	100% (SVC coil off)	100% (SVC coil on)	No difference in mean DFT	

Abbreviations: DC, dual-coil; SC, single-coil.

have been attributed to the proximal SVC coil.[42–45] This is largely due to exaggerated fibrotic ingrowth and dense vascular adhesions that form around the defibrillation coil[46] and its position near the angulation of the innominate vein and SVC junction[47] (**Fig. 1**). During extraction, necessary manual traction forces on the lead are transmitted to the innominate-SVC angle, increasing the risk of potentially catastrophic vascular injury[45,48] and mortality.[49,50] In Hauser and colleagues'[51] analysis of the US Food and Drug Administration's (FDA's) Manufacturer User Defined Experience (MAUDE) database for adverse events related to lead extraction, 70% of all deaths and life-threatening injuries were caused by lacerations in the SVC, innominate vein and right atrium. In a multicenter cohort of 2176 ICD lead extractions at experienced, high-volume centers, dual-coil leads were 2.6 times more difficult to extract, even after adjusting for age, implant duration, extraction indication, back-filled coils, fixation mechanism, and number of leads removed. Moreover, all deaths and major complications occurred exclusively among patients with dual-coil leads, despite longer lead implant durations in the single-coil leads.[50] In another single-center cohort of over 5000 lead extractions, dual-coil leads were also associated with a 2.7-fold higher 30-day mortality compared with single-coil leads.[49] Therefore, the current literature suggests that extraction of dual-coil leads may be associated with more challenging extraction procedures and poorer outcomes. As life expectancy prolongs, and repeat pocket interventions make patients increasingly susceptible to hardware failure and/or infection, lead extraction becomes an increasingly important consideration in the management of device patients.

Mortality

The most recently published study comparing outcomes in single- versus dual-coil ICD leads was based on the Israeli ICD Registry. In this cohort of 6343 patients, there was no difference in mortality between the 2 lead designs.[29] However, mean follow-up was only 1.6 years. Conversely, when data were pooled from 4 other studies on a total of 97,843 patients over a follow-up period of 35 to 72 months, all-cause mortality was significantly lower with single-coil leads (hazard ratio [HR] 0.91; 95% CI: 0.86-0.95; $P<.0001$).[14] This was primarily driven by data from the ALTITUDE study, the largest collection of data comparing all-cause mortality in almost 13,000 patients with single- and dual-coil leads[13] (**Fig. 2**). Although the survival analysis in these studies was adjusted for several covariates, residual confounding could not be

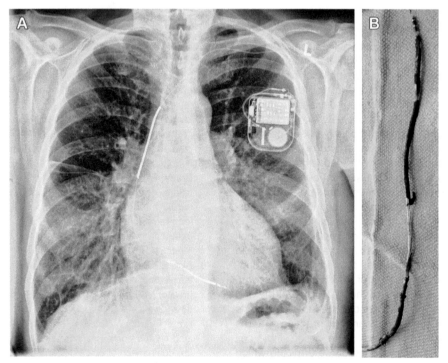

Fig. 1. (*A*): Chest radiograph showing a dual-coil ICD lead. (*B*) Dual-coil ICD lead following transvenous extraction. Note the fibrous encapsulation along the lead, most notably around the RV and SVC coils.

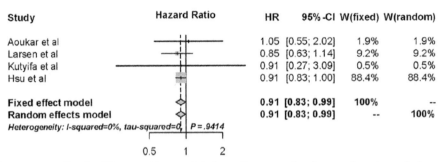

Fig. 2. All-cause mortality by ICD type. Forest plot from Kumar and colleagues' meta-analysis summarizing estimated HR for all-cause mortality in single-coil versus dual-coil ICD leads. The plot shows lower estimates of all-cause mortality with single-coil ICDs. (*From* Kumar P, Baker M, Gehi A. Comparison of single-coil and dual-coil implantable defibrillators: a meta-analysis. JACC Clin Electrophysiol 2017;3(1):12–9; with permission.)

excluded. Because patients were not randomized to single- or dual-coil leads, the difference in mortality between the 2 lead designs could be attributed to factors such as selection bias, where sicker patients with more advanced heart failure may have received dual-coil leads. As discussed previously, the higher mortality rate seen with dual-coil leads may also be attributed to long-term lead-related complications and poor outcomes associated with lead extraction. This theory is supported by the finding that the difference in mortality was noted several years after the initial implant procedure.

SUMMARY

The historical preference of dual-coil leads dates back to an era of abdominal devices and high DFTs. With the advent of high energy left pectoral active cans and biphasic defibrillation waveforms, a 1 to 2 J advantage with a dual-coil lead is far less clinically meaningful if current devices are already able to achieve 10 to 20 J safety margins with an RV coil alone. This is particularly true if the trade-off is a higher risk of death and/or catastrophic vascular complication with lead extraction. This may, in part, explain the survival benefit reported with single-coil leads among large cohort studies. Therefore, with modern ICD technology, the current data support the use of single-coil leads in routine de novo left pectoral implants. Single-coil leads may also be an appropriate first choice in young patients who may face longer life expectancies and a higher risk of lead failure or infection. Based on the results of the ALTITUDE study and the National Cardiovascular Data Registry's (NCDR) ICD data, it appears that practice patterns are already tipping back in favor of single-coil leads.[13,52] Studies focused on determining which patient populations may benefit from dual-coil leads are needed.

REFERENCES

1. Russo AM, Stainback RF, Bailey SR, et al. ACCF/HRS/ AHA/ASE/HFSA/SCAI/SCCT/SCMR 2013 appropriate use criteria for implantable cardioverter-defibrillators and cardiac resynchronization therapy: a report of the American College of Cardiology Foundation appropriate use criteria task force, Heart Rhythm Society, American Heart Association, American Society of Echocardiography, Heart Failure Society of America, Society for Cardiovascular Angiography and Interventions, Society of Cardiovascular Computed Tomography, and Society for Cardiovascular Magnetic Resonance. Heart Rhythm 2013;10(4):e11–58.
2. Bennett M, Parkash R, Nery P, et al. Canadian Cardiovascular Society/Canadian Heart Rhythm Society 2016 implantable cardioverter-defibrillator guidelines. Can J Cardiol 2017;33(2):174–88.
3. Mirowski M, Mower MM, Reid PR, et al. Implantable automatic defibrillators: their potential in prevention of sudden coronary death. Ann N Y Acad Sci 1982;382:371–80.
4. Mirowski M, Reid PR, Mower MM, et al. Termination of malignant ventricular arrhythmias with an implanted automatic defibrillator in human beings. N Engl J Med 1980;303(6):322–4.
5. Brady PA, Friedman PA, Trusty JM, et al. High failure rate for an epicardial implantable cardioverter-defibrillator lead: implications for long-term follow-up of patients with an implantable cardioverter-defibrillator. J Am Coll Cardiol 1998;31(3):616–22.
6. Almassi GH, Olinger GN, Wetherbee JN, et al. Long-term complications of implantable cardioverter defibrillator lead systems. Ann Thorac Surg 1993;55(4): 888–92.
7. Korte T, Jung W, Spehl S, et al. Incidence of ICD lead related complications during long-term follow-up: comparison of epicardial and endocardial electrode systems. Pacing Clin Electrophysiol 1995; 18(11):2053–61.

8. Gold MR, Foster AH, Shorofsky SR. Lead system optimization for transvenous defibrillation. Am J Cardiol 1997;80(9):1163–7.

9. Bardy GH, Dolack GL, Kudenchuk PJ, et al. Prospective, randomized comparison in humans of a unipolar defibrillation system with that using an additional superior vena cava electrode. Circulation 1994;89(3):1090–3.

10. Gold MR, Olsovsky MR, Pelini MA, et al. Comparison of single- and dual-coil active pectoral defibrillation lead systems. J Am Coll Cardiol 1998;31(6):1391–4.

11. Favale S, Dicandia CD, Tunzi P, et al. A prospective, randomized, comparison in patients between a pectoral unipolar defibrillation system and that using an additional inferior vena cava electrode. Pacing Clin Electrophysiol 1999;22(8):1140–5.

12. Kudenchuk PJ, Bardy GH, Dolack GL, et al. Efficacy of a single-lead unipolar transvenous defibrillator compared with a system employing an additional coronary sinus electrode. A prospective, randomized study. Circulation 1994;89(6):2641–4.

13. Hsu JC, Saxon LA, Jones PW, et al. Utilization trends and clinical outcomes in patients implanted with a single- vs a dual-coil implantable cardioverter-defibrillator lead: insights from the ALTITUDE study. Heart Rhythm 2015;12(8):1770–5.

14. Sunderland N, Kaura A, Murgatroyd F, et al. Outcomes with single-coil versus dual-coil implantable cardioverter defibrillators: a meta-analysis. Europace 2017. [Epub ahead of print].

15. Baccillieri MS, Gasparini G, Benacchio L, et al. Multicentre comparison of shock efficacy using single- vs. Dual-coil lead systems and Anodal vs. cathodaL polarITY defibrillation in patients undergoing transvenous cardioverter-defibrillator implantation. The MODALITY study. J Interv Card Electrophysiol 2015;43(1):45–54.

16. Larsen JM, Hjortshoj SP, Nielsen JC, et al. Single-coil and dual-coil defibrillator leads and association with clinical outcomes in a complete Danish nationwide ICD cohort. Heart Rhythm 2016;13(3):706–12.

17. Kutyifa V, Huth Ruwald AC, Aktas MK, et al. Clinical impact, safety, and efficacy of single- versus dual-coil ICD leads in MADIT-CRT. J Cardiovasc Electrophysiol 2013;24(11):1246–52.

18. Gold MR, Olsovsky MR, DeGroot PJ, et al. Optimization of transvenous coil position for active can defibrillation thresholds. J Cardiovasc Electrophysiol 2000;11(1):25–9.

19. Gold M, Val-Mejias J, Leman RB, et al. Optimization of superior vena cava coil position and usage for transvenous defibrillation. Heart Rhythm 2008;5(3):394–9.

20. Manolis AS, Chiladakis J, Maounis TN, et al. Two-coil versus single-coil transvenous cardioverter defibrillator systems: comparative data. Pacing Clin Electrophysiol 2000;23(11 Pt 2):1999–2002.

21. Schulte B, Sperzel J, Carlsson J, et al. Dual-coil vs single-coil active pectoral implantable defibrillator lead systems: defibrillation energy requirements and probability of defibrillation success at multiples of the defibrillation energy requirements. Europace 2001;3(3):177–80.

22. Rinaldi CA, Simon RD, Geelen P, et al. A randomized prospective study of single coil versus dual coil defibrillation in patients with ventricular arrhythmias undergoing implantable cardioverter defibrillator therapy. Pacing Clin Electrophysiol 2003;26(8):1684–90.

23. Libero L, Lozano IF, Bocchiardo M, et al. Comparison of defibrillation thresholds using monodirectional electrical vector versus bidirectional electrical vector. Ital Heart J 2001;2(6):449–55.

24. Kumar P, Baker M, Gehi A. Comparison of single-coil and dual-coil implantable defibrillators: a meta-analysis. JACC Clin Electrophysiol 2017;3(1):12–9.

25. Lubinski A, Lewicka-Nowak E, Zienciuk A, et al. Comparison of defibrillation efficacy using implantable cardioverter-defibrillator with single- or dual-coil defibrillation leads and active can. Kardiol Pol 2005;63(3):234–41 [discussion:242–33].

26. Pires LA, Johnson KM. Intraoperative testing of the implantable cardioverter-defibrillator: how much is enough? J Cardiovasc Electrophysiol 2006;17(2):140–5.

27. Healey JS, Gula LJ, Birnie DH, et al. A randomized-controlled pilot study comparing ICD implantation with and without intraoperative defibrillation testing in patients with heart failure and severe left ventricular dysfunction: a substudy of the RAFT trial. J Cardiovasc Electrophysiol 2012;23(12):1313–6.

28. Strickberger SA, Klein GJ. Is defibrillation testing required for defibrillator implantation? J Am Coll Cardiol 2004;44(1):88–91.

29. Leshem E, Suleiman M, Laish-Farkash A, et al. Contemporary rates and outcomes of single- vs. dual-coil implantable cardioverter defibrillator lead implantation: data from the Israeli ICD Registry. Europace 2017;19(9):1485–92.

30. Healey JS, Hohnloser SH, Glikson M, et al. Cardioverter defibrillator implantation without induction of ventricular fibrillation: a single-blind, non-inferiority, randomised controlled trial (SIMPLE). Lancet 2015;385(9970):785–91.

31. Phan K, Ha H, Kabunga P, et al. Systematic review of defibrillation threshold testing at de novo implantation. Circ Arrhythm Electrophysiol 2016;9(4):e003357.

32. Gold MR, Higgins S, Klein R, et al. Efficacy and temporal stability of reduced safety margins for ventricular defibrillation: primary results from the Low Energy Safety Study (LESS). Circulation 2002;105(17):2043–8.

33. Gold MR, Val-Mejias J, Cuoco F, et al. Comparison of fixed tilt and tuned defibrillation waveforms: the

PROMISE study. J Cardiovasc Electrophysiol 2013; 24(3):323–7.

34. Varma N, Efimov I. Right pectoral implantable cardioverter defibrillators: role of the proximal (SVC) coil. Pacing Clin Electrophysiol 2008;31(8):1025–35.

35. Epstein AE, Kay GN, Plumb VJ, et al. Elevated defibrillation threshold when right-sided venous access is used for nonthoracotomy implantable defibrillator lead implantation. The Endotak investigators. J Cardiovasc Electrophysiol 1995;6(11):979–86.

36. Friedman PA, Rasmussen MJ, Grice S, et al. Defibrillation thresholds are increased by right-sided implantation of totally transvenous implantable cardioverter defibrillators. Pacing Clin Electrophysiol 1999;22(8):1186–92.

37. Gold MR, Shih HT, Herre J, et al. Comparison of defibrillation efficacy and survival associated with right versus left pectoral placement for implantable defibrillators. Am J Cardiol 2007;100(2):243–6.

38. Varma N, Schaerf R, Kalbfleisch S, et al. Defibrillation thresholds with right pectoral implantable cardioverter defibrillators and impact of waveform tuning (the Tilt and Tune trial). Europace 2017;19(11): 1810–7.

39. Stajduhar KC, Ott GY, Kron J, et al. Optimal electrode position for transvenous defibrillation: a prospective randomized study. J Am Coll Cardiol 1996;27(1):90–4.

40. Gradaus R, Breithardt G, Bocker D. ICD leads: design and chronic dysfunctions. Pacing Clin Electrophysiol 2003;26(2 Pt 1):649–57.

41. Kennergren C, Bjurman C, Wiklund R, et al. A single-centre experience of over one thousand lead extractions. Europace 2009;11(5):612–7.

42. Bracke FA, Meijer A, Van Gelder LM. Malfunction of endocardial defibrillator leads and lead extraction: where do they meet? Europace 2002;4(1):19–24.

43. Malecka B, Kutarski A, Grabowski M. Is the transvenous extraction of cardioverter-defibrillator leads more hazardous than that of pacemaker leads? Kardiol Pol 2010;68(8):884–90.

44. Cooper JM, Stephenson EA, Berul CI, et al. Implantable cardioverter defibrillator lead complications and laser extraction in children and young adults with congenital heart disease: implications for implantation and management. J Cardiovasc Electrophysiol 2003;14(4):344–9.

45. Bracke F. Complications and lead extraction in cardiac pacing and defibrillation. Neth Heart J 2008; 16(Suppl 1):S28–31.

46. Segreti L, Di Cori A, Soldati E, et al. Major predictors of fibrous adherences in transvenous implantable cardioverter-defibrillator lead extraction. Heart Rhythm 2014;11(12):2196–201.

47. Koplan BA, Weiner S, Gilligan D, et al. Clinical and electrical performance of expanded polytetrafluoroethylene-covered defibrillator leads in comparison to traditional leads. Pacing Clin Electrophysiol 2008;31(1):47–55.

48. Maytin M, Epstein LM. The challenges of transvenous lead extraction. Heart 2011;97(5):425–34.

49. Brunner MP, Cronin EM, Duarte VE, et al. Clinical predictors of adverse patient outcomes in an experience of more than 5000 chronic endovascular pacemaker and defibrillator lead extractions. Heart Rhythm 2014;11(5):799–805.

50. Epstein LM, Love CJ, Wilkoff BL, et al. Superior vena cava defibrillator coils make transvenous lead extraction more challenging and riskier. J Am Coll Cardiol 2013;61(9):987–9.

51. Hauser RG, Katsiyiannis WT, Gornick CC, et al. Deaths and cardiovascular injuries due to device-assisted implantable cardioverter-defibrillator and pacemaker lead extraction. Europace 2010;12(3): 395–401.

52. Pokorney SD, Parzynski M, Daubert JP, et al. Temporal trends in and factors associated with use of single- versus dual-coil implantable cardioverter-defibrillator leads: data from the NCDR ICD registry. JACC Clin Electrophysiol 2017;3(6):612–9.

53. Aoukar PS, Poole JE, Johnson GW, et al. No benefit of a dual coil over a single coil ICD lead: evidence from the sudden cardiac death in heart failure trial. Heart Rhythm 2013;10(7):970–6.

54. Ellis C, Hurt J. Single-coil versus dual-coil ICD lead shock efficacy in a large ICD registry. J Innov Card Rhythm Management 2012;3:953–8.

55. Rub N, Schweitzer O, Mewis C, et al. Addition of a defibrillation electrode in the low right atrium to a right ventricular lead does not reduce ventricular defibrillation thresholds. Pacing Clin Electrophysiol 2004;27(3):346–51.

Causes and Prevention of Inappropriate Implantable Cardioverter-Defibrillator Shocks

Nitin Kulkarni, MD, Mark S. Link, MD*

KEYWORDS

- Implantable cardioverter-defibrillator ● Inappropriate shocks ● Electromagnetic interference

KEY POINTS

- Implantable cardioverter-defibrillators (ICDs) deliver inappropriate therapy with a reported incidence between 2% and 20% a year.
- Nonphysiologic sensing may be caused by external electromagnetic sources, device-related issues, or supraventricular arrhythmias.
- Electromagnetic sources reported to result in inappropriate shocks include monopolar electrosurgery used during surgery; MRI; close proximity to leaking alternating current from various sources, including power equipment and arc welding; and being exposed to an electrical stun gun.
- Device-related causes of inappropriate shocks are physiologic, such as T-wave oversensing or sensing of diaphragmatic myopotentials, or pathologic, such as oversensing of lead noise.
- Advances in ICD programming have decreased but not eliminated inappropriate shocks.

INTRODUCTION

The use of implantable cardioverter-defibrillators (ICDs) as a primary prevention therapy has been shown to reduce mortality in patients after cardiac arrest and also with left ventricular systolic dysfunction.[1] However, these devices are not without morbidity. In addition to periprocedural complications, patients are also at risk of receiving inappropriate therapies, which include inappropriate shocks and antitachycardic pacing (ATP). ICD shocks have been associated with the development of psychological disorders, poor quality of life, and increased risk of death when compared with patients who do not receive any therapy.[2] Given the morbidity and potential mortality associated with inappropriate shocks, significant advances have been made in ICD programming to minimize inappropriate therapies with the publication of several landmark trials.[3–5]

This article reviews the epidemiology and etiology of inappropriate ICD shocks, the adverse effects of ICD shocks, and strategies to minimize the risk of ICD therapies.

EPIDEMIOLOGY

The rates of inappropriate shocks reported in clinical trials are significant. In the Multicenter Automatic Defibrillator Implantation II (MADIT II) trial, 11.5% of the patients experienced an inappropriate shock, with inappropriate shocks accounting for 31.2% of all shocks during the 2-year follow-up.[6] Similar rates were found in an analysis of the Sudden Cardiac Death in Heart Failure (SCD-HeFT) trial, in which 17.4% of the patients

Division of Cardiology, Department of Internal Medicine, University of Texas Southwestern Medical Center, 5323 Harry Hines Boulevard, Dallas, TX 75390-9047, USA
* Corresponding author.
E-mail address: mark.link@utsouthwestern.edu

Card Electrophysiol Clin 10 (2018) 67–74
https://doi.org/10.1016/j.ccep.2017.11.006

experienced inappropriate shocks during a median follow-up of 3.8 years, and inappropriate shocks accounted for at least 32.3% of all ICD shocks.[7] Even higher percentage of patients were noted have experienced inappropriate shocks in the Prophylactic Defibrillator Implantation in Patients with Nonischemic Dilated Cardiomyopathy (DEFINITE) trial, with 49 of the 229 patients (21.4%) in the ICD arm experiencing inappropriate shocks during a mean follow-up of 29 months.[8]

Rates of inappropriate shocks reported in registry and cohort studies tend to be more variable and at times markedly lower compared with incidence rates in clinical trials. A Dutch study of 1544 patients who had ICDs implanted from 1996 to 2004 found 13% of patients received inappropriate shocks during 41 months of follow-up.[9] A similar rate was found in a large US observational study of 186,000 patients, where the 5-year incidence rate of inappropriate shocks was 16%.[10] In contrast, a Danish study looking at a prospective cohort of 1609 patients with ischemic heart disease and primary prevention ICDs found an inappropriate shocks incidence rate of 2.6% during mean follow-up of 1.9 years.[11] Additionally, a retrospective multicenter study in Spain of 1012 patients also found an inappropriate shocks incidence rate of 6.8% during a mean follow-up of 2.7 years.[12] However, an analysis of the patients enrolled in Boston Scientific's remote monitoring system (LATITUDE) found that 41% of first shocks were deemed inappropriate.[13] A major limitation in assessing the trends of inappropriate shocks over time using cohort or registry data is that often these studies report a rate of inappropriate shocks over a certain time period rather than an annual rate. Heterogeneity in device programming over time may account for the wide variance in incidence rates in "real-world" studies.

The advent of the subcutaneous ICD (S-ICD) was an opportunity to obviate some of the complications associated with a transvenous ICD system (pneumothorax, lead fracture, lead perforation, lead dislodgement, and device-associated endocarditis) in eligible patients. The rates of inappropriate shocks with the S-ICD system seem to be comparable with the rates of transvenous ICD. In a large Dutch cohort of 581 patients, 8.3% of patients received inappropriate shocks during a mean follow-up of 21 months.[14] In a multicenter prospective trial assessing safety and efficacy of S-ICDs, 13.1% of patients received inappropriate shocks over a mean follow-up of 11 months.[15]

ETIOLOGIES OF INAPPROPRIATE SHOCKS

Etiologies of inappropriate shocks are conceptualized into framework consisting of three groups: (1) environmental causes leading to electromagnetic interference and inappropriate sensing of external noise, (2) device-related causes from inappropriate sensing of physiologic or pathologic signals, and (3) supraventricular arrhythmias. Environmental causes of inappropriate shocks are from inappropriate sensing of electromagnetic signals in the environment. These include monopolar electrosurgery used during surgery[16]; MRI[17]; close proximity to leaking alternating current from various sources, including power equipment (**Fig. 1**) and arc welding[18]; and being exposed to an electrical stun gun.[19] Device-related causes of inappropriate shocks are categorized based on the cause of inappropriate sensing: physiologic, such as T-wave oversensing (**Fig. 2**) or sensing of diaphragmatic myopotentials (**Fig. 3**); or

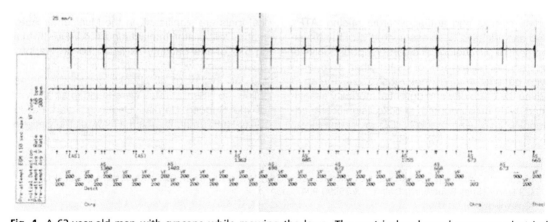

Fig. 1. A 63-year-old man with syncope while mowing the lawn. The ventricular channel senses an electrical signal from the electric lawnmower.

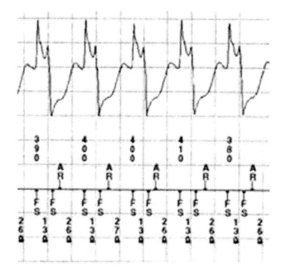

Fig. 2. T-wave oversensing in a 43-year-old patient with hypertrophic cardiomyopathy.

pathologic, such as oversensing of lead noise. Finally, patients can develop supraventricular tachycardia (SVT) or atrial fibrillation (AF) or atrial flutter (AFl) with rapid ventricular rates greater than the detection rate cutoffs (**Fig. 4**). If SVT discriminators fail or are ineligible to be applied because of detection in ventricular fibrillation (VF) zone, this can lead to inappropriate ICD shocks.

Based on the analysis of the MADIT II, the overwhelming cause of inappropriate shocks is supraventricular arrhythmias. AF/AFl/SVT accounts for 80% of inappropriate shocks in the MADIT II

cohort, with abnormal sensing accounting for the remainder.[6] These findings are similar to what are found in registry data. In the Dutch cohort of 1544 patients with ICD, misdiagnosis of supraventricular arrhythmias was the cause in 76% of patients with inappropriate shocks.[9] In a large US observational study, the most common reasons for inappropriate shocks were AF, AFl, SVT, and sinus tachycardia (accounting for 88% of inappropriate shocks), with inappropriate sensing accounting for only 9% of inappropriate shocks.

Although AF is also a predictor of inappropriate shocks in patients with S-ICDs, the most common cause of inappropriate shocks in subjects with these devices is T-wave oversensing (**Fig. 5**), which accounted for 73% of inappropriate shocks in a large Dutch cohort, followed by supraventricular arrhythmias (18%).[14] Predictors of inappropriate shocks in this patient cohort include a history of hypertrophic cardiomyopathy (hazard ratio [HR], 4.6; 95% confidence interval [CI], 1.6–13.9) and a history of AF (HR, 2.4; 95% CI, 1.1–5.2). The high rate of inappropriate shocks caused by cardiac signal oversensing emphasizes the importance of appropriate patient selection for this novel technology.

Given that supraventricular arrhythmias are the most common cause of inappropriate shocks in patients with transvenous ICDs, it is not surprising that a history of supraventricular arrhythmias, specifically AF, is one of the strongest predictors of receiving inappropriate shocks, a finding that is consistent across multiple studies.[6,9,12] Aggressive strategies using ICD programming, changes

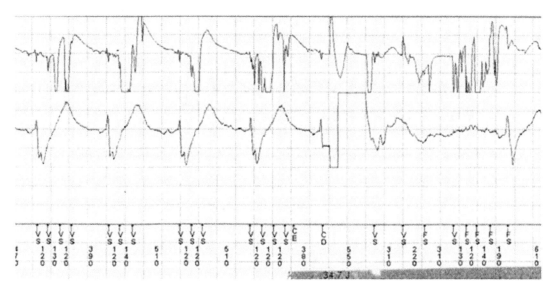

Fig. 3. Lead fracture in a 36-year-old man with arrhythmogenic right ventricular dysplasia. An insulation break exposes the electrical conducting wire to myopotentials.

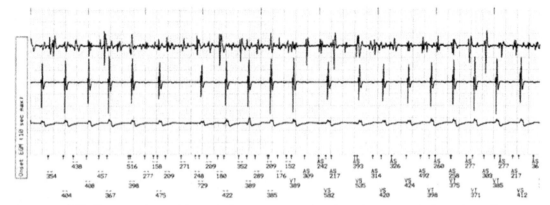

Fig. 4. Atrial fibrillation with a rapid ventricular response causing detection in ventricular tachycardia zone.

in medication regimen, or even ablative therapies should be considered in patients with a history of inappropriate shocks caused by supraventricular arrhythmias to prevent future events.

CONSEQUENCES OF IMPLANTABLE CARDIOVERTER-DEFIBRILLATOR SHOCKS

Although ICDs have been well established as a life-saving intervention in patients at risk of sustained

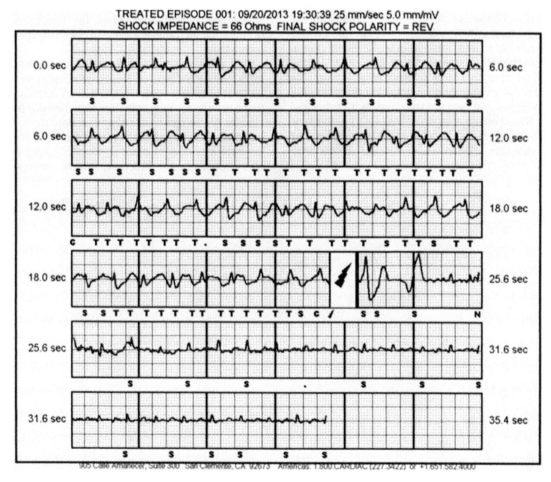

Fig. 5. A 35-year-old man with hypertrophic cardiomyopathy who received an S-ICD shock while exercising because of T-wave oversensing.

ventricular tachycardia (VT) or VF, the therapy is not without consequence. In a substudy of the SCD-HeFT trial, patients who had received an ICD shock were noted to have a decrease in quality of life as characterized by worsening perceived emotional, social, and physical function when compared with patients without ICD shocks.[20] This reduction in quality of life has also been found in a substudy of the Coronary Artery Bypass Graft (CABG) Patch trial.[21] Additionally, patients who experience inappropriate shocks within first 12 months of implant have more clinic visits, greater hospitalization rates, and overall higher rates of health care utilization.[22]

However, most concerning is the association of ICD shocks with increased mortality. First initially reported by Poole and colleagues[7] in 2008, the authors observed that patients in the SCD-HeFT cohort who received an appropriate ICD shock were at a significantly higher risk of death than those without ICD shocks (HR, 5.68; CI, 3.97–8.12). Those who received inappropriate ICD shocks were also at a higher risk of death when compared with those who did not receive any shocks (HR, 1.98; CI, 1.29–3.05). These findings have been consistent in a study of the MADIT II cohort, in which subjects with appropriate and inappropriate ICD shocks were noted to have a higher risk of death than those with ICD shocks (HR, 3.36; CI, 2.04–5.55; and HR, 2.29; CI, 1.11–4.71, respectively).[6] This increased mortality signal with inappropriate shocks has been noted in a large Dutch registry in which patients with inappropriate shocks had a 60% increase in mortality.[9]

It is of yet unclear the role of ICD shocks in worsening mortality. ICD shocks themselves may play a pathologic role in clinical deterioration, because high-voltage shocks may lead to worsening cardiac contractility.[23] A meta-analysis of ICD programming trials found that therapy reduction programming (higher detection rates and longer detection intervals) when compared with conventional programming lead to a reduction in mortality (HR, 0.74; CI, 0.61–0.91).[24] This study supports the causation theory, given that a reduction in shocks in randomized control trials lead to a reduction in mortality.

Alternatively, patients experiencing appropriate shocks secondary to VT/VF represent a high-risk and sicker subset of patients, and hence higher mortality rates. Patients experiencing inappropriate shocks are more likely to have rapid AF, which is also associated with increased mortality.[25,26] In case-control study of patients with ICD enrolled in Boston Scientific's remote monitoring system (LATITUDE),[13] the authors found that patients who had inappropriate shocks caused by AF/AFI were at increased risk of death (HR, 1.61; CI, 1.17–2.21), but not those who had inappropriate shocks secondary to sinus tachycardia/SVT (HR, 0.97; CI, 0.68–1.37) or inappropriate sensing (HR, 0.91; CI, 0.50–1.67), suggesting that the substrate, rather than the shock itself, is leading to worsening clinical outcomes.

Nevertheless, given that harm signal associated with ICD shocks, both appropriate and inappropriate strategies to minimize shocks are not only worth pursuing, but part of good clinical care.

PREVENTION OF APPROPRIATE AND INAPPROPRIATE IMPLANTABLE CARDIOVERTER-DEFIBRILLATOR SHOCKS

Patients with ICD shocks offer an opportunity for intervention to help prevent future recurrences. Preventative strategies for inappropriate shocks secondary to arrhythmias include ICD reprogramming to using therapy-reduction strategies, implementing medical therapy, referring patients to cardiac rehabilitation (often underused), and referring patients for ablation, whether it be for SVT, AF, or AV junction ablation (not discussed here). Patients with ICD shocks secondary to oversensing require device reprogramming or lead revision.

Implantable Cardioverter-Defibrillator Programming

A multitude of clinical trials have shown a consistent strategy in ICD programming that leads to a reduction in ICD shocks, and these strategies are recommended in an expert consensus statement endorsed by the Heart Rhythm Society, European Heart Rhythm Association, Asia-Pacific Heart Rhythm Society, and Sociedad Latinoamericana de Estimulacian Cardiaca y Electrofiologia.[27] These strategies are divided into three categories: (1) prolonging detection, (2) implementing ATP to terminate VT, and (3) using discriminator algorithms to distinguish SVT from VT.

Prevention Parameters Evaluation (PREPARE) study was the first to show clinical benefits of prolonging arrhythmia detection.[3] A historical cohort with conventional detection programming (12 of 16 intervals or 18 of 24 intervals) was compared with a treatment arm of 700 patients primary prevention ICD with prolonged arrhythmia detection (30 of 40 intervals), and the authors found significant reduction in ICD shocks in the treatment arm (9% vs 17%) with no difference in syncope. These findings were then replicated in two prospective randomized clinical trials. Both the Role of Long Detection Window Programming in Patients with Left Ventricular Dysfunction (RELEVANT; n = 324)[28] and the much larger Avoid Delivering

Therapies for Non-Sustained Arrhythmias in ICD Patients III (ADVANCE III; n = 1902)[4] showed that prolonged arrhythmia detection (30 of 40 interval) led to reductions in ICD shocks and heart failure hospitalizations, without an increased risk of syncope. Additionally, in both studies the treatment arm had a significant reduction in the incidence of inappropriate shocks (in ADVANCE III: incident rate ratio of 0.55; 95% CI, 0.36–0.85). Lastly, although the delayed and high-rate therapy arms in Multicenter Automatic Defibrillator Implantation Trial: Reduce Inappropriate Therapy (MADIT-RIT) did not show a difference in appropriate or inappropriate shocks, there were significant reductions in appropriate and inappropriate antitachycardia pacing, and no difference in rates of syncope between the treatment and control groups.[5]

Contemporary ICDs use discrimination algorithms to help distinguish sinus tachycardia and SVT from VT. The three main algorithms used are (1) onset, (2) stability, and (3) morphology. Onset is used to distinguish sinus tachycardia from VT by assess the beginning of tachycardia. Sinus tachycardia exhibits a "warm up" phenomenon with gradual shortening of the R-R interval, whereas VT has an abrupt start with sudden shortening of the R-R interval. The stability algorithm is used to distinguish AF from VT, by assessing the R-R interval regularity, with AF having irregular R-R intervals and VT regular R-R intervals. Lastly, the morphology algorithm uses a stored template of the ventricular electrogram during sinus rhythm, and compares the percentage match of the stored template to the morphology during tachycardia, with a poorly matching template being classified as VT and a reasonably matching template classified as SVT. Patients who develop aberrant conduction during tachycardia can inadvertently have SVT misclassified as VT and receive an inappropriate shock with this algorithm. The evidence for the use of discriminator algorithms largely comes from observational data. An analysis of 106,513 patients enrolled in Medtronic's remote monitoring system (CARELINK) found that use of SVT discriminators reduced all-cause shocks (HR, 0.83; 95% CI, 0.70–0.97).[29] Additionally, one small randomized controlled trial of 149 patients with history of VT/VF found a significant reduction in inappropriate therapy with use of discrimination algorithms.[30] Despite the lack of robust data, it is worth noting that major ICD programming trials had SVT discriminators turned on and it is difficult to distinguish what role the discriminator algorithms played in the reduction of therapies in these trials.[4,5] Furthermore, the use of these algorithms is endorsed by the expert consensus statement on ICD programming.[27]

Medical Therapy

Because a predominance of inappropriate shocks are secondary to atrial arrhythmias, medical therapy for better rate or rhythm control plays a cornerstone in treatment to prevent future shocks. In a prospective randomized control trial of 412 patients with secondary-prevention ICDs, subjects were randomized to β-blocker alone, sotalol, or amiodarone plus β-blocker.[31] When compared with β-blockers alone, the combination of amiodarone plus β-blocker was found to significantly reduce the rate of any shock (HR, 0.27; 95% CI, 0.14–0.52) and inappropriate shocks (HR, 0.22; 95% CI, 0.07–0.64). Sotalol was also better at reducing all shocks (HR, 0.61; 95% CI, 0.37–1.01) and inappropriate shocks (HR, 0.61; 95% CI, 0.29–1.30) compared with β-blockers alone but not as effective as the combination amiodarone and β-blocker.

Among β-blockers, there are data to suggest that carvedilol is better than metoprolol for the reduction of inappropriate therapy. In a substudy of the Multicenter Automatic Defibrillator Implantation With Cardiac Resynchronization Therapy (MADIT-CRT) trial, Ruwald and colleagues[32] found that patients on carvedilol had the lowest rates of inappropriate ATP (HR, 0.66; 95% CI, 0.48–0.90) and inappropriate shocks (HR, 0.54; 95% CI, 0.36–0.80) when compared with patients on metoprolol. It may be that carvedilol is the β-blocker of choice in patients experiencing inappropriate ICD shocks.

Cardiac Rehabilitation

An often underused treatment modality, cardiac rehabilitation has been associated with improvement in quality of life and lower rates of hospitalizations in patients with chronic heart failure.[33,34] Interestingly, cardiac rehabilitation has also been associated with lower rates of ICD shocks. In a recently published meta-analysis including six studies with a total of 1603 patients, Pandey and colleagues[35] found that the use of exercise training reduced the risk of ICD therapy (odds ratio, 0.47; 95% CI, 0.24–0.91). Exercise therapy leads to improvements in cardiorespiratory fitness, which is associated with a favorable reduction in sympathetic nervous system activity,[36] and to lower rates of recurrent of AF.[37] These mechanisms may account for a reduction in ICD shocks seen with cardiac rehabilitation.

SUMMARY

ICDs have a proven benefit for sudden cardiac death protection in selected patient populations.

However, they are not without risk. Beyond the procedural complications associated with implantation, patients remain at risk of inappropriate shocks leading to a wide range of adverse clinical events. It is of utmost importance that implanting physicians prevent inappropriate shocks (initial episodes and recurrences) with optimal ICD programming, medical therapy, and referring patients to cardiac rehabilitation or ablation.

REFERENCES

1. Epstein AE, DiMarco JP, Ellenbogen KA, et al. ACC/AHA/HRS 2008 guidelines for device-based therapy of cardiac rhythm abnormalities: a report of the American College of Cardiology/American Heart Association Task Force on Practice Guidelines (Writing Committee to Revise the ACC/AHA/NASPE 2002 Guideline Update for Implantation of Cardiac Pacemakers and Antiarrhythmia Devices): developed in collaboration with the American Association for Thoracic Surgery and Society of Thoracic Surgeons. Circulation 2008;117(21):e350–408.

2. Borne RT, Varosy PD, Masoudi FA. Implantable cardioverter-defibrillator shocks: epidemiology, outcomes, and therapeutic approaches. JAMA Intern Med 2013;173(10):859–65.

3. Wilkoff BL, Williamson BD, Stern RS, et al. Strategic programming of detection and therapy parameters in implantable cardioverter-defibrillators reduces shocks in primary prevention patients: results from the PREPARE (Primary Prevention Parameters Evaluation) study. J Am Coll Cardiol 2008;52(7):541–50.

4. Gasparini M, Proclemer A, Klersy C, et al. Effect of long-detection interval vs standard-detection interval for implantable cardioverter-defibrillators on antitachycardia pacing and shock delivery: the ADVANCE III randomized clinical trial. JAMA 2013;309(18):1903–11.

5. Moss AJ, Schuger C, Beck CA, et al. Reduction in inappropriate therapy and mortality through ICD programming. N Engl J Med 2012;367(24):2275–83.

6. Daubert JP, Zareba W, Cannom DS, et al. Inappropriate implantable cardioverter-defibrillator shocks in MADIT II: frequency, mechanisms, predictors, and survival impact. J Am Coll Cardiol 2008;51(14):1357–65.

7. Poole JE, Johnson GW, Hellkamp AS, et al. Prognostic importance of defibrillator shocks in patients with heart failure. N Engl J Med 2008;359(10):1009–17.

8. Kadish A, Dyer A, Daubert JP, et al. Prophylactic defibrillator implantation in patients with nonischemic dilated cardiomyopathy. N Engl J Med 2004;350(21):2151–8.

9. van Rees JB, Borleffs CJ, de Bie MK, et al. Inappropriate implantable cardioverter-defibrillator shocks: incidence, predictors, and impact on mortality. J Am Coll Cardiol 2011;57(5):556–62.

10. Saxon LA, Hayes DL, Gilliam FR, et al. Long-term outcome after ICD and CRT implantation and influence of remote device follow-up: the ALTITUDE survival study. Circulation 2010;122(23):2359–67.

11. Weeke P, Johansen JB, Jørgensen OD, et al. Mortality and appropriate and inappropriate therapy in patients with ischaemic heart disease and implanted cardioverter-defibrillators for primary prevention: data from the Danish ICD Register. Europace 2013;15(8):1150–7.

12. Fernandez-Cisnal A, Arce-León Á, Arana-Rueda E, et al. Analyses of inappropriate shocks in a Spanish ICD primary prevention population: predictors and prognoses. Int J Cardiol 2015;195:188–94.

13. Powell BD, Saxon LA, Boehmer JP, et al. Survival after shock therapy in implantable cardioverter-defibrillator and cardiac resynchronization therapy-defibrillator recipients according to rhythm shocked. The ALTITUDE survival by rhythm study. J Am Coll Cardiol 2013;62(18):1674–9.

14. Olde Nordkamp LR, Brouwer TF, Barr C, et al. Inappropriate shocks in the subcutaneous ICD: incidence, predictors and management. Int J Cardiol 2015;195:126–33.

15. Weiss R, Knight BP, Gold MR, et al. Safety and efficacy of a totally subcutaneous implantable-cardioverter defibrillator. Circulation 2013;128(9):944–53.

16. Crossley GH, Poole JE, Rozner MA, et al. The Heart Rhythm Society (HRS)/American Society of Anesthesiologists (ASA) Expert Consensus Statement on the perioperative management of patients with implantable defibrillators, pacemakers and arrhythmia monitors: facilities and patient management this document was developed as a joint project with the American Society of Anesthesiologists (ASA), and in collaboration with the American Heart Association (AHA), and the Society of Thoracic Surgeons (STS). Heart Rhythm 2011;8(7):1114–54.

17. Beinart R, Nazarian S. Effects of external electrical and magnetic fields on pacemakers and defibrillators: from engineering principles to clinical practice. Circulation 2013;128(25):2799–809.

18. Akhtar M, Bhat T, Tantray M, et al. Electromagnetic interference with implantable cardioverter defibrillators causing inadvertent shock: case report and review of current literature. Clin Med Insights Cardiol 2014;8:63–6.

19. Lakkireddy D, Khasnis A, Antenacci J, et al. Do electrical stun guns (TASER-X26) affect the functional integrity of implantable pacemakers and defibrillators? Europace 2007;9(7):551–6.

20. Mark DB, Anstrom KJ, Sun JL, et al. Quality of life with defibrillator therapy or amiodarone in heart failure. N Engl J Med 2008;359(10):999–1008.

21. Namerow PB, Firth BR, Heywood GM, et al. Quality-of-life six months after CABG surgery in patients randomized to ICD versus no ICD therapy: findings from the CABG Patch Trial. Pacing Clin Electrophysiol 1999;22(9):1305–13.

22. Bhavnani SP, Giedrimiene D, Coleman CI, et al. The healthcare utilization and cost of treating patients experiencing inappropriate implantable cardioverter defibrillator shocks: a propensity score study. Pacing Clin Electrophysiol 2014;37(10):1315–23.

23. Stein KM, Devereux RB, Hahn RT, et al. Effect of transthoracic shocks on left ventricular function. Resuscitation 2005;66(3):309–15.

24. Tan VH, Wilton SB, Kuriachan V, et al. Impact of programming strategies aimed at reducing nonessential implantable cardioverter defibrillator therapies on mortality: a systematic review and meta-analysis. Circ Arrhythm Electrophysiol 2014;7(1):164–70.

25. Kannel WB, Wolf PA, Benjamin EJ, et al. Prevalence, incidence, prognosis, and predisposing conditions for atrial fibrillation: population-based estimates. Am J Cardiol 1998;82(8A):2N–9N.

26. January CT, Wann LS, Alpert JS, et al. 2014 AHA/ACC/HRS guideline for the management of patients with atrial fibrillation: executive summary: a report of the American College of Cardiology/American Heart Association Task Force on practice guidelines and the Heart Rhythm Society. Circulation 2014; 130(23):2071–104.

27. Wilkoff BL, et al. 2015 HRS/EHRA/APHRS/SOLAECE expert consensus statement on optimal implantable cardioverter-defibrillator programming and testing. J Arrhythm 2016;32(1):1–28.

28. Gasparini M, Menozzi C, Proclemer A, et al. A simplified biventricular defibrillator with fixed long detection intervals reduces implantable cardioverter defibrillator (ICD) interventions and heart failure hospitalizations in patients with non-ischaemic cardiomyopathy implanted for primary prevention: the RELEVANT [Role of long dEtection window programming in patients with LEft VentriculAr dysfunction, Non-ischemic eTiology in primary prevention treated with a biventricular ICD] study. Eur Heart J 2009;30(22):2758–67.

29. Fischer A, Ousdigian KT, Johnson JW, et al. The impact of atrial fibrillation with rapid ventricular rates and device programming on shocks in 106,513 ICD and CRT-D patients. Heart Rhythm 2012;9(1):24–31.

30. Dorian P, Philippon F, Thibault B, et al. Randomized controlled study of detection enhancements versus rate-only detection to prevent inappropriate therapy in a dual-chamber implantable cardioverter-defibrillator. Heart Rhythm 2004;1(5):540–7.

31. Connolly SJ, Dorian P, Roberts RS, et al. Comparison of beta-blockers, amiodarone plus beta-blockers, or sotalol for prevention of shocks from implantable cardioverter defibrillators: the OPTIC Study: a randomized trial. JAMA 2006;295(2):165–71.

32. Ruwald MH, Abu-Zeitone A, Jons C, et al. Impact of carvedilol and metoprolol on inappropriate implantable cardioverter-defibrillator therapy: the MADIT-CRT trial (multicenter automatic defibrillator implantation with cardiac resynchronization therapy). J Am Coll Cardiol 2013;62(15):1343–50.

33. Flynn KE, Piña IL, Whellan DJ, et al. Effects of exercise training on health status in patients with chronic heart failure: HF-ACTION randomized controlled trial. JAMA 2009;301(14):1451–9.

34. O'Connor CM, Whellan DJ, Lee KL, et al. Efficacy and safety of exercise training in patients with chronic heart failure: HF-ACTION randomized controlled trial. JAMA 2009;301(14):1439–50.

35. Pandey A, Parashar A, Moore C, et al. Safety and efficacy of exercise training in patients with an implantable cardioverter-defibrillator a meta-analysis. JACC EP 2017;3(2):117–26.

36. Billman GE. Aerobic exercise conditioning: a non-pharmacological antiarrhythmic intervention. J Appl Physiol (1985) 2002;92(2):446–54.

37. Pathak RK, Elliott A, Middeldorp ME, et al. Impact of CARDIOrespiratory FITness on arrhythmia recurrence in obese individuals with atrial fibrillation: the CARDIO-FIT study. J Am Coll Cardiol 2015;66(9): 985–96.

When is Device-Detected Atrial Fibrillation Actionable?

Jeremiah Wasserlauf, MD, MS[a],
Rod S. Passman, MD, MSCE, FHRS[b],*

KEYWORDS

- Atrial fibrillation • Cardiac implanted electronic devices • Pacemaker • Defibrillator
- Thromboembolism • Stroke

KEY POINTS

- Atrial high-rate episodes (AHREs) are commonly encountered and predict increased thromboembolic risk at durations of 24 hours or less. Shorter cutoffs have been less consistently associated with risk.
- There is no consensus on a single threshold that merits anticoagulation or other treatment. Very short episodes may not require action beyond continued monitoring.
- A more effective approach to risk stratification may integrate atrial fibrillation (AF) features, such as density, duration, and burden, with thromboembolic risk scores, such as CHA_2DS_2-VASc, and other markers of atrial myopathy or hypercoagulability.
- Studies are ongoing to address the use of oral anticoagulation for subclinical AF alone detected by cardiac implanted electronic devices, as well as tailored anticoagulation in response to AHREs in those with a known history of AF.

Atrial fibrillation (AF) is a common cardiac arrhythmia affecting between 2.9 and 7.7 million adults in the United States.[1–3] This prevalence is predicted to increase to between 5.6 and 15.9 million people by 2050. The annual incremental cost of AF has been estimated at $8705 per patient, costing the United States a total of $26.0 billion per year.[4]

AF can occur with or without symptoms, and can lead to hospitalization, dementia, congestive heart failure, and arterial thromboembolism.[5,6] AF is associated with a nearly fivefold increase in stroke.[7] Moreover, strokes that occur in patients with AF are associated with larger infarct size, greater disability, and a higher risk of early death.[8,9] Stroke risk can be more precisely estimated using the risk prediction scores of $CHADS_2$ (ie, congestive heart failure, hypertension, age $\geq$75 years, diabetes mellitus, prior stroke or transient ischemic attack [TIA] or thromboembolism [doubled])[10] and CHA_2DS_2-VASc (congestive heart failure, hypertension, age $\geq$75 years [doubled], diabetes mellitus, prior stroke or TIA or thromboembolism [doubled], vascular disease, age 65–74 years, sex category).[11,12] Oral anticoagulation with warfarin or novel oral anticoagulant (NOAC) is indicated for patients with a CHA_2DS_2-VASc score of 2 or greater and has been demonstrated to reduce the risk of ischemic stroke.[13–17]

Current guidelines recommend that selection of antithrombotic therapy be made irrespective of

Disclosures: No relevant disclosures (J. Wasserlauf). Medtronic: research support, consulting fees (R.S. Passman).
[a] Division of Cardiology, Northwestern University Feinberg School of Medicine, 646 North St. Clair, Suite 600, Chicago, IL 60611, USA; [b] Division of Cardiology, Northwestern University Feinberg School of Medicine, 251 East Huron Street, Suite 8-503, Chicago, IL 60611, USA
* Corresponding author.
E-mail address: r-passman@northwestern.edu

whether the AF pattern is paroxysmal (episodes shorter than 7 days), persistent (episodes longer than 7 days), or permanent (cases in which restoration and/or maintenance of sinus rhythm have been abandoned).[18] There is currently no consensus, however, on how to manage a fourth pattern of subclinical AF detected by cardiac implanted electronic devices (CIEDs) in patients without history of clinical AF (**Fig. 1**). Awareness of these atrial high-rate episodes (AHREs) has increased alongside increased use of CIEDs,[5] yet there is a paucity of data to guide management in this scenario because patients with CIED-only documented AF have not been included in clinical trials of anticoagulants and other AF therapies. This article provides an overview of device-detected AHREs and outlines the current body of literature, as well as evolving areas of investigation.

PREVALENCE AND ACCURACY OF ATRIAL HIGH-RATE EPISODES

Episodes of AF can frequently be asymptomatic, which can have major clinical implications because at least a quarter of AF-related strokes present as the first manifestation of AF. Even in patients with an existing diagnosis of AF, most episodes can occur without symptoms.[19–21] Implanted devices represent an increasingly important source of data on these subclinical AF episodes because approximately 400,000 CIEDs are implanted each year in the United States, and there are more than 3 million patients currently living with CIEDs.[22]

In patients without history of AF, the prevalence of AHREs has been observed to be between 10% and more than 50%, depending on the population studied.[23–27] Despite a lack of symptoms, patients with subclinical AF remain at risk for major complications.[28] Indeed, AF detection rates of 30% at 3 years have been reported in patients who

presented with cryptogenic stroke and no history of AF.[29,30]

Several investigators have reported on the accuracy of AHREs in the diagnosis of atrial tachyarrhythmias (ATs), demonstrating excellent sensitivity in most series. One study of 40 subjects with tachycardia-bradycardia syndrome and permanent pacemakers found mode switching algorithms to be 98.1% sensitive and 100% specific for the diagnosis of ATs compared with Holter monitor data. The algorithms detected 98.9% of the total duration of AF and 96.4% of the total duration of atrial flutter.[31] Another study of 2 models of implanted devices found that the devices detected 100% of sustained AT episodes and 95.3% of the net AT duration observed on Holter recordings of 40 subjects. Appropriate detection of normal sinus rhythm at termination of AT occurred in 83.7% and 92.1% of episodes in the 2 devices, respectively.[32] Although these studies included subjects with dual-chamber devices, an RR interval-based algorithm used in single-chamber ventricular devices also performed with high sensitivity and specificity in a study based on Holter databases.[33]

The specificity of device AT detection seems to improve with increasing duration and rate of episodes, with a study by Pollak and colleagues[34] finding that only 18% of recorded AHREs episodes of less than 10 seconds confirmed true AT compared with 89% of episodes greater than 5 minutes. Only 18% of AHREs with rates less than 250/min corresponded to true ATs compared with 57% of episodes with rates greater than 250/min. However, not all recorded AHREs represent true ATs, even when selecting for elevated rate and extended duration.[35] In the study by Pollak and colleagues,[34] 12% of the stored episodes with a rate greater than 250/min and duration greater than 5 minutes were still false-positives. In the ASSERT (The Asymptomatic Atrial

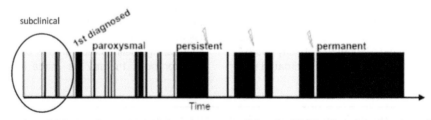

Fig. 1. Progression of AF over time: a typical chaotic pattern of time in AF (*black*) and time in sinus rhythm (*gray*) over time (x-axis). AF progresses from undiagnosed to first diagnosed, paroxysmal, persistent, to permanent. Episodes of AF before the first clinical diagnosis are increasingly recognized in patients with CIEDs. Flashes indicate cardioversions as examples for therapeutic interventions that influence the natural time course of the arrhythmia. (*Adapted from* Kirchhof P, Auricchio A, Bax J, et al. Outcome parameters for trials in atrial fibrillation: recommendations from a consensus conference organized by the German Atrial Fibrillation Competence NETwork and the European Heart Rhythm Association. Europace 2007;9(11):1008; with permission)

Fibrillation and Stroke Evaluation in Pacemaker Patients and the Atrial Fibrillation Reduction Atrial Pacing) trial, 17.3% of AHREs greater than 6 minutes in duration were false-positives. When the duration threshold was extended to 30 minutes, 6 hours, and 24 hours, false-positives dropped to 6.8%, 3.3%, and 1.8%, respectively.[36] This relationship has led to the exclusion of subjects with very short AHREs (<5 min) from most trials, despite frequent occurrence of these episodes in practice. It should also be considered that, although AHREs do accurately measure ATs, the use of various atrial rate cutoffs may select for some ATs that may not be associated with stroke.[37]

In patients without an indication for CIEDs, insertable cardiac monitors (ICMs) are an alternative modality for monitoring of AF. These subcutaneous implantable devices continuously record an ECG using a circular memory buffer, and automatically detect AF and other cardiac arrhythmias.[38] In a prospective study, ICMs correctly identified 37 of 38 subjects with AF detected by Holter monitor (sensitivity 97.4%), and 97 of 100 subjects without Holter-detected AF (97% specificity).[39] Another study followed 154 subjects who received an ICM with remote monitoring and recordings were independently reviewed to adjudicate true-positives and false-positives. During a mean follow-up time of 12.1 months, true AF was detected in 45 subjects (29%) compared with 9 (6%) false-positives; however, false bradycardia detection for undersensing occurred in 44 (29%) subjects and false tachycardia detection for oversensing occurred in 4 (3%); therefore, false recognition of bradyarrhythmias remains a particularly common issue.[40]

ATRIAL HIGH-RATE EPISODES AND STROKE RISK

Although multiple series published over the past 2 decades have confirmed an observation of increased stroke risk associated with AHREs, the duration of AHRE needed to increase risk has varied widely across studies from as short as 5 minutes to as long as 24 hours (**Table 1**). Although cutoffs offer some risk prediction, the duration of AHRE associated with stroke is likely not constant among all patients, and may depend on the extent of other thromboembolic risk factors. One alternative to a single cutoff of AHRE duration would be a combination of AHRE presence and duration incorporated with established thromboembolic risk factors. This was evaluated in a 2009 retrospective study by Botto and colleagues.[41] In this study, subjects with dual chamber pacemakers and a history of symptomatic ATs were assessed based on a $CHADS_2$ score combined with duration of AF, as

classified in 3 groups: AF less than 5 minutes (AF-free), AF greater than 5 minutes (AF-5 minutes) but less than 24 hours, and AF greater than 24 hours (AF-24 hours). Using this system, 2 subpopulations were identified with significantly different risks of thromboembolic events: 0.8% versus 5% ($P = .035$). The former group consisted of subjects who were AF-free with $CHADS_2$ less than or equal to 2, or AF-5 minutes with $CHADS_2$ less than or equal to 1, or AF-24 hours with $CHADS_2$ equal to 0. The latter group comprised the remaining combinations of $CHADS_2$ score and AF duration. This observation supports the hypothesis that the cutoff duration of AHRE that is associated with thromboembolic risk may depend on additional risk factors rather than being constant among all patients.

The temporal relationship between AF and stroke is also not well understood. In a TRENDS substudy (The Relationship Between Daily Atrial Tachyarrhythmia Burden From Implantable Device Diagnostics and Stroke Risk)[42] in which 20 of 40 subjects with stroke and systemic embolism were found to have AHREs detected before their event, 9 did not have any AHREs in the 30 days preceding the event. Fourteen of the 20 subjects with AHREs were not in AF at diagnosis of stroke or systemic embolism, and the last AHREs in these 14 subjects occurred 168 ± 199 days before stroke or systemic embolism. In the ASSERT trial,[43] 18 of 51 subjects with stroke or systemic embolism experienced AHREs before their event, of whom only 4 had AHREs detected within 30 days before stroke or systemic embolism, and only 1 of these subjects was experiencing an AHRE at the time of the stroke. In the 14 subjects with AHREs detected more than 30 days before stroke or systemic embolism, the median interval from the most proximal episode was 339 days (25th to 75th percentile, 211–619 days).

In a 2012 study of subjects with thromboembolic events and AHRE by Shanmugam and colleagues,[44] 73% of subjects with detected AHREs were not experiencing an AHRE at the time of their event, with a mean of 46.7 ± 71.9 days between the last detected AHRE and a thromboembolic event.

There are several possibilities that may explain why the occurrence of AHREs and stroke do not always correlate temporally. Subjects found to have AHREs and stroke in these studies had multiple vascular risk factors and may have had coincident strokes from causes other than cardioemboli due to atrial arrhythmias. This is particularly true when considering that strokes were not specifically adjudicated as being cardioembolic in any of these studies. In addition, strokes were often combined with TIAs and other cardiovascular events in

Table 1
Studies of atrial high-rate episodes and thromboembolic risk

Study (Author, Year)	Type of CIED	Study Type and Follow-up	Population Studied	History of AT (Yes, No, or Both)	AHRE Definition or Duration Analyzed	Stroke Incidence	Other Outcomes
MOST (Glotzer et al,[69] 2003)	PPM	• Ancillary study of RCT • Median 27 mo	• n = 312 • Sinus node dysfunction • Sinus rhythm at implantation	Both	• Definition: atrial rate 220 BPM for 10 beats • Only episodes ≥5 min analyzed	• 8 (2.2%/y) strokes in AHRE group • 2 (0.58%/y) strokes in non-AHRE group	• AHREs independently associated with • Total mortality (HR 2.48, 95% CI 1.25–4.91; P = .0092) • Death or nonfatal stroke (HR 2.79, 95% CI 1.51–5.15; P = .0011) • AF (HR 5.93, 95% CI 2.88–12.2; P = .0001)
Capucci et al,[70] 2005	PPM	• Prospective multicenter observational study • Median 22 mo	• n = 725 • Bradycardia • Symptomatic atrial tachyarrhythmias	Yes	• AHRE >5 min • AHRE >1 d	• 7 (0.6%/y) total patients with ischemic stroke (AHRE status not reported)	• AHRE >5 min = not associated with embolic events • AHRE >1 d = adjusted HR of 3.1 (95% CI 1.1–10.5; P = .044) for ischemic stroke, TIA, or peripheral arterial embolism
TRENDS (Glotzer et al,[71] 2009)	PPM, ICD, or CRT	• Prospective multicenter observational study • Mean 1.4 y	• n = 2486 • 1 or more stroke risk factors	Both	• Zero burden • Low burden (<5.5 h) • High burden (≥5.5 h)	• 20 (0.59%/y) total patients with stroke (AHRE status not reported)	• Adjusted TE risk (vs zero burden): • Low burden (<5.5 h) = HR 0.98 (95% CI 0.34–2.82; P = .97) • High burden (≥5.5 h) = 2.20 (95% CI 0.96–5.05, P = .06)
ASSERT (Healey et al,[26] 2012)	PPM or ICD	• Prospective multicenter observational analysis (with an ancillary RCT) • Mean 2.5 y	• n = 2580 • Age ≥65 y • History of hypertension on medical treatment	No	• Definition: atrial rate ≥190 BPM for >6 min.	• 10 (1.5%/y) patients with stroke in AHRE group • 36 (0.62%/y) patients with stroke in AHRE-free group	• AHRE = adjusted HR 2.50 (95% CI 1.28–4.89; P = .008) for primary outcome of stroke and systemic embolism

Study	Device	Study design	Population	Definition	Strokes	Outcome
Shanmugam et al,[44] 2012	CRT	• Ancillary analysis of 2 prospective multicenter observational studies • Median 370 d	• n = 560 • Heart failure • Sinus rhythm at enrollment	Both	• Definition: atrial rate >180 BPM exceeding 14 min in 24 h • AHRE >3.8 h/d.	• 4 (0.36%/y) ischemic strokes (AHRE status not reported)	AHRE >3.8 h over a day = adjusted HR 9.4 (95% CI 1.8–47.0; P = .006) for TE
SOS AF (Boriani et al,[72] 2014)	PPM, ICD, or CRT	• Pooled analysis of 3 prospective multicenter observational studies • Median 24 mo	• n = 10,016	Both	• Definition: atrial rate >175 BPM lasting ≥20 s • AHRE burden ≥5 min • AHRE burden ≥1 h • AHRE burden ≥6 h • AHRE burden ≥12 h • AHRE burden ≥23 h	• 24 strokes (0.27%/y) in patients with ≥1h AHRE burden • 2 strokes (0.08%/y) in patients with ≥5 min to <1 h AHRE burden	AHRE burden ≥1 h vs <1 h = adjusted HR 2.11 (95% CI 1.22–3.64; P = .008) for ischemic stroke
RATE (Swiryn et al,[35] 2016)	PPM or ICD	• Prospective multicenter registry study • Median 22.9 mo	• n = 5379 • Patients ≥18 y of age • PPM or ICD implanted within prior 45 d • Excluded if permanent AF or episode of AF documented in preceding 3 mo	Both (excluding permanent AF or AF in preceding 3 mo)	• Definition: ≥3 consecutive PACs. • Short AHRE = onset and offset within 1 EGM. • Long AHRE = onset and/or offset not in the same EGM.	Not reported	Long AHRE: • PPM patients: no independent association with composite outcome • ICD patients: adjusted OR 1.57 (P = .006) for composite outcome Short AHRE: Not associated with adverse events
ASSERT follow-up study (Van Gelder et al,[63] 2017)	PPM or ICD	• Follow-up analysis of a prospective multicenter observational analysis • Mean 2.5 y	• n = 2455 • Age ≥65 y • History of hypertension on medical treatment	No	• Definition: atrial rate ≥190 BPM for >6 min • No AHRE • AHRE >6 min – 6h • AHRE >6h – 24h • AHRE ≥24h	Not reported	AHRE >24h = adjusted HR 3.24 (95% CI 1.51–6.95, P = .003) for ischemic stroke or systemic embolism

Abbreviations: BPM, beats per minute; CRT, cardiac resynchronization therapy; EGM, electrogram; HR, hazard ratio; ICD, implantable cardioverter-defibrillator; MOST, MOde selection trial; OR, odds ratio; PAC, premature atrial complex; PPM, permanent pacemaker; RATE, Registry of Atrial Tachycardia and Atrial Fibrillation Episodes; RCT, randomized controlled trial; SOS AF, Stroke preventiOn Strategies based on Atrial Fibrillation information from implanted devices; TE, thromboembolism; TRENDS, The Relationship Between Daily Atrial Tachyarrhythmia Burden From Implantable Device Diagnostics and Stroke Risk.

composite study endpoints. Stroke incidence rates were generally low and demonstrated modest increases in absolute risk by AHRE status, or were not reported at all (see **Table 1**). The association between AHREs and stroke may also not be directly causal but rather with AHREs as a marker of an inflammatory, prothrombotic state[45,46] or underlying atrial myopathy with disturbed flow characteristics (**Fig. 2**).[47,48]

By contrast, a Veterans Administration case-crossover analysis of subjects with implanted devices and acute stroke demonstrated that the risk of stroke is significantly increased for 30 days following an episode of AF, with a warfarin-adjusted odds ratio of 4.2 (95% CI 5.39–73.1) compared with a control period of 91 to 120 days preceding the event.[49] Further analysis of the ASSERT data demonstrated an unadjusted hazard ratio of 5.6 for stroke occurring within 30 days of an AF episode, though the risk was attenuated after adjusting for baseline differences.

Thus, most patients with AHREs who suffer a stroke are not experiencing an AHRE at the time of diagnosis; however, the period following AHREs and overall presence of AHREs is associated with a significant increase in stroke risk.

CLINICAL MANAGEMENT OF ATRIAL HIGH-RATE EPISODES

Detection of AHREs seems to decrease the time to diagnosis and management of AF. This is facilitated by the existence of remote monitoring, which has been shown to shorten the time to detection of AHREs compared with in-office monitoring. In a study by Lazarus,[50] remote monitoring resulted in a mean interval of 26 days from last follow-up to occurrence of events notified by remote monitoring, which corresponds to a theoretic decrease in detection time of 154 and 64 days compared with routine 6- and 3-month follow-up, although clinical events included not only arrhythmias but also system-status and configuration-related events. Consistent reductions in time to detection of actionable events have also been reported in subsequent studies.[51–53]

Additionally, remote monitoring has been associated with a trend toward fewer strokes[52,54]; a significant reduction in hospitalization for atrial arrhythmia, stroke, or both[54]; and prompting of health care encounters in which anticoagulation and other treatments are initiated.[51] Based on these data and the Veteran's Administration study, which demonstrated a 30-day period of increased risk of stroke following an AHRE, there is good reason to consider anticoagulation on the basis of AHREs. Yet, patients with AHREs alone are not generally included in studies of oral anticoagulant therapy, and there are no data from randomized trials showing a benefit of anticoagulation in this setting without history of clinical AF. The IMPACT trial randomized 2718 subjects with dual-chamber and biventricular defibrillators to start and stop anticoagulation based on remote monitoring compared with usual management and anticoagulation determined by standard criteria.[55] The primary endpoint was a composite of stroke, systemic embolism, and major bleeding. The trial was stopped after 2 years for futility. There were 945 subjects who developed AHREs, of whom 264 met study anticoagulation criteria. Rates of stroke, systemic embolism, and major bleeding did not differ

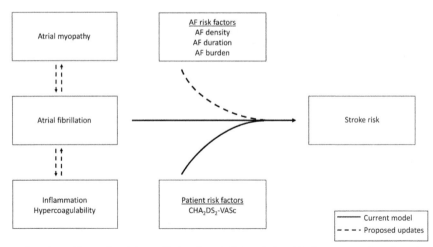

Fig. 2. Future directions for stroke risk prediction in AF. The relationship between AF and stroke may not be directly causal, and may eventually be refined by incorporating other markers of inflammation, hypercoagulability, or atrial myopathy along with specific features of AF episodes and traditional thromboembolic risk factors.

between groups. Although the investigators concluded that anticoagulation based on remote monitoring did not prevent thromboembolism, there were several important limitations of this study. This was a study exclusively of heart failure subjects; thus the results cannot be extrapolated to other AF populations. The intervention assessed was not simply the use of anticoagulation for AHREs but a complex strategy of remote monitoring combined with a risk-based algorithm for oral anticoagulation. When focusing specifically on the use of anticoagulation, there was only 72.2% compliance with anticoagulation in the intervention arm among eligible subjects, compared with the already favorable use of oral anticoagulation in 60% of the control arm. In addition, 80.9% of anticoagulation was accomplished with vitamin K antagonist therapy rather than NOACs. This is important when considering that the time between initiation of vitamin K antagonists and the establishment of therapeutic levels of anticoagulation may be several days as opposed to rapidly acting NOACs. The composite endpoint also consisted of thromboembolism and bleeding, which could offset each other with increased use of anticoagulation and contribute to a nonsignificant difference in the primary endpoint.

Two additional studies have been designed to further address this question and are currently recruiting. ARTESiA (Apixaban for the Reduction of Thrombo-Embolism in Patients With Device-Detected Sub-Clinical Atrial Fibrillation, NCT01938248) is a randomized controlled trial of aspirin 81 mg daily compared against apixaban in subjects with CIEDs, AHRE greater than or equal to 6 minutes but less than or equal to 24 hours, age greater than or equal to 55 years, and risk factors for stroke. The 2 primary endpoints are a composite of stroke and systemic embolism, and major bleeding. This trial has an estimated enrollment of 4000 subjects and anticipated mean follow-up time of 3 years.

NOAH (non–vitamin K antagonist Oral anticoagulants in patients with Atrial High rate episodes, NCT02618577) is a randomized controlled trial of edoxaban compared with aspirin 100 mg or placebo (depending on other indications for antiplatelet therapy) in subjects with CIEDs, AHRE greater than or equal to 6 minutes, age greater than or equal to 65 years, and a CHA_2DS_2-VASc score of 2 or more. The estimated enrollment is 3400 subjects with anticipated follow-up time of 28 months. These 2 studies would be the first to assess the important question of whether modern anticoagulant therapy

carries a benefit for AHREs in a similar fashion to clinical AF.

An equally important question is whether CIEDs can be used to withdraw anticoagulation in patients with clinical AF. This includes patients who have undergone ablation or cardioversion, or are managed on antiarrhythmic medication. Current guidelines recommend continued anticoagulation following rhythm control as dictated by underlying stroke risk,[18] an approach that has been advocated due to the absence of a permanent cure for AF, high long-term recurrence rates following cardioversion alone, high burden of asymptomatic episodes, and conflicting data on the relationship between AF timing, duration, and stroke. Despite these clear recommendations, it is not uncommon for patients to have their anticoagulation stopped following successful AF ablation, although this may be an unsafe practice in patients with a CHA_2DS_2-VASC score of 2 or higher.[56,57] However, cessation of anticoagulation in select patients with no AF or low AF burden recorded by CIEDs has been safely demonstrated. Mascarenhas and colleagues[58] placed ICMs in 70 subjects with a high CHA_2DS_2-VASC score and HAS-BLED (Hypertension, Abnormal renal/liver function, Stroke, Bleeding history or predisposition, labile international normalized ratio [INR], Elderly [age $\geq$65 years], Drugs/alcohol concomitantly) score. There were 53 subjects who maintained normal sinus rhythm or less than 1% AF burden for 3 months, and elected to discontinue oral anticoagulation. No adverse events occurred over a follow-up period of nearly 2 years. A similar study was conducted in 65 subjects following catheter ablation with a $CHADS_2$ score of 1 to 3 who were free from AF after a 3-month period and underwent implantation of an ICM. The day following implantation, oral anticoagulation was discontinued. Of the 65 subjects, 41 had an AF burden less than 1 hour per day and were able to remain off of anticoagulation and no thromboembolic events occurred.[59]

The ability to monitor patients remotely and treat with rapidly acting NOACs allows for the additional possibility of a pill-in-pocket strategy for anticoagulation that may limit the risks of lifelong exposure to anticoagulation in patients with known AF without affecting stroke risk. This type of targeted anticoagulation would likely improve medication adherence during the period of highest risk and improve cost-effectiveness.[60] In the REACT.COM pilot study (The Rhythm Evaluation for Anticoagulation with Continuous Monitoring), subjects on NOACs with nonpermanent AF and a $CHADS_2$ score of 1 or 2 stopped taking their NOAC after a 60-day period with no AF episodes greater than or equal to 1 hour.[61] NOACs were reinitiated for 30 days following any AF episode greater than or equal to 1 hour diagnosed through daily ICM transmissions. Over a median follow-up of 14 months, only 31% of subjects had any threshold AF event and a 94% reduction in the time on NOAC was observed compared with chronic anticoagulation without any observed strokes. There were 2 possible and 1 definite TIAs that all occurred in subjects with a CHADS$_2$ score of 1 receiving aspirin 81 mg daily and all in the absence of a threshold AF event in the preceding 12 months. The Tailored Anticoagulation for Non-Continuous Atrial Fibrillation trial (TACTIC-AF) is a similar pilot study including subjects with nonpermanent AF and dual-chamber pacemakers or ICDs, with CHADS$_2$ scores of 1 to 3 on NOACs, and no history of stroke.[62] Subjects were reinitiated on their NOAC therapy for 30 days in response to a continuous AHRE greater than 6 minutes or a total AHRE burden greater than 6 hours over 24 hours. The study showed a 74.3% reduction in time on NOAC without any adverse thromboembolic events. The safety of a targeted-anticoagulation strategy in a population with known AF would need rigorous evaluation in the form of a randomized clinical trial against the current standard of continuous anticoagulation. In the case of subclinical AHREs, there is not a universally accepted standard against which to compare pill-in-pocket anticoagulation; however, to be feasible, such a strategy would require capability for point-of-care notification of arrhythmias, which would necessitate near real-time patient notification of threshold events using smartphone-based AF detection and communication via wearable or implantable AF-sensitive devices.

SUMMARY AND FUTURE DIRECTIONS

AHREs are frequently encountered in clinical practice and can be associated with an increase in risk of stroke, though the absolute increase in stroke risk seems lower than that of clinically detected AF. Numerous unanswered questions about their management remain.

There is no consensus on the optimal criteria for identifying the patients with AHREs who are at increased risk of stroke. Most studies have focused risk stratification on a threshold of duration of AHREs, with significant cutoffs that have generally been observed at 24 hours or less. Shorter episodes have not been associated with stroke risk in the most recent series, such as duration of 1 electrogram or shorter in the RATE (Registry of Atrial Tachycardia and Atrial Fibrillation Episodes) registry,[35] or 6 minutes to 24 hours in the ASSERT

follow-up study.[63] This suggests that very short episodes may not require action beyond continued monitoring. Given the progressive nature of AF, any decision to withhold anticoagulation based on a specific AF duration would still require close surveillance to assess for future episode prolongation. A more effective approach to risk stratification may integrate AF duration and thromboembolic risk scores such as CHADS$_2$ or CHA$_2$DS$_2$-VASc,[41] or other markers of atrial myopathy or hypercoagulability. Markers of coagulation and fibrinolysis,[64,65] myocyte strain and injury, renal function, and inflammation have already been associated with stroke risk,[66] and may eventually play a role in refining or personalizing risk prediction in AF.

Oral anticoagulation offers effective protection against stroke in AF and is variably used in practice for treatment of AHREs. There is clinical equipoise for the use of oral anticoagulation for CIED-detected subclinical AF alone, which is consistent with current professional society guidelines, which do not contain any specific recommendations for the use of oral anticoagulation for AHREs.[6,13] Randomized controlled trials are ongoing to study the effect of NOACs in patients with AHREs of 6 minutes or longer and risk factors for stroke. A patient-directed approach to anticoagulation in response to AHREs is now possible due to the existence of wireless continuous rhythm monitoring, along with rapidly acting NOACs, and may someday take shape to allow a pill-in-pocket strategy only in response to a prolonged AF episode. For such a strategy to be successful, further understanding of the causative role of AF in stroke and the temporal association between the two would need to be further elucidated.

Finally, the historical designations of AF as paroxysmal, persistent, and permanent have been shown to correlate poorly with clinical burden of AF.[67] Furthermore, whether AF duration, burden, or density is a better measure of stroke risk is still unknown[68] and requires further investigation. The recognition of subclinical, CIED-detected AF challenges the view of AF as a dichotomous variable, one that is entirely present or absent, and has important implications in the diagnosis and management of patients with known AF and those with AF risk factors.

REFERENCES

1. Go AS, Hylek EM, Phillips KA, et al. Prevalence of diagnosed atrial fibrillation in adults: national implications for rhythm management and stroke prevention: the AnTicoagulation and Risk Factors in Atrial Fibrillation (ATRIA) Study. JAMA 2001; 285(18):2370–5.

2. Miyasaka Y, Barnes ME, Gersh BJ, et al. Secular trends in incidence of atrial fibrillation in Olmsted County, Minnesota, 1980 to 2000, and implications on the projections for future prevalence. Circulation 2006;114(2):119–25.

3. Colilla S, Crow A, Petkun W, et al. Estimates of current and future incidence and prevalence of atrial fibrillation in the U.S. adult population. Am J Cardiol 2013;112(8):1142–7.

4. Kim MH, Johnston SS, Chu BC, et al. Estimation of total incremental health care costs in patients with atrial fibrillation in the United States. Circ Cardiovasc Qual Outcomes 2011;4(3):313–20.

5. Go AS, Mozaffarian D, Roger VL, et al. Heart disease and stroke statistics–2014 update: a report from the American Heart Association. Circulation 2014;129(3):e28–292.

6. Kirchhof P, Benussi S, Kotecha D, et al. 2016 ESC Guidelines for the management of atrial fibrillation developed in collaboration with EACTS. Eur Heart J 2016;37(38):2893–962.

7. Wolf PA, Abbott RD, Kannel WB. Atrial fibrillation as an independent risk factor for stroke: the Framingham Study. Stroke 1991;22(8):983–8.

8. Saxena R, Lewis S, Berge E, et al. Risk of early death and recurrent stroke and effect of heparin in 3169 patients with acute ischemic stroke and atrial fibrillation in the International Stroke Trial. Stroke 2001;32(10):2333–7.

9. Kimura K, Minematsu K, Yamaguchi T, Japan Multicenter Stroke Investigators' Collaboration (J-MUSIC). Atrial fibrillation as a predictive factor for severe stroke and early death in 15,831 patients with acute ischaemic stroke. J Neurol Neurosurg Psychiatry 2005;76(5):679–83.

10. Gage BF, Waterman AD, Shannon W, et al. Validation of clinical classification schemes for predicting stroke: results from the National Registry of Atrial Fibrillation. JAMA 2001;285(22):2864–70.

11. Lip GY, Nieuwlaat R, Pisters R, et al. Refining clinical risk stratification for predicting stroke and thromboembolism in atrial fibrillation using a novel risk factor-based approach: the euro heart survey on atrial fibrillation. Chest 2010;137(2):263–72.

12. Mason PK, Lake DE, DiMarco JP, et al. Impact of the CHA2DS2-VASc score on anticoagulation recommendations for atrial fibrillation. Am J Med 2012; 125(6):603.e1-6.

13. January CT, Wann LS, Alpert JS, et al. 2014 AHA/ ACC/HRS guideline for the management of patients with atrial fibrillation: a report of the American College of Cardiology/American Heart Association Task Force on Practice Guidelines and the Heart Rhythm Society. J Am Coll Cardiol 2014;64(21): e1–76.

14. Indredavik B, Rohweder G, Lydersen S. Frequency and effect of optimal anticoagulation before onset of ischaemic stroke in patients with known atrial fibrillation. J Intern Med 2005;258(2):133–44.

15. Patel MR, Mahaffey KW, Garg J, et al. Rivaroxaban versus warfarin in nonvalvular atrial fibrillation. N Engl J Med 2011;365(10):883–91.

16. Granger CB, Alexander JH, McMurray JJ, et al. Apixaban versus warfarin in patients with atrial fibrillation. N Engl J Med 2011;365(11):981–92.

17. Connolly SJ, Ezekowitz MD, Yusuf S, et al. Dabigatran versus warfarin in patients with atrial fibrillation. N Engl J Med 2009;361(12):1139–51.

18. Calkins H, Hindricks G, Cappato R, et al. 2017 HRS/ EHRA/ECAS/APHRS/SOLAECE expert consensus statement on catheter and surgical ablation of atrial fibrillation. Heart Rhythm 2017;14(10):e275–444.

19. Page RL, Wilkinson WE, Clair WK, et al. Asymptomatic arrhythmias in patients with symptomatic paroxysmal atrial fibrillation and paroxysmal supraventricular tachycardia. Circulation 1994;89(1):224–7.

20. Strickberger SA, Ip J, Saksena S, et al. Relationship between atrial tachyarrhythmias and symptoms. Heart Rhythm 2005;2(2):125–31.

21. Quirino G, Giammaria M, Corbucci G, et al. Diagnosis of paroxysmal atrial fibrillation in patients with implanted pacemakers: relationship to symptoms and other variables. Pacing Clin Electrophysiol 2009;32(1):91–8.

22. Buch E, Boyle NG, Belott PH. Pacemaker and defibrillator lead extraction. Circulation 2011;123(11): e378–380.

23. Defaye P, Dournaux F, Mouton E. Prevalence of supraventricular arrhythmias from the automated analysis of data stored in the DDD pacemakers of 617 patients: the AIDA study. The AIDA Multicenter Study Group. Automatic interpretation for diagnosis assistance. Pacing Clin Electrophysiol 1998;21(1 Pt 2): 250–5.

24. Cheung JW, Keating RJ, Stein KM, et al. Newly detected atrial fibrillation following dual chamber pacemaker implantation. J Cardiovasc Electrophysiol 2006;17(12):1323–8.

25. Orlov MV, Ghali JK, Araghi-Niknam M, et al. Asymptomatic atrial fibrillation in pacemaker recipients: incidence, progression, and determinants based on the atrial high rate trial. Pacing Clin Electrophysiol 2007;30(3):404–11.

26. Healey JS, Connolly SJ, Gold MR, et al. Subclinical atrial fibrillation and the risk of stroke. N Engl J Med 2012;366(2):120–9.

27. Ziegler PD, Glotzer TV, Daoud EG, et al. Detection of previously undiagnosed atrial fibrillation in patients with stroke risk factors and usefulness of continuous monitoring in primary stroke prevention. Am J Cardiol 2012;110(9):1309–14.

28. Flaker GC, Belew K, Beckman K, et al. Asymptomatic atrial fibrillation: demographic features and prognostic information from the Atrial Fibrillation

Follow-up Investigation of Rhythm Management (AFFIRM) study. Am Heart J 2005;149(4):657–63.

29. Sanna T, Diener HC, Passman RS, et al. Cryptogenic stroke and underlying atrial fibrillation. N Engl J Med 2014;370(26):2478–86.

30. Brachmann J, Morillo CA, Sanna T, et al. Uncovering atrial fibrillation beyond short-term monitoring in cryptogenic stroke patients: three-year results from the cryptogenic stroke and underlying atrial fibrillation trial. Circ Arrhythm Electrophysiol 2016;9(1): e003333.

31. Passman RS, Weinberg KM, Freher M, et al. Accuracy of mode switch algorithms for detection of atrial tachyarrhythmias. J Cardiovasc Electrophysiol 2004; 15(7):773–7.

32. Purerfellner H, Gillis AM, Holbrook R, et al. Accuracy of atrial tachyarrhythmia detection in implantable devices with arrhythmia therapies. Pacing Clin Electrophysiol 2004;27(7):983–92.

33. Deshmukh A, Brown ML, Higgins E, et al. Performance of atrial fibrillation detection in a new single-chamber ICD. Pacing Clin Electrophysiol 2016;39(10):1031–7.

34. Pollak WM, Simmons JD, Interian A Jr, et al. Clinical utility of intraatrial pacemaker stored electrograms to diagnose atrial fibrillation and flutter. Pacing Clin Electrophysiol 2001;24(4 Pt 1):424–9.

35. Swiryn S, Orlov MV, Benditt DG, et al. Clinical implications of brief device-detected atrial tachyarrhythmias in a cardiac rhythm management device population: results from the registry of atrial tachycardia and atrial fibrillation episodes. Circulation 2016;134(16):1130–40.

36. Kaufman ES, Israel CW, Nair GM, et al. Positive predictive value of device-detected atrial high-rate episodes at different rates and durations: an analysis from ASSERT. Heart Rhythm 2012;9(8): 1241–6.

37. Fuchs T, Torjman A. Atrial tachycardia in patients with cryptogenic stroke: is there a need for anticoagulation? Isr Med Assoc J 2015;17(11):669–72.

38. Tomson TT, Passman R. Current and emerging uses of insertable cardiac monitors: evaluation of syncope and monitoring for atrial fibrillation. Cardiol Rev 2017;25(1):22–9.

39. Sanders P, Purerfellner H, Pokushalov E, et al. Performance of a new atrial fibrillation detection algorithm in a miniaturized insertable cardiac monitor: results from the reveal LINQ usability study. Heart Rhythm 2016;13(7):1425–30.

40. Maines M, Zorzi A, Tomasi G, et al. Clinical impact, safety, and accuracy of the remotely monitored implantable loop recorder Medtronic Reveal LINQTM. Europace 2017. [Epub ahead of print].

41. Botto GL, Padeletti L, Santini M, et al. Presence and duration of atrial fibrillation detected by continuous monitoring: crucial implications for the risk of

thromboembolic events. J Cardiovasc Electrophysiol 2009;20(3):241–8.

42. Daoud EG, Glotzer TV, Wyse DG, et al. Temporal relationship of atrial tachyarrhythmias, cerebrovascular events, and systemic emboli based on stored device data: a subgroup analysis of TRENDS. Heart Rhythm 2011;8(9):1416–23.

43. Brambatti M, Connolly SJ, Gold MR, et al. Temporal relationship between subclinical atrial fibrillation and embolic events. Circulation 2014;129(21): 2094–9.

44. Shanmugam N, Boerdlein A, Proff J, et al. Detection of atrial high-rate events by continuous home monitoring: clinical significance in the heart failure-cardiac resynchronization therapy population. Europace 2012;14(2):230–7.

45. Inoue H, Nozawa T, Okumura K, et al. Prothrombotic activity is increased in patients with nonvalvular atrial fibrillation and risk factors for embolism. Chest 2004;126(3):687–92.

46. Lim HS, Willoughby SR, Schultz C, et al. Effect of atrial fibrillation on atrial thrombogenesis in humans: impact of rate and rhythm. J Am Coll Cardiol 2013; 61(8):852–60.

47. Watson T, Shantsila E, Lip GY. Mechanisms of thrombogenesis in atrial fibrillation: Virchow's triad revisited. Lancet 2009;373(9658):155–66.

48. Goldberger JJ, Arora R, Green D, et al. Evaluating the atrial myopathy underlying atrial fibrillation: identifying the arrhythmogenic and thrombogenic substrate. Circulation 2015;132(4):278–91.

49. Turakhia MP, Ziegler PD, Schmitt SK, et al. Atrial fibrillation burden and short-term risk of stroke: case-crossover analysis of continuously recorded heart rhythm from cardiac electronic implanted devices. Circ Arrhythm Electrophysiol 2015;8(5): 1040–7.

50. Lazarus A. Remote, wireless, ambulatory monitoring of implantable pacemakers, cardioverter defibrillators, and cardiac resynchronization therapy systems: analysis of a worldwide database. Pacing Clin Electrophysiol 2007;30(Suppl 1):S2–12.

51. Ricci RP, Morichelli L, Santini M. Remote control of implanted devices through Home Monitoring technology improves detection and clinical management of atrial fibrillation. Europace 2009;11(1): 54–61.

52. Varma N, Epstein AE, Irimpen A, et al. Efficacy and safety of automatic remote monitoring for implantable cardioverter-defibrillator follow-up: the lumos-T safely reduces routine office device follow-up (TRUST) trial. Circulation 2010; 122(4):325–32.

53. Crossley GH, Boyle A, Vitense H, et al, CONNECT Investigators. The CONNECT (Clinical Evaluation of Remote Notification to Reduce Time to Clinical Decision) trial: the value of wireless remote monitoring

with automatic clinician alerts. J Am Coll Cardiol 2011;57(10):1181–9.

54. Mabo P, Victor F, Bazin P, et al. A randomized trial of long-term remote monitoring of pacemaker recipients (the COMPAS trial). Eur Heart J 2012;33(9):1105–11.

55. Martin DT, Bersohn MM, Waldo AL, et al. Randomized trial of atrial arrhythmia monitoring to guide anticoagulation in patients with implanted defibrillator and cardiac resynchronization devices. Eur Heart J 2015;36(26):1660–8.

56. Sjalander S, Holmqvist F, Smith JG, et al. Assessment of use vs discontinuation of oral anticoagulation after pulmonary vein isolation in patients with atrial fibrillation. JAMA Cardiol 2017;2(2):146–52.

57. Themistoclakis S, Corrado A, Marchlinski FE, et al. The risk of thromboembolism and need for oral anticoagulation after successful atrial fibrillation ablation. J Am Coll Cardiol 2010;55(8):735–43.

58. Mascarenhas DA, Farooq MU, Ziegler PD, et al. Role of insertable cardiac monitors in anticoagulation therapy in patients with atrial fibrillation at high risk of bleeding. Europace 2016;18(6):799–806.

59. Zuern CS, Kilias A, Berlitz P, et al. Anticoagulation after catheter ablation of atrial fibrillation guided by implantable cardiac monitors. Pacing Clin Electrophysiol 2015;38(6):688–93.

60. Steinhaus DA, Zimetbaum PJ, Passman RS, et al. Cost effectiveness of implantable cardiac monitor-guided intermittent anticoagulation for atrial fibrillation: an analysis of the REACT.COM pilot study. J Cardiovasc Electrophysiol 2016;27(11):1304–11.

61. Passman R, Leong-Sit P, Andrei AC, et al. Targeted anticoagulation for atrial fibrillation guided by continuous rhythm assessment with an insertable cardiac monitor: the rhythm evaluation for anticoagulation with continuous monitoring (REACT.COM) pilot study. J Cardiovasc Electrophysiol 2016;27(3):264–70.

62. Waks J, Passman R, Thosani A, et al. Intermittent anticoagulation guided by continuous atrial fibrillation burden monitoring using dual chamber pacemakers and implantable cardioverter-defibrillators – results from the Tailored Anticoagulation for Non-Continuous Atrial Fibrillation (TACTIC-AF) pilot study. Heart Rhythm Society annual scientific sessions; 2017.

63. Van Gelder IC, Healey JS, Crijns HJ, et al. Duration of device-detected subclinical atrial fibrillation and occurrence of stroke in ASSERT. Eur Heart J 2017;38(17):1339–44.

64. Ohara K, Inoue H, Nozawa T, et al. Accumulation of risk factors enhances the prothrombotic state in atrial fibrillation. Int J Cardiol 2008;126(3):316–21.

65. Lip GY, Lane D, Van Walraven C, et al. Additive role of plasma von Willebrand factor levels to clinical factors for risk stratification of patients with atrial fibrillation. Stroke 2006;37(9):2294–300.

66. Hijazi Z, Oldgren J, Siegbahn A, et al. Biomarkers in atrial fibrillation: a clinical review. Eur Heart J 2013;34(20):1475–80.

67. Charitos EI, Purerfellner H, Glotzer TV, et al. Clinical classifications of atrial fibrillation poorly reflect its temporal persistence: insights from 1,195 patients continuously monitored with implantable devices. J Am Coll Cardiol 2014;63(25 Pt A):2840–8.

68. Charitos EI, Stierle U, Ziegler PD, et al. A comprehensive evaluation of rhythm monitoring strategies for the detection of atrial fibrillation recurrence: insights from 647 continuously monitored patients and implications for monitoring after therapeutic interventions. Circulation 2012;126(7):806–14.

69. Glotzer TV, Hellkamp AS, Zimmerman J, et al. Atrial high rate episodes detected by pacemaker diagnostics predict death and stroke: report of the Atrial Diagnostics Ancillary Study of the MOde Selection Trial (MOST). Circulation 2003;107(12):1614–9.

70. Capucci A, Santini M, Padeletti L, et al. Monitored atrial fibrillation duration predicts arterial embolic events in patients suffering from bradycardia and atrial fibrillation implanted with antitachycardia pacemakers. J Am Coll Cardiol 2005;46(10):1913–20.

71. Glotzer TV, Daoud EG, Wyse DG, et al. The relationship between daily atrial tachyarrhythmia burden from implantable device diagnostics and stroke risk: the TRENDS study. Circ Arrhythm Electrophysiol 2009;2(5):474–80.

72. Boriani G, Glotzer TV, Santini M, et al. Device-detected atrial fibrillation and risk for stroke: an analysis of >10,000 patients from the SOS AF project (Stroke preventiOn Strategies based on Atrial Fibrillation information from implanted devices). Eur Heart J 2014;35(8):508–16.

His Bundle Pacing
Is It Ready for Prime Time?

Fatima M. Ezzeddine, MD, Gopi Dandamudi, MD, FHRS*

KEYWORDS

- His bundle pacing • Ventricular pacing • Pacing strategies • Bundle branch block

KEY POINTS

- His bundle pacing is emerging as a viable pacing strategy in daily clinical practice. Several investigators have shown both feasibility and positive clinical outcomes with His bundle pacing.
- Clinical benefits include lack of pacing induced dyssynchrony, correction of bundle branch blocks, improvement in heart failure symptoms and left ventricular systolic function.
- With improvement in delivery tools and lead designs, His bundle pacing is likely to become a common pacing strategy in the near future.

INTRODUCTION

Long-term right ventricular apical pacing (RVAP) has been associated with detrimental effects, including increased risk for heart failure (HF), atrial fibrillation, (AF), and death.[1–4] Most of these adverse effects result from ventricular dyssynchrony related to perturbed ventricular depolarization. In addition, biventricular pacing (BiVp) has limited benefits in patients with non–left bundle branch block (LBBB) and severely reduced ejection fraction (EF); 20% to 30% of patients seem to not respond to cardiac resynchronization therapy (CRT).[5,6] Consequently, alternative pacing strategies that mimic natural physiology are desired. Recently, permanent His bundle pacing (PHBP) has emerged as a true physiologic form of ventricular pacing that has been shown in recent years to be safe and feasible in clinical practice. Because it induces ventricular contraction by exciting the intrinsic conduction system, it has the benefit of reducing or eliminating both interventricular and intraventricular dyssynchrony.

BACKGROUND

The bundle of His was first described in 1893 by Wilhelm His Jr, a Swiss anatomist and cardiologist.[7] He described it as a muscle bundle connecting the auricular and ventricular septal walls. Damage to the conducting cells forming the bundle of His caused asynchrony in the beat of the auricle and ventricle, referred to as heart block. His bundle recordings were first performed by Alanis and colleagues[8] on isolated perfused hearts of dogs and cats and were published in 1958. In 1969, Scherlag and colleagues[9] published the first His bundle recordings performed in human beings using intravascular catheters. A year later, Narula and colleagues[10] demonstrated the possibility for achieving temporary HBP in humans using a multipolar catheter positioned at the atrioventricular (AV) junction above the septal leaflet of the tricuspid valve.

The bundle of His is a chordlike structure that traverses from the compact AV node through the membranous interventricular septum and measures around 20 mm in length and 4 mm in diameter. The membranous septum is formed between the junction of 2 valve commissures. On the left side, it is the commissure between the right and noncoronary cusps of the aortic valve; on the right side, it is the commissure between the septal and anterior leaflets of the tricuspid valve. The bundle of His traverses at the junction between these commissures and is covered by fibrous annular tissue.[11] In 1919, Kaufman and Rothberger[12] first proposed the concept of

Indiana University School of Medicine, 1801 North Senate Boulevard, Suite 4000, Indianapolis, IN 46032, USA
* Corresponding author.
E-mail address: gdandamu@iu.edu

Card Electrophysiol Clin 10 (2018) 87–98
https://doi.org/10.1016/j.ccep.2017.11.009
1877-9182/18/© 2017 Elsevier Inc. All rights reserved.

functional longitudinal dissociation of the His bundle. Purkinje cells were found to conduct predominantly in a longitudinal rather than transverse direction, and predestined fibers within the His bundle conducted to each fascicle. James and Sherf[13] studied the structure of the human His bundle under both light and electron microscopy and found that the AV node is made of conducting cells organized by twisting collagen strands that funnel into a more parallel orientation in the His bundle. The Purkinje cells were also longitudinally oriented and separated by collagen septa. These longitudinal bundles had sparse interspersed transverse connections. This concept of longitudinal dissociation was redemonstrated by Narula14 in 1977. Patients with LBBB and baseline prolonged HV intervals were paced slightly distal in the proximal His bundle, resulting in narrowing of the QRS. The following year, El-Sherif and colleagues[15] noted that distal HBP, in patients with acute right bundle branch block (RBBB) after a myocardial infarction and patients with chronic LBBB, resulted in normalization of the QRS complex with a shorter stimulus to the ventricular interval compared with the intrinsic HV interval.[15] This theory was also demonstrated in canine experiments in which conduction delay within the His bundle was associated with the appearance of a BBB following anterior septal artery ligation.

PHYSIOLOGY

Broadly speaking, PHBP can be divided into 2 subgroups: selective HBP (SHBP) and nonselective HBP (NSHBP) (**Fig. 1**). SHBP occurs when the pacing stimulus to the QRS onset is equal to

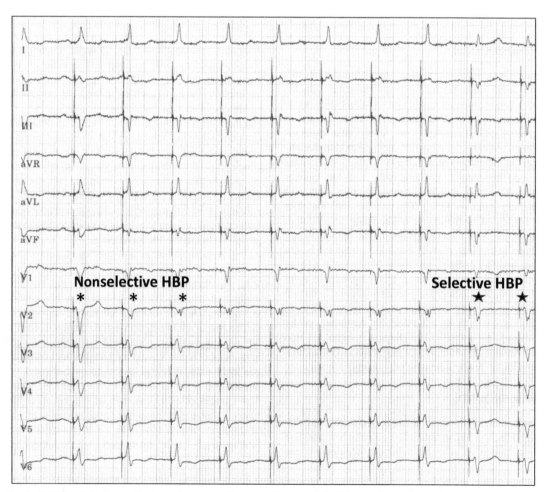

Fig. 1. A 12-lead electrocardiogram demonstrating recruitment of the His bundle as the pacing output is reduced gradually. The first 8 paced complexes demonstrate NHBP. In lead V2, subtle differences between the first 3 paced complexes (*asterisk*) can be seen because of variable fusion. The final 2 paced beats are SHBP (*star*). Note the isoelectric segment following the pacing stimulus and a narrow QRS complex with no fusion.

the intrinsic HV interval with no fusion with local myocardium at the pacing output selected (ie, a clear isoelectric segment in all 12 leads between the pacing stimulus and QRS onset and the QRS morphology is identical to the baseline intrinsic QRS morphology). NSHBP is defined as His-bundle capture with local myocardial fusion at the pacing output selected and with the pacing stimulus to QRS onset being shorter than the intrinsic HV interval. Given the interaction of nearby ventricular myocardium with His capture, NSHBP can be influenced by the output as well as the local anatomy. However, responses with NSHBP can be variable. In some cases, with high current output preferential recruitment of the His bundle occurs and output reduction can result in QRS widening with variable fusion and ultimately result in fixed septal capture only. In other cases, NSHBP is seen with higher outputs and the QRS narrows with lower outputs and can result in SHBP at very low outputs.

In 2005, Kawashima and Sasaki[16] published the results of an autopsy studying the macroscopic anatomy of the AV bundle in 105 elderly human hearts. They described 3 anatomic variations and focused on its location relative to the membranous part of the ventricular septum. They described 3 types of anatomy and their prevalence.

1. Type I seen in 47% of the specimens: AV bundle ran along the lower border of the membranous septum and was usually covered with a thin layer of myocardial fibers.
2. Type II seen in 32% of the specimens: AV bundle was discretely separated from the membranous septum and was insulated by thick myocardial fibers.
3. Type III seen in 21% of the specimens: AV bundle was naked and ran beneath the endocardium with no insulation from the surrounding myocardial fibers.

These anatomic variations can explain the various clinical responses observed with PHBP. The most common response is SHBP pacing at low output pacing and fusion at higher outputs. This type of response can be explained by the type I anatomy.[17] In some cases, fusion with local myocardium is always obtained regardless of what the pacing output is; this is consistent with a type II anatomy.[17] Lastly, in about 10% to 15% of cases, SHBP is easily achieved even at higher pacing outputs; this is consistent with a type III anatomy.[17]

Several mechanisms have been postulated to explain QRS narrowing in patients with BBBs undergoing PHBP. The concept of longitudinal dissociation described earlier supports the idea of bypassing proximal blocks as a potential mechanism behind HBP-mediated QRS narrowing. In addition, output dependence seems to play a role in overcoming a conduction block. Applying increasing stimulus strength can recruit fibers closely bordering the abnormal myocardium causing functional block and reproduce native conduction through the His-Purkinje system.[14] A third proposed mechanism explaining HBP-mediated QRS narrowing relies on the idea of virtual electrode polarization.[18] The delivery of a charge to an area creates virtual electrodes with depolarized and hyperpolarized regions surrounding the pacing tip, which can lead to the recovery of diseased local tissue from inexcitability.[18] Conduction propagation can also be theorized by the source-sink concept; propagating wave front (source) acts as a depolarizing current source for the adjacent repolarized tissue (the sink).[19] For conduction to be successful, the source current must be sufficient to bring the sink to its activation threshold. In some cases, HBP results in partial QRS narrowing without complete normalization; this can be explained by distal or complex blocks within the His-Purkinje system, anatomic variations, lead placement, or a combination of these factors.

IMPLANT TECHNIQUE

Current implant techniques use Medtronic products (Medtronic, Inc, Minneapolis, Minnesota) that are specifically designed for the procedure. They involve the use of a fixed-curve sheath (C315His, Medtronic, Inc) or a steerable catheter (C304, Medtronic, Inc).[20] A Medtronic Select Secure 3830 lead is advanced through either of these sheaths, and His-bundle mapping with the lead is performed using unipolar configuration (**Fig. 2**). Alternatively, a standard EP catheter can be used to localize the His before mapping with the pacing lead. The His bundle can be mapped to a region with the triangle of Koch (can extend from the upper lip of the coronary sinus ostium to the summit of the septum adjacent to the septal leaflet of the tricuspid valve). The 3830 lead is a dedicated bipolar, steroid-eluting, lumenless lead, which is 4.1F in diameter. It has an exposed active helix, which is 1.8 mm in length.

Once a His-bundle electrogram is recorded, pacing is performed in the unipolar configuration. After confirming His bundle recruitment, the lead is screwed into place with 6 to 8 clockwise rotations, ensuring that the torque is transmitted through the sheath to the lead tip. The sheath is pulled back until the proximal pole is well exposed and pacing is performed to assess His-bundle

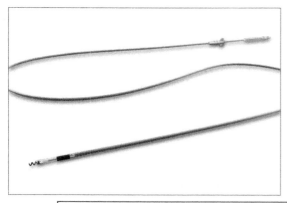

3830 Lead Specifications:

- 4.1 FR lead body diameter
- Bipolar
- Fixed screw helix
- Steroid eluting
- Polyurethane outer insulation
- Cable inner conductor

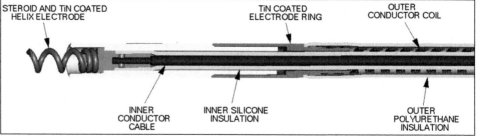

STEROID AND TiN COATED HELIX ELECTRODE

TiN COATED ELECTRODE RING

OUTER CONDUCTOR COIL

INNER CONDUCTOR CABLE

INNER SILICONE INSULATION

OUTER POLYURETHANE INSULATION

Cross-sectional view of a Medtronic 3830 lead

Fig. 2. A Select Secure 3830 pacing lead. Note the solid core of the lead and the inability to use an inner stylet. (*Courtesy of* Medtronic, Inc., Minneapolis, MN; Reproduced with permission of Medtronic, Inc.)

capture. It is important to document when His bundle recruitment is lost and when septal capture is lost (ie, 2 different thresholds in both unipolar and bipolar configurations). This ensures that the correct pacing output is programmed to reliably capture the His Purkinje system. The pulse width is usually set at 1 millisecond to ensure safety margins while minimizing battery drain. The average capture thresholds tend to be higher than RV pacing, and the mean R-wave amplitudes are lower because of the fibrous structure of the His bundle. When His-bundle injury current occurs, lower capture thresholds have been noted[21] (**Fig. 3**). It must also be noted that in order to avoid far-field atrial oversensing, R-wave sensing greater than 1 mV is recommended. A backup RV pacing lead is not routinely implanted when performing HBP. A backup RV lead may be needed in cases when there is pacemaker dependency and His/RV capture thresholds are greater than 2 V. A follow-up to check pacemaker function is recommended at 1 to 3 weeks and at 2 months to assess His-bundle capture thresholds and ventricular sensing.[23] Remote follow-up is crucial to assess long-term function of the device system. Capture management algorithms are usually turned off, as evoked responses during His-bundle capture are often delayed and of reduced strength.

CLINICAL BENEFITS

The detriments of RVAP have been well known for some time. Several trials performed in the past 2 decades have cemented the fact that a high degree of RVAP can lead to an increased incidence of AF and HF. Sweeney and colleagues[3] demonstrated the adverse effects of ventricular pacing, including the increased incidence of HF and AF in the pacemaker population. Also, Wilkoff and colleagues[2] demonstrated that unnecessary RV pacing can result in significant adverse outcomes, including increased HF hospitalizations. Recently, Kiehl and colleagues[24] demonstrated the incidence of pacing-induced cardiomyopathy in patients with baseline preserved left ventricular (LV) EFs to be more than 12% during a mean follow-up of 4 years. Two independent predictors were identified in this cohort: a lower preimplant LVEF and increased RV pacing burden. Interestingly, RV pacing greater than 20% seemed to differentiate patients who had a higher risk for developing pacing-induced cardiomyopathy. In 2000, Deshmukh and colleagues[25] described the first clinical trial with PHBP in patients with chronic AF and tachycardia-induced cardiomyopathy. Following AV junction ablation, PHBP was achieved in most patients with improvement in LV function. Since then, several investigators around the world have published their

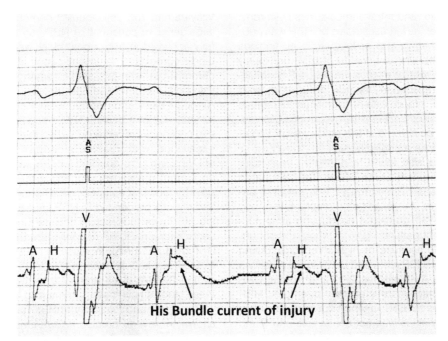

Fig. 3. Tracing is from the Pacing System Analyzer (PSA) at the time of the pacemaker implant. The pacing lead is connected in a unipolar fashion and connected to the atrial channel on the PSA for better delineation of His-bundle electrograms. The patient is in 2:1 infranodal block as demonstrated by local His-bundle activation followed by failure to conduct to the ventricles. His-bundle current of injury is also observed once the lead is screwed in (*arrows*).[22] A, local atrial electrograms; H, local His electrograms; V, local ventricular electrograms.

experience with HBP and the field has gradually advanced with favorable results noted.

The clinical benefits of PHBP include AV and interventricular/intraventricular synchronization using the native conduction system; potential for less injury to the tricuspid valve, as the lead tip may lie in the right atrium without crossing the valve[26–28]; and improvement in clinical outcomes, such as reduction in HF due to chronic RV pacing.[29] PHBP has also been shown to be clinically effective in patients with chronic LBBB by recruiting distal conduction fibers and restoring electrical and mechanical resynchronization[30,31]

In an early study performed by Padeletti and colleagues[32] in patients with narrow QRS noneligible for CRT, temporary HBP did not improve LV function as compared with alternate RV pacing sites; it was suggested that it might be inferior to LV pacing. In contrast to these findings, subsequent studies demonstrated consistent beneficial effects of HBP. Several studies evaluated the hemodynamic and clinical benefits of HBP over RVAP. Occhetta and colleagues[33] performed a randomized crossover study in 16 of 18 patients with chronic AF undergoing AV junction ablation and randomized them to 6 months of RV pacing versus para-Hisian HBP. Para-Hisian pacing resulted in improvement in New York Heart

Association (NYHA) functional class, quality-of-life scores, and 6-minute walk test. Kronborg and colleagues[34] showed that stable direct HBP (DHBP) or para-Hisian pacing was feasible in 85% of patients with narrow QRS and high-grade AV block and lead to normalization of the ventricular activation pattern with statistically significantly less LV dyssynchrony as compared with RV pacing. Catanzariti and colleagues[35] also examined HBP effects acutely and found that it prevented interventricular and intraventricular asynchrony either on the same day as the procedure or on the following day. These beneficial effects of improved ventricular contractile performance persisted after 2 years of follow-up.[36] This reduced asynchronous pacing induced LVEF depression and mitral regurgitation in comparison with RVAP. Similarly, Zanon and colleagues[37] conducted a crossover midterm study in which patients underwent 3 months of DHBP and then 3 months of RVAP. Myocardial perfusion was found to be significantly better during DHBP than during RVAP. In a study by Pastore and colleagues,[38] 37 patients with normal cardiac function had PHBP with an apical RV backup lead and underwent 3 months of HBP followed by 3 months of RVAP. Switching from HBP to RVAP resulted in a significant increase in systolic and diastolic electromechanical delays and consequent interventricular and intraventricular dyssynchrony. Finally, one of the largest studies on HBP was published by Sharma and colleagues[29]; its findings supported the clinical benefits of HBP previously examined in smaller studies, namely, HF hospitalization was reduced in the HBP group compared with the RVP group, with no significant difference in mortality noted between the two groups. However, it should be noted that this study was not powered to detect a mortality benefit.

PHBP was also found to normalize ventricular activation in patients with BBBs. Barba-Pichardo and colleagues[39] attempted HBP in selected patients referred for pacemaker implantation and found that HBP corrected conduction abnormalities in 73% of patients (32% of whom did not undergo PHBP because of high thresholds during initial testing). HBP corrected BBBs in the presence of complete AV block resulting in a normal QRS complex. A few years later, they attempted HBP in candidates for CRT in whom LV stimulation via the coronary sinus was not achievable and found that DHBP corrected conduction in 13 of the 16 patients (81%) selected.[40] In 9 patients, DHBP successfully resulted in definitive resynchronization with improvement in functional class and parameters of LV function.[39] Similarly, Lustgarten and colleagues[41] assessed DHBP in patients with standard indications for biventricular pacing, and noted that it resulted in a significantly narrower QRS as compared with native conduction and BiVp (mean QRS duration: native 171 milliseconds, DHBP 148 milliseconds, and BiVp 158 milliseconds, $P<.0001$). This finding of electrical resynchronization was revisited by the same group of researchers again in a crossover comparison study assessing the feasibility of, and the clinical response to, PHBP as an alternative to BiVp in CRT-indicated patients.[30] It was found that HBP can elicit 6-month CRT clinical responses similar to those of BiVp. Therefore, HBP can be considered an alternative to CRT if the traditional method of LV resynchronization via the coronary sinus fails. Recently, Huang and colleagues[42] published their experience with PHBP in patients with AF and rapid ventricular rates despite medical therapy. They underwent successful PHBP and AV nodal ablation. They were able to demonstrate improvement in LVEFs and LV end-diastolic dimensions. Moreover, the degree of response was greater in those patients with higher degree of LV dysfunction at baseline. Ajijola and colleagues[31] recently published their experience with PHBP in patients with LV systolic dysfunction and LBBBs who were CRT eligible. They were able to demonstrate correction of LBBB with PHBP in 16 of 21 patients and also improvement in ejection fractions in most of these patients.

Vijayaraman and colleagues[43] demonstrated in a large series of patients that HBP can be successfully achieved in both nodal block and infranodal block contexts. The investigators were able to demonstrate chronic stable pacing thresholds with both selective and nonselective HBP in both AV nodal block and infranodal block patients, with minimal use of a backup RV pacing lead. Sharma and colleagues recently published their multicenter experience in patients who underwent HBP instead of LV pacing (who qualified for CRT therapy based on current guidelines). Patients either had failed prior LV lead placement or were nonresponders or had directly proceeded to HBP instead of LV pacing. HBP was successfully achieved in 90% of patients with significant narrowing of QRS duration (157 ms to 118 ms), increase in LVEF (from 30% to 44%) and improvement in New York Heart Association (NYHA) class (from 2.8 to 1.8). Some of these studies have been summarized in **Table 1**.

The safety and feasibility of HBP has also been shown in several studies. Vijayaraman and colleagues[43] noted that catheter manipulation during HBP caused injury to the His bundle in 7.8% of patients undergoing PHBP with resultant RBBB in most cases. However, complete spontaneous resolution of the RBBB occurred in most of the cases; RBBB persisted in 2.5% of the cases (all normalized with HBP).[44] Furthermore, Sharma and colleagues[29] found that PHBP without a mapping catheter or a backup RV lead was successfully achieved in 80% of patients. Pacing thresholds were higher; fluoroscopy times were similar in these individuals to those of the RV pacing group, and no increased risks were noted when the procedure was performed by experienced operators. Frank dislodgement of the pacing lead in the His-bundle position is quite rare (<1%) based on the collective experiences of several high-volume implant operators. Occasional complete heart block can also occur immediately after the lead is screwed in, but this is also transient in most cases. Normal conduction usually resumes within a few minutes. Sharma and colleagues[29] recently demonstrated that an increase in capture threshold occurred in 7% of patients and loss of bundle branch recruitment in 7% of patients over a mean follow-up period of 14 months in patients who had a CRT indication but underwent HBP instead.

CASE EXAMPLES

1. A 64- year old woman presented with sudden cardiac arrest (successfully resuscitated from ventricular fibrillation) and intermittent heart block 3 years ago. The workup for other causes was negative (no ischemia, negative

Table 1
Recent clinical publications on permanent His bundle pacing

Study Population	Design	n	Findings
NYHA class III HF symptoms, LBBB >120 ms, EF <35%, failed LV lead placement (*Europace* 2013)[40]	Nonrandomized, nonconsecutive	16	HBP success: 56%; follow-up: 31 mo Mean LVEF improvement from 29% to 36%, one NYHA class improvement
HBP vs RV pacing in preserved EF population (*Heart Rhythm* 2015)[29]	Unselected population, consecutive pts	192	HBP success: 80%; follow-up: 2 y Reduction in HF hospitalizations in pts with >40% ventricular pacing (2% vs 15% favoring HBP)
HBP vs BiVp in CRT-eligible patients, NYHA class II to III, mean EF 25% (*Heart Rhythm* 2015)[30]	Patient blinded, crossover design	29	HBP success: 72%; 57% completed crossover analysis at 1 y; no difference in NYHA class, 6-min walk, LVEF improvement between both groups
HBP in lieu of CRT, NYHA class II to IV, QRS >120 ms, EF <35% (*Heart Rhythm* 2017)[31]	Nonrandomized	21	HBP success: 76%; significant improvement in mean QRS duration (180–129 ms), NYHA class (III–II), LVEF (from 27%–41%)
HBP in patients undergoing AVJ ablation for AF and with either preserved or reduced LVEF (JAHA 2017)[42]	Nonrandomized, consecutive pts	52	HBP success: 81%; median follow-up of 20 mo; no change in QRS (107 vs 105 ms), significant EF improvement (30% to 50%), decreases in BNP levels, LV end-diastolic dimensions, and BNP levels, improvement >1 class in NYHA functional status
HBP in patients with failed LV/nonresponders in lieu of LV lead (*Heart Rhythm* 2017)[44]	Nonrandomized,	95	HBP success: 90%; mean follow-up of 14 mo, significant improvement in mean QRS duration (157–118 ms), LVEF (30% to 44%), and NYHA class (2.8–1.8)

Abbreviations: AVJ, AV junction; BNP, brain natriuretic peptide; JAHA, *Journal of the American Heart Association*; pts, patients.

cardiovascular MRI). Genetic testing (including SCN5A mutations) was negative. Her LVEF was 54% at the time. She underwent successful implantation of a dual-chamber implantable cardioverter-defibrillator. Over the next 1.5 years, she started to develop progressive shortness of breath, HF symptoms; a 2-dimensional echocardiogram demonstrated an LVEF of 40%. Pacing-induced cardiomyopathy was suspected, and upgrade to HBP or CRT therapy with an LV lead (in case HBP was not successful) (**Fig. 4**) was discussed. She consented to it. On the day of the procedure, her intrinsic rhythm demonstrated high-grade AV block with an LBBB (**Fig. 5**). HBP resulted in correction of her heart block and LBBB (**Fig. 6**). Note the T waves change acutely due to cardiac memory. A CRT- Defibrillator was used with the His lead plugged into the LV port and an LV-RV offset maximally extended, resulting

in functional noncapture of the RV stimulus. HBP thresholds were 1 V at 1 millisecond. Three weeks later, her electrocardiogram (ECG) demonstrated normalization of her T waves and NSHBP (minimal fusion) (**Fig. 7**). Three months after the procedure, her LVEF normalized to 55% with resolution of her HF symptoms.

2. A 56-year-old woman with a history of nonischemic cardiomyopathy, LBBB, and reduced LVEF was referred for consideration for CRT-D therapy. She had been developing progressive shortness of breath and had NYHA class III HF symptoms. Two years before presentation, she also received chemotherapy for breast cancer. She had a wide LBBB at baseline (**Fig. 8**) and consented for HBP or LV lead placement if HBP could not be accomplished. Her LVEF was 20% before implantation. She underwent successful PHBP with recruitment of her LBBB

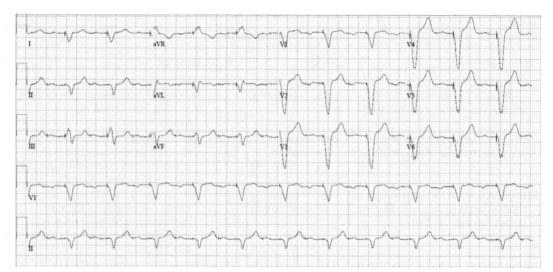

Fig. 4. A 64 year old with RVAP after presenting with sudden cardiac arrest (VF) in the setting of intermittent high-grade AV block.

(**Fig. 9**). The ECG demonstrated SHBP with no local fusion. HBP thresholds were 0.75 V at 1 millisecond. At 3 months, her RV pacing output was reduced to minimal values to reduce battery drain. Her HF symptoms improved dramatically (from NYHA class III to I), and her EF improved to 40% at 6 months.

LIMITATIONS

Certain problems unique to HBP are faced with conventional active fixation pacing leads, including a higher pacing threshold owing to the fibrous structure of the His bundle and due to current limitations in lead design and delivery. In

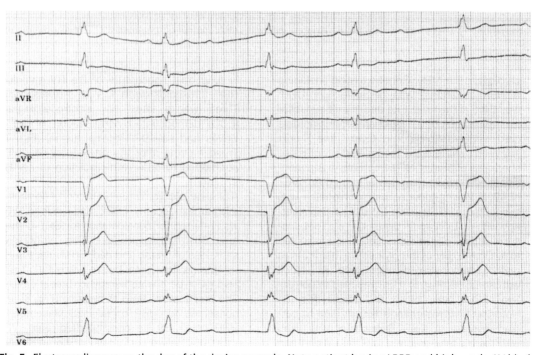

Fig. 5. Electrocardiogram on the day of the device upgrade. Note patient having LBBB and high-grade AV block.

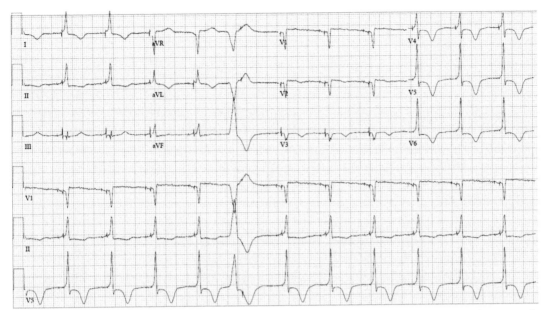

Fig. 6. PHBP with recruitment of the LBBB. Note the deep T-wave inversions seen with pacing due to cardiac memory.

addition, higher pacing thresholds can lead to increased battery drain and shorter battery longevity compared with traditional RV pacing. Other limitations of PHBP include inability to perform lead implantation in 10% to 20% of patients, particularly in patients with dilated and remodeled atria or other structural heart disease, which makes mapping of the His bundle and delivery of the lead difficult. Ventricular undersensing, atrial oversensing on the ventricular channel, and atrial capture can also occur and need to be carefully avoided or excluded at the time of implantation. Long-term randomized safety and efficacy data are yet to be determined.

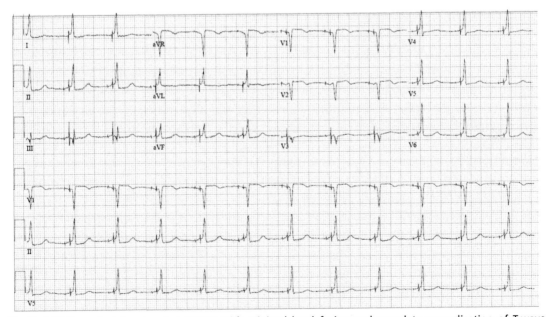

Fig. 7. ECG 3 weeks later showing NSHBP with minimal local fusion and complete normalization of T-wave inversions.

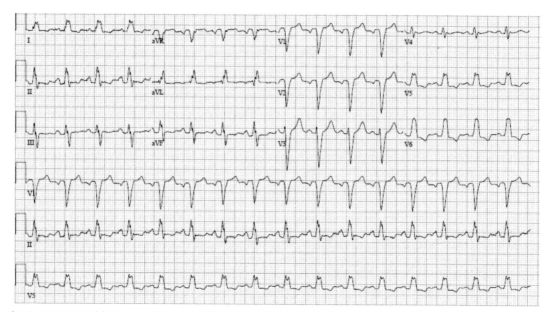

Fig. 8. A 56-year-old woman with wide LBBB and nonischemic cardiomyopathy, NYHA class III symptoms, and a LVEF of 20%.

FUTURE DIRECTIONS

Despite all the promising (theoretic and practical) benefits of HBP, it is still not widely adopted in clinical practice partly because of the perception that it is technically challenging and that long-term randomized data are unavailable at this time. There are still many unanswered questions to be addressed through large-scale randomized studies. The His

Optimized Pacing Evaluated for Heart Failure trial (HOPE-HF, clinical trials.gov ID: NCT02671903)[45] is an ongoing double-blinded crossover study assessing the effect of HBP on exercise capacity in patients with HF who are candidates for CRT. Another ongoing trial studying HBP versus Coronary Sinus Pacing for Cardiac Synchronization Therapy (HIS-SYNC, clinical trials.gov ID: NCT02700425)[46] is being conducted in a randomized systematic

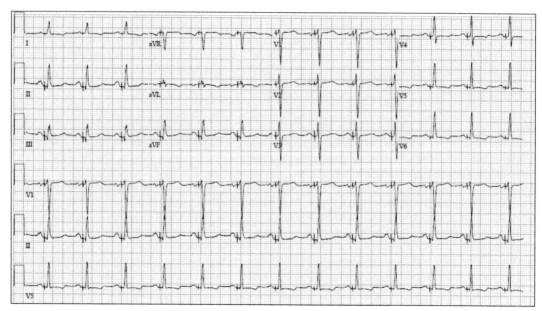

Fig. 9. Complete normalization of LBBB with SHBP and improvement of NYHA class from III to I. LVEF improved to 40% at 6 months.

manner and should provide answers regarding the utility of PHBP in patients with LBBB who currently qualify for CRT therapy. With the demonstration of clinical risks and benefits through such randomized trials and continued technological advances, PHBP is likely to gain more acceptance and find its way as a permanent fixture in cardiac pacing. Along with trials, concomitant investment into lead designs and delivery systems need to occur to make PHBP a part of routine clinical practice.

REFERENCES

1. Lamas GA, Lee KL, Sweeney MO, et al. Ventricular pacing or dual-chamber pacing for sinus-node dysfunction. N Engl J Med 2002;346:1854–62.
2. Wilkoff BL, Cook JR, Epstein AE, et al. Dual-chamber pacing or ventricular backup pacing in patients with an implantable defibrillator: the dual chamber and VVI implantable defibrillator (DAVID) trial. JAMA 2002;288:3115–23.
3. Sweeney MO, Hellkamp AS, Ellenbogen KA, et al. Adverse effect of ventricular pacing on heart failure and atrial fibrillation among patients with normal baseline QRS duration in a clinical trial of pacemaker therapy for sinus node dysfunction. Circulation 2003;107:2932–7.
4. Barsheshet A, Moss AJ, Mcnitt S, et al. Long-term implications of cumulative right ventricular pacing among patients with an implantable cardioverter-defibrillator. Heart Rhythm 2011;8(2):212–8.
5. Moss AJ, Hall WJ, Cannom DS, et al. Cardiac-resynchronization therapy for the prevention of heart-failure events. N Engl J Med 2009;361:1329–38.
6. Auricchio A, Prinzen FW. Non-responders to cardiac resynchronization therapy. Circ J 2011;75:521–7.
7. Kasper D, Fauci A, Hauser S. Harrisson's principles of internal medicine. 19th edition. New York: McGraw-Hill Professional; 2015.
8. Alanis J, Gonzalez H, Lopez E. The electrical activity of the bundle of His. J Physiol 1958;142:127–40.
9. Scherlag BJ, Lau SH, Helfant RH, et al. Catheter technique for recording His bundle activity in man. Circulation 1969;39:13–8.
10. Narula OS, Scherlag BJ, Javier RP, et al. Analysis of the A-V conduction defect in complete heart block utilizing His bundle electrograms. Circulation 1970; 41:437–48.
11. Kapa S, Bruce CJ, Friedman PA, et al. Advances in cardiac pacing: beyond the transvenous right ventricular apical lead. Cardiovasc Ther 2010;28(6):369–79.
12. Kaufmann R, Rothberger CJ. Beiträge zur entstehungsweise extrasystolischer allorhythmien. Zeitschrift F ür Die Gesamte Experimentelle Medizin 1919;9:104–22.
13. James TN, Sherf L. Fine structure of the His bundle. Circulation 1971;44:9–28.
14. Narula OS. Longitudinal dissociation in the His bundle. Bundle branch block due to asynchronous conduction within the His bundle in man. Circulation 1977;56(6):996–1006.
15. El-Sherif N, Amay-Y-Leon F, Schonfield CL, et al. Normalization of bundle branch block patterns by distal His bundle pacing. Clinical and experimental evidence of longitudinal dissociation in the pathologic His bundle. Circulation 1978;57:473–83.
16. Kawashima T, Sasaki H. A macroscopic anatomical investigation of atrioventricular bundle locational variation relative to the membranous part of the ventricular septum in elderly human hearts. Surg Radiol Anat 2005;27:206–13.
17. Dandamudi G, Vijayaraman P. The complexity of the His bundle: understanding its anatomy and physiology through the lens of the past and the present. Pacing Clin Electrophysiol 2016;39(12):1294–7.
18. Cheng Y, Mowrey KA, Van Wagoner DR, et al. Virtual electrode-induced reexcitation: a mechanism of defibrillation. Circ Res 1999;85(11):1056–66.
19. Xie Y, Sato D, Garfinkel A, et al. So little source, so much sink: requirements for afterdepolarizations to propagate in tissue. Biophys J 2010;99:1408–15.
20. Dandamudi G, Vijayaraman P. How to perform permanent His bundle pacing in routine clinical practice. Heart Rhythm 2016;13(6):1362–6.
21. Vijayaraman P, Dandamudi G, Worsnick S, et al. Acute His-bundle injury current during permanent His-bundle pacing predicts excellent pacing outcomes. Pacing Clin Electrophysiol 2015;38(5):540–6.
22. Vijayaraman P, Dandamudi G, Ellenbogen KA. Electrophysiological observations of acute His bundle injury during permanent His bundle pacing. J Electrocardiol 2016;49(5):664–9.
23. Vijayaraman P, Dandamudi G. How to perform permanent His bundle pacing: tips and tricks. Pacing Clin Electrophysiol 2016;39(12):1298–304.
24. Kiehl EL, Makki T, Kumar R, et al. Incidence and predictors of right ventricular pacing-induced cardiomyopathy in patients with complete atrioventricular block and preserved left ventricular systolic function. Heart Rhythm 2016;13(12):2272–8.
25. Deshmukh P, Casavant D, Romanyshyn M, et al. Permanent direct His bundle pacing: a novel approach to cardiac pacing in patients with normal His-Purkinje activation. Circulation 2000;101(8): 869–77.
26. Vijayaraman P, Dandamudi G, Bauch T, et al. Imaging evaluation of implantation site of permanent direct His bundle pacing lead. Heart Rhythm 2014;11:529–30.
27. de Sa C, Hardin NJ, Crespo EM, et al. Autopsy evaluation of the implantation site of a permanent direct His bundle pacing lead. Circ Arrhythm Electrophysiol 2012;5:244–6.
28. Bauch T, Vijayaraman P, Dandamudi G, et al. Three-dimensional printing for in vivo visualization

of His bundle pacing leads. Am J Cardiol 2015;116: 485–6.

29. Sharma PS, Dandamudi G, Naperkowski A, et al. Permanent His-bundle pacing is feasible, safe, and superior to right ventricular pacing in routine clinical practice. Heart Rhythm 2015;12(2):305–12.

30. Lustgarten DL, Crespo EM, Arkhipova-Jenkins I, et al. His-bundle pacing versus biventricular pacing in cardiac resynchronization therapy patients: a crossover design comparison. Heart Rhythm 2015; 12(7):1548–57.

31. Ajijola OA, Upadhyay GA, Macias C, et al. Permanent His-bundle pacing for cardiac resynchronization therapy: initial feasibility study in lieu of left ventricular lead. Heart Rhythm 2017;14(9):1353–61.

32. Padeletti L, Lieberman R, Schreuder J, et al. Acute effects of His bundle pacing versus left ventricular and right ventricular pacing on left ventricular function. Am J Cardiol 2007;100(10):1556–60.

33. Occhetta E, Bortnik M, Magnani A, et al. Prevention of ventricular desynchronization by permanent para-Hisian pacing after atrioventricular node ablation in chronic atrial fibrillation. J Am Coll Cardiol 2006; 47(10):1938–45.

34. Kronborg MB, Mortensen PT, Gerdes JC, et al. His and para-His pacing in AV block: feasibility and electrocardiographic findings. J Interv Card Electrophysiol 2011;31(3):255–62.

35. Catanzariti D, Maines M, Cemin C, et al. Permanent direct his bundle pacing does not induce ventricular dyssynchrony unlike conventional right ventricular apical pacing. J Interv Card Electrophysiol 2006; 16(2):81–92.

36. Catanzariti D, Maines M, Manica A, et al. Permanent His-bundle pacing maintains long-term ventricular synchrony and left ventricular performance, unlike conventional right ventricular apical pacing. Europace 2013;15(4):546–53.

37. Zanon F, Bacchiega E, Rampin L, et al. Direct His bundle pacing preserves coronary perfusion compared with right ventricular apical pacing: a prospective, cross-over mid-term study. Europace 2008;10(5):580–7.

38. Pastore G, Aggio S, Baracca E, et al. Hisian area and right ventricular apical pacing differently affect left atrial function: an intra-patients evaluation. Europace 2014;16(7):1033–9.

39. Barba-Pichardo R, Moriña-Vázquez P, Fernández-Gómez JM, et al. Permanent His-bundle pacing: seeking physiological ventricular pacing. Europace 2010;12(4):527–33.

40. Barba-Pichardo R, Manovel Sánchez A, Fernández-Gómez JM, et al. Ventricular resynchronization therapy by direct His-bundle pacing using an internal cardioverter defibrillator. Europace 2013;15(1):83–8.

41. Lustgarten DL, Calame S, Crespo EM, et al. Electrical resynchronization induced by direct His-bundle pacing. Heart Rhythm 2010;7(1):15–21.

42. Huang W, Su L, Wu S, et al. Benefits of permanent His bundle pacing combined with atrioventricular node ablation in atrial fibrillation patients with heart failure with both preserved and reduced left ventricular ejection fraction. J Am Heart Assoc 2017;6(4).

43. Vijayaraman P, Naperkowski A, Ellenbogen KA, et al. Electrophysiologic insights into site of atrioventricular block: lessons from permanent His bundle pacing. JACC Clin Electrophysiol 2015;1(6):571–81.

44. Sharma PS, Dandamudi G, Herweg B, et al. Permanent His bundle pacing as an alternative to biventricular pacing for cardiac resynchronization therapy: a multi-center experience. Heart Rhythm 2017. [Epub ahead of print].

45. Available at: https://clinicaltrials.gov/ct2/show/NCT02671903. Accessed May 2, 2017.

46. Available at: https://clinicaltrials.gov/ct2/show/NCT02700425. Accessed May 2, 2017.

Management of Perioperative Anticoagulation for Device Implantation

Merrill H. Stewart, MD, Daniel P. Morin, MD, MPH, FHRS*

KEYWORDS

- Perioperative anticoagulation • Pacemaker • Implantable cardioverter defibrillator • Hematoma
- Device complications • Antiplatelets

KEY POINTS

- Implantation of cardiac implantable electronic devices is on the rise, and an increasing number of these are implanted in the setting of anticoagulation or antiplatelet agents.
- Device site hematoma is a major consequence resulting in increasing cost, morbidity, and mortality for the patient.
- In patients at moderate to high risk of thromboembolic consequences, continuation of vitamin K–antagonist therapy has been shown to result in decreased hematoma formation compared with temporary cessation and perioperative heparin bridging.
- Dual antiplatelet usage also results in significant bleeding risk; however, certain situations necessitate uninterrupted therapy.
- Temporary interruption of direct oral anticoagulants seems safe but more research is needed in this area.

Cardiac implantable electronic devices (CIEDs) represent a commonly used and increasingly prevalent technology, with more than 1 million pacemakers (PPMs) and 300,000 implantable cardioverter-defibrillators (ICDs) placed worldwide in 2009. That year, the United States led the world in implantation numbers, with 225,567 PPMs and 133,262 ICDs.[1] Patients with CIEDs frequently have comorbidities that necessitate anticoagulation or antiplatelet medications. For example, 23% to 24% of patients receiving PPMs and 32% to 37% of those receiving ICDs are taking warfarin around the time of implantation.[2,3] Because anticoagulation and antiplatelet therapy potentially place the patient at increased risk for bleeding at the time of implantation, a commonly encountered clinical dilemma is identifying the best management strategy for these agents at time of the procedure. A thorough analysis of this problem requires having an understanding of the overall and patient-specific risks of thrombotic complications during the absence of anticoagulation or antiplatelet agents, and then balancing these risks with the increased risk of bleeding when performing device implantation in the presence of these agents.

Disclosure Statement: M.H. Stewart has no disclosures. Speaker's bureau for Boehringer-Ingelheim and Medtronic, and research grants from Boston Scientific (ISRCRM400003) and Medtronic (CR-1726) (D.P. Morin).
John Ochsner Heart and Vascular Institute, Ochsner Clinical School, University of Queensland School of Medicine, 1514 Jefferson Highway, New Orleans, LA 70121, USA
* Corresponding author.
E-mail address: Dmorin@ochsner.org

Card Electrophysiol Clin 10 (2018) 99–109
https://doi.org/10.1016/j.ccep.2017.11.008

SCOPE OF THE PROBLEM

Although perhaps seemingly benign, device-site hematomas (see examples in **Fig. 1**) and bleeding complications have a significant effect on patient morbidity and mortality. These complications increase hospitalization time, reoperation rate, and risk of infection, while prolonging duration off anticoagulation, thus increasing thromboembolic risk.[4,5] An early review of 3164 device implantations found an average hematoma incidence rate of 4.9%.[6] A single hematoma almost doubles the risk of infection, and if reintervention is required, the chance of infection is increased more than 15-fold.[7] Hematoma or bleeding complications increase the cost of implanting an ICD by $6995 (in 2006 dollars) and add on average 3 days to the index hospitalization.[8] If infection does occur, it increases mortality 4.4- to 7.7-fold (an absolute increase of 3.9% to 9.6%), with an incremental cost per admission of $14,360–$16,498.[9]

One of the difficulties encountered in studying pocket hematomas during device implantation is the variability of definition. A hematoma is defined by its diameter; elevation above the surrounding skin; or whether it requires further operative intervention, anticoagulation cessation, or blood transfusion. Understandably, hematoma-related morbidity rises with size and subsequent intervention, but the variability in definition makes interstudy comparisons difficult. The Bridge or Continue Coumadin for Device Surgery Randomized Controlled Trial (BRUISE CONTROL) trial, discussed later, defined a hematoma as one requiring further surgery, prolongation of hospitalization, or interruption of anticoagulation.[10] By comparison, an earlier small randomized study by Tolosana and colleagues[11] defined a hematoma simply as a mass protruding greater than 2 cm above the pulse generator. Most recently, published trials have settled on the BRUISE definition, with a "significant" hematoma being one requiring a change in therapy (ie, blood transfusion, exploration, pressure dressing, or hospitalization).[12–14]

THROMBOEMBOLIC RISK

An individual's risk of bleeding must be weighed against their risk of thromboembolism in the setting of cessation of anticoagulation. Then, the relative severity of complication should also be considered. There is significant variation among vascular thromboembolic (VTE) complications, ranging from peripheral embolism, to transient ischemic attack (TIA), to disabling stroke. Bleeding complications can range from superficial hematomas to potentially fatal pericardial tamponade. With some variation, most studies define high risk for VTE as an annual thromboembolic risk of >4% to 5%. This includes patients with atrial fibrillation with $CHADS_2$ (congestive heart failure, hypertension, age $\geq$75 years, diabetes mellitus, and stroke or TIA) score greater than or equal to 2, a mechanical valve in the mitral position, or recent venous thromboembolism.[15,16] An annual stroke risk of 5% translates into a daily risk of 0.014%, which if anticoagulation is held for a week perioperatively equates to a VTE rate of 0.1%. However, these risk calculations indicate aggregate risk over a typical year, and the prothrombotic milieu of the postoperative state likely temporarily

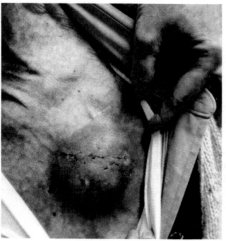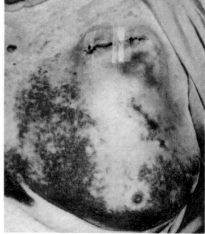

Fig. 1. Examples of device site hematoma after ICD implantation.

increases the risk. In a study examining 1293 episodes of warfarin cessation for procedures in 1024 patients with predominantly atrial fibrillation, of whom approximately 50% had CHADS scores greater than or equal to 2, the average stroke rate was 0.7%, substantially higher than predicted based on their annual risk alone.[17] In another interesting series of 406 PPM implantations, for which anticoagulation and antiplatelet agents were held in all patients, there was a 2.7% thromboembolic event rate. Of note, in that series fewer than 50% of patients with atrial fibrillation were taking an anticoagulant before the procedure, indicating that baseline medical management was suboptimal.[18] These studies suggest a nonnegligible thromboembolic risk during the periprocedural period.

TO BRIDGE OR NOT TO BRIDGE

As recently as 2012, guidelines recommended perioperative bridging with low-molecular-weight heparin (LMWH) or unfractionated heparin (UFH) in patients who required oral anticoagulant (OAC) cessation for surgery and were at high risk of thromboembolism.[19] The goal was to minimize thromboembolic complications while the level of OAC was subtherapeutic immediately before and after the procedure, while allowing for hemostasis during the procedure.

There was concern, however, that the short-term hemostatic benefits of anticoagulation cessation could be offset by the dangers of subsequent heparinization. A retrospective review in 2004 examined 3164 device procedures (PPMs and ICDs), of which 1069 were performed during temporary cessation of anticoagulation before the procedure. Warfarin was held in all patients, and heparin bridging administered postoperatively at high doses (either a 2500–5000 IU bolus following the procedure, followed by continuous infusion with a target activated partial thromboplastin time 40–60 seconds; continuous infusion without bolus started at 12 hours after procedure; UFH 12,500 IU twice a day; or LMWH 1 mg/kg twice a day), or low doses (subcutaneous UFH 10,000–15,000 IU daily, LMWH with dalteparin 2500 IU or enoxaparin 20 mg daily, or continuous infusion of heparin 400–600 IU/h). There was an overall bleeding risk of 4.9%. Among those bridged with high-dose heparin, there was an 11.6% risk of bleeding, compared with 2.9% in the low-dose category ($P<.001$).[6] The overall rate of thromboembolic events was low (0.13%–0.44%), but this was not reported by individual treatment category.

As an alternative to heparin bridging, in 1998 Goldstein and colleagues[20] published a small series demonstrating safety of PPM implantation during continuous therapeutic warfarin. There were no complications in this series of 37 patients, which was limited by its small size. Another small series by al-Khadra[21] in 2003 showed similar results, with only one hematoma among 47 patients on therapeutic warfarin at the time of implantation. Despite these data, the predominant strategy at the time remained heparin bridging for those at high thromboembolic risk, and anticoagulant cessation for those at low risk.

In another attempt to mitigate the risks of heparin bridging, a 2000 study randomized patients with high thromboembolic risk undergoing device implantation to heparin resumption at either 6 or 24 hours postdevice, and compared these patients with a low-risk control group who were not given perioperative heparin. They noted a 23% (6/26) incidence of pocket hematoma when heparin was used at 6 hours compared with 17% (4/23) at 24 hours, and only a 2% (2/115) incidence in the control group.[22] Only one thromboembolic event occurred in the low-risk group.

Several subsequent studies examined patients undergoing device implantation, exploring all three approaches of holding OAC, continuing OAC during the procedure, or holding OAC and bridging perioperatively with heparin (**Table 1**).[5,12,14,23–28] Generally, only those at moderate to high thromboembolic risk were bridged with heparin. Most studies considered as high risk those patients with a mechanical valve in the mitral position, chronic atrial fibrillation with additional risk factors, recent stroke or TIA, or recent venous thrombosis. Unfortunately, there was no universal agreement of thromboembolic risk assessment between studies. There also was significant variation between end points, with differing definitions of pocket hematomas and bleeding. The primary OAC used for most studies was a vitamin K antagonist (VKA); the direct OACs (DOACs) are addressed separately later. Formal recommendations have also been released by the American College of Chest Physicians, as shown in **Table 2**.

Among the studies examining VKA, which were primarily observational, there was increased risk of bleeding associated with heparin use. Studies varied more with regard to the level of risk found to be associated with oral anticoagulation continuation when compared with cessation. Several representational studies are summarized next.

Giudici and colleagues[25] examined 1025 device implantations in patients on chronic VKA OAC. Anticoagulation was stopped at the physician's discretion in 555 patients, whereas 470 patients had anticoagulation continued, with a mean international normalized rate (INR) of 2.6. The hematoma rate was

Table 1
Bleeding complication rate by anticoagulation strategy

Trial	Patients (n)	Trial Type	Heparin Bridging (%)	Continued VKA Therapy (%)	VKA Cessation (%)	No Anticoagulation (%)
Goldstein et al,[20] 1998	150	Obs.	—	2/37 (5.4)	—	2/113 (1.8)
Michaud et al,[22] 2000	192	Obs.	10/49 (20.4)	1/28 (3.6)	—	2/115 (1.7)
al-khadra,[21] 2003	47	Obs.	—	1/47 (2.1)	—	—
Giudici et al,[25] 2004	1025	Obs.	—	9/470 (1.9)	9/555 (1.6)	—
Tischenko et al,[23] 2009	272	Obs.	9/38 (23.7)	9/117 (7.7)	—	5/117 (4.3)
Tolosana etal,[11] 2009	101	RCT	4/51 (7.8)	4/50 (8.0)	—	—
Ahmed et al,[14] 2010	459	Obs.	7/123 (5.7)	1/222 (0.5)	2/114 (1.8)	—
Ghanbari et al,[24] 2010	123	Obs.	—	6/29 (20.7)	1/20 (5.0)	3/74 (4.0)
Tompkins et al,[12] 2010	713	Obs.	22/154 (14.3)	3/46 (6.5)	11/258 (4.3)	3/255 (1.2)
Cheng et al,[13] 2011	100	RCT	2/7 (28.6)	0/50 (0)	1/43 (2.3)	—
Li et al,[27] 2011	766	Obs.	14/199 (7)	12/324 (3.7)	5/243 (2.1)	—
Cano et al,[26] 2012	419	Obs.	30/208 (14)	3/129 (2.3)	0/82 (0)	—
Birnie et al,[10] 2013	681	RCT	54/338 (16)	12/343 (3.5)	—	—

Abbreviations: Obs., observational; RCT, randomized controlled trial; VKA, vitamin K antagonist.

similar in the anticoagulated group (15/555) versus the unanticoagulated group (12/470). There was only one thromboembolic complication, a stroke, in the unanticoagulated group.

Tischenko and colleagues[23] retrospectively compared 117 patients on therapeutic VKA at the time of device implantation with 177 matched control subjects not on VKA at baseline, and then also examined 38 individuals who had VKA discontinued and underwent LMWH bridging. There were nine (7.7%) hematomas in the continued VKA group, five (4.3%) hematomas in those who were never

Table 2
Risk stratification for perioperative thromboembolism from American College of Chest Physicians

Risk Group	Indication for Anticoagulation		
	Mechanical Heart Valve	Atrial Fibrillation	VTE
High	• Mitral valve prosthesis • Cage-ball or tilting disk aortic valve prosthesis • Recent (<6 mo) stroke/TIA	• CHADS2 score of 5 or 6 • Recent (<3 mo) stroke/TIA • Rheumatic valvular heart disease	• Recent (<3 mo) VTE • Severe thrombophilia[a]
Moderate	• Bileaflet aortic valve prosthesis and one of more of the following: atrial fibrillation, prior stroke/TIA, hypertension, diabetes, congestive heart failure, age >75 y	• CHADS2 score of 3 or 4	• VTE in the past 3–12 mo • Nonsevere thrombophilia (eg, factor V Leiden or prothrombin mutation) • Recurrent VTE • Active cancer
Low	• Bileafleaflet aortic valve prosthesis without atrial fibrillation and no other risk factors for stroke	• CHADS2 score of 0–2 (assuming no prior stroke of TIA)	• VTE >12 mo without other risk factors

Suggestions released by the American College of Chest Physicians.
[a] Severe thrombophilia includes protein C, protein S, or antithrombin deficiency; antiphosopholipid antibody; multiple abnormalities.
From Douketis JD, Spyropoulos AC, Spencer FA, et al. Perioperative management of antithrombotic therapy: antithrombotic therapy and prevention of thrombosis, 9th ed: American College of Chest Physicians evidence-based clinical practice guidelines. Chest 2012;141(2 Suppl):e330S; with permission.

anticoagulated, and nine (23.7%) hematomas in the bridging group (P = .01 LMWH vs VKA continuation). There were no thromboembolic complications in this study.

Ahmed and colleagues[14] reviewed 459 patients of similar thromboembolic risk undergoing device implantation, among whom 222 had VKA continued, 123 had VKA interrupted with LMWH or intravenous (IV) UFH bridging, and 114 had VKA held without bridging. There was one (0.45%) hematoma in the VKA continuation group, seven (5.7%) in the heparin bridging group, and two (1.75%) in the group who had anticoagulation held perioperatively (P = .004 for bridging vs VKA continuation). There were four (3.5%) thromboembolic complications (TIAs) in the group who had VKA withheld, one (0.8%) TIA in the bridging group, and no TIAs in the group on continued VKA (P = .01 for VKA withheld vs VKA continued). The low incidence of pocket hematoma in this study was likely related to their strict definition of hematoma: severe pain, prolonged hospitalization, discontinuation of anticoagulation, or operative intervention. This study did have a larger incidence of thromboembolic complications in the interrupted group than seen in other series.

Li and colleagues[27] studied 766 patients undergoing device implantation, of whom 243 had VKA discontinued, 324 had VKA continued, and 199 had VKA discontinued with heparin bridging. The average CHADS$_2$ score was identical among the three groups, although more patients in the heparin bridging category had mechanical mitral valves (35% vs 13% and 4%). There were five (2.1%) hematomas in the VKA-withheld group, 12 (3.7%) in the VKA-continued group, and 14 (7.0%) in the heparin group (P = .029 for heparin vs other groups). There were two thromboembolic events in the study: one stroke each in the heparin-bridged group and the OAC-continued group, with no strokes in the OAC-discontinued group.

BEFORE OR AFTER

Although these studies demonstrated increased bleeding risk associated with the use of heparin, it was unknown whether it was the preoperative or postoperative heparin that had a greater influence on bleeding risk. One hypothesis was that any preoperative anticoagulant effect at the time of the procedure would be mitigated by intraprocedural hemostasis measures, and thus would have less effect on postoperative complications, such as hematomas.[10] Robinson and colleagues[29] retrospectively reviewed four separate heparin-bridging protocols that were used serially at one

institution over 2 years. The study included 148 patients, all with an indication for chronic OAC. VKA was held in all patients, and LMWH was used either preoperatively (pre/no post), postoperatively (no pre/post), both (pre/post), or neither (no pre/no post). Hematoma rates for the various protocols were as follows: pre/no post (8%), no pre/no post (9%), pre/post (22%), and no pre/post (29%). Thus, there was a significantly different incidence of bleeding depending on whether or not LMWH was used postoperatively (23% vs 8%; P = .01).

EARLY RANDOMIZED CONTROLLED TRIALS

Although the bulk of studies evaluating the use of heparin and OAC in the context of device placement were observational, a few early randomized trials attempted to address the issue in a more structured fashion. Tolosana and colleagues[11] randomized 101 patients at high thromboembolic risk undergoing PPM or ICD implantation to either VKA discontinuation with IV UFH started 24 hours after procedure, or to VKA continuation during the procedure. There were four (7.8%) hematomas in the heparin group and four (8%) hematomas in the VKA continuation group, with no VTE events in either group (P = 1.00). Although this study did not demonstrate a difference in the rate of hematoma formation as prior studies had, VKA continuation was shown to be as safe as heparin bridging. This study was underpowered to detect a difference in VTE events.

Cheng and colleagues[13] conducted a slightly different study of 100 patients at moderate and high thromboembolic risk, randomizing them to VKA continuation during device implantation or VKA interruption. Among those randomized to interruption (n = 50), those at high risk (n = 7) had heparin bridging before and after, and those at moderate risk (n = 43) received no heparin. There were no hematomas or bleeding complications in the VKA continuation group, whereas there were two (29%) hematomas among those whose warfarin suspension was bridged with heparin. The study's one thromboembolic event occurred in a moderate-risk patient randomized to VKA interruption. This study, although small, suggested safety of VKA continuation, and was in line with prior observational studies that showed increased bleeding risk associated with heparin.

META-ANALYSES

Three large meta-analyses were published in 2012, attempting to gather the observational and randomized data from trials comparing bridging heparin with VKA OAC continuation. These analyses ranged from 6 to 13 studies (with substantial overlap), covering 1032 to 5978 patients. Two of the analyses compared only those with an uninterrupted-VKA group and a heparin-bridging group,[15,30] whereas the third analysis included studies evaluating antiplatelet agents and those without a heparin-bridging arm.[31] A few common issues were encountered, such as the lack of uniformity among studies in their definition of those at high thromboembolic risk. In addition, there was variation in the definition of bleeding complications, such as the size of a reportable hematoma, and variation in the timing and dosing of heparin before and after the procedure.

Feng and colleagues[15] reviewed six studies with 1032 patients and found a significant reduction in pocket hematoma in the VKA-continuation group compared with the heparin-bridging group (odds ratio [OR], 0.29; $P<.00001$). There was no statistical difference in thromboembolic complications, with only three events among all studies (OR, 0.48; $P = .48$). Ghanbari and colleagues[30] reviewed eight studies, adding two randomized controlled trials to the six studies examined in Feng and colleagues,[15] and again found significantly lower bleeding (hematoma plus extracardiac bleeding) in the VKA-continuation group (OR, 0.30; $P<.01$). They also found no difference in thromboembolic events, with only 5 total out of 2321 patients (OR, 0.65; $P = .58$).[30]

BRIDGE OR CONTINUE COUMADIN FOR DEVICE SURGERY RANDOMIZED CONTROLLED TRIAL

Two early randomized controlled trials had demonstrated the safety and noninferiority of VKA continuation in the setting of device implantation. However, observational studies and meta-analyses suggested VKA continuation was actually safer than heparin bridging, with no effect on thromboembolic events. To attempt to show the superiority of VKA continuation, a larger randomized trial was developed.

In 2013, Birnie and colleagues[10] released the results of the BRUISE CONTROL trial. At 17 medical centers across Canada and one in Brazil, the study randomized 668 patients in a 1:1 fashion to either warfarin continuation or warfarin interruption with heparin bridging. Eligible participants had an annual thromboembolic risk of 5% or more, were taking warfarin, and required nonemergent placement of a cardiac rhythm device (PPM or ICD). The study was not blinded for the patient, but to blind the investigators each patient was designated two teams: one that implanted

the device and was in charge of follow-up programming; and a separate team blinded to anticoagulation treatment who managed postoperative complications and follow-up. Patients randomized to the heparin bridging arm had warfarin stopped 5 days before the procedure and heparin (LMWH or UFH) started at least 3 days before the procedure when the INR decreased to a subtherapeutic level. The bridging anticoagulation was held before the procedure (24 hours with LMWH or 4 hours for IV UFH). Heparin was resumed 24 hours after the procedure either as LMWH or IV UFH. The primary end point was a clinically significant pocket hematoma, defined as a hematoma requiring further surgery, prolongation of hospitalization, or cessation of VKA. With an initial planned enrollment of 984 patients, the study was ended prematurely in 2013 following a prespecified interim analysis at 66% of goal enrollment. At the end of the study there were 12 of 343 (3.5%) hematomas in the warfarin continuation group, and 54 of 338 (16%) in the heparin-bridging group (relative risk, 0.19; $P<.001$). There were two thromboembolic events in the warfarin-continuation group (one stroke, one TIA) and none in the heparin-bridging group. Incidentally, both thromboembolic events occurred in patients who unintentionally had subtherapeutic INRs on the day of the procedure (INR, 1.0 and 1.2).[10]

BRUISE CONTROL was the first randomized controlled trial to show significantly decreased hematoma risk when OAC in the form of warfarin was maintained at therapeutic levels during a procedure, when compared with heparin bridging. This trial validated the results of earlier observational studies and meta-analyses. Given the low incidence of thromboembolic events when comparing these two strategies, evaluating any potential difference in these outcomes requires studying a much larger population.

ADDITIONAL COMPLICATIONS

Although most bleeding events associated with PPM or ICD implantation are pocket hematomas, there are other potential hemorrhagic complications to consider. Retroperitoneal bleeding, gastrointestintal bleeding, pericardial tamponade, and access site hematomas have all been described.[10,13,26–28,32,33] Their frequency, however, is typically much less than 1%. They are also not separately considered in most meta-analyses.[15,24,31] Thus, it is not known whether different anticoagulation strategies pose differential risk to non-pocket-hematoma hemorrhagic complications.

FORGOING ANTICOAGULATION ALTOGETHER

Although thromboembolic risk is increased during device implantation, the absolute risk remains low because of typically short perioperative period. Perhaps because of these low event rates, prior meta-analyses have failed to show any difference in thromboembolic risk between VKA continuation and interruption with bridging.[15,30] Still unanswered, however, was the question of actual risk of forgoing anticoagulation altogether in high-risk populations. That is, how protective was VKA continuation or bridging from a thromboembolic risk perspective?

One prior meta-analysis examining patients whose anticoagulation was discontinued without heparin bridging did not show any difference in thromboembolic risk.[31] However, of the four studies used to create this cohort, only two listed baseline thromboembolic risk, three out of four were observational (with the resultant possibility of selection bias), and at least one was predominantly moderate-risk patients who had VKA discontinued without heparin bridging.[12–14,25] Another more recently published meta-analysis in the wake of the BRUISE CONTROL study did demonstrate an increased thromboembolic risk associated with VKA cessation without heparin bridging compared with heparin bridging (OR, 2.56; P = .02).[34] These results were driven by two studies, one of which consisted of almost entirely venous thrombotic complications. The other study by Ahmed and colleagues[14] did show significantly increased TIAs when VKA was held without heparin bridging in a population with similar baseline thromboembolic risk. In a randomized study from Finland, 213 moderate-to-high-risk patients had VKA continued during device implantation or interrupted for 3 days without heparin bridging. There was no difference in bleeding risk or hematoma rate, but there was one significant stroke in the VKA-interrupted group.[35]

Although not extensively studied in the CIED patient population, perioperatively forgoing anticoagulation altogether was the focus of the recently published Bridging Anticoagulation in Patients who Require Temporary Interruption of Warfarin Therapy for an Elective Invasive Procedure or Surgery (BRIDGE) trial. The BRIDGE trial randomized 1884 patients to bridging anticoagulation or placebo. All patients had warfarin OAC interrupted for 5 days preoperatively and restarted 24 hours after the procedure. There was no difference in thromboembolic events between bridging LMWH and no bridging (0.3% vs 0.4%; P = .01 for noninferiority). Similar to CIED trials, they found more

bleeding with bridging anticoagulation (3.2% vs 1.3%; P = .005). Although those at highest risk of thromboembolism (ie, stroke/TIA within 12 weeks) were excluded, the BRIDGE population still was a substantially high-risk group, with a mean CHADS score of 2.35.[36]

The BRIDGE trial suggests that there exists a threshold for safe interruption of anticoagulation without bridging, and it may be lower than previously thought. Nonetheless, given the potential severity of thromboembolic events, and now the demonstrated safety of VKA continuation, confident cessation of anticoagulation in intermediate-to-high-risk patients requires more robust data.

LOW-RISK PATIENTS

In patients at low risk for thromboembolism who are on OAC and undergoing surgery, the most recent societal guidelines (see **Table 2**) recommend anticoagulation cessation without bridging therapy.[19] Most studies examining various other perioperative anticoagulation strategies have considered only those patients at high risk. When patients at low risk are considered, they typically have served as a nonbridging control for a higher-risk group.[13,26] However, although their annual thromboembolic risk may be low, this risk increases during the perioperative period, and anticoagulation cessation and reinitiation may also make them temporarily prothrombotic.[37,38] Thus, continuing VKA during device surgery in low-risk patients is something that could be considered. Cano and colleagues[39] recently published a prospective study of 278 patients, of whom 117 were considered to be at high thromboembolic risk and 161 were at low risk. VKA was continued in all patients. There were no thromboembolic events in either group, and a 4.3% hematoma rate in the high-risk group compared with 1.9% in the low-risk group (P = .28). With a low hematoma rate comparable with nonanticoagulated cohorts in other studies and no thromboembolic events, this article suggests further study is needed into this particular patient population.

DIRECT ORAL ANTICOAGULANTS

Since the first trial demonstrating efficacy and safety of dabigatran in 2009, DOAC usage has steadily increased (**Fig. 2**).[40–43] A total of 4591 patients in the Randomized Evaluation of Long-Term Anticoagulation Therapy (RE-LY) trial, which compared dabigatran with warfarin, had at least one invasive procedure during the trial period. Dabigatran was stopped an average of 49 hours before surgery, warfarin 5 days before, and 17%

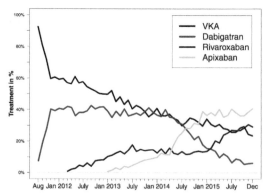

Fig. 2. First time initiation of anticoagulation, percentage of total by type: VKA, dabigatran, rivaroxaban, or apixaban. (*From* Staerk L, Fosbol EL, Gadsboll K, et al. Non-vitamin K antagonist oral anticoagulation usage according to age among patients with atrial fibrillation: temporal trends 2011–2015 in Denmark. Sci Rep 2016;6:31477; with permission.)

of dabigatran patients received perioperative heparin versus 28.5% of the warfarin cohort ($P<.001$). Dabigatran was restarted once adequate hemostasis had been achieved, and warfarin was restarted according to local practice. There were similar rates of perioperative bleeding in the warfarin group (4.6%) versus the dabigatran 150 mg (5.1%; $P = .58$), or 110 mg groups (3.8%; $P = .28$), with no difference in thromboembolic events.[44]

Only a few observational series examining the role of DOACs in cardiac rhythm device implantation have been published thus far. Most trials involved dabigatran, because of its commercial release before that of the other agents. An early series of 25 patients who had dabigatran stopped on average 16 hours before the procedure and restarted 17 hours later showed only one bleeding event and no thromboembolic events.[45] Larger cases series (n = 133, n = 236) comparing uninterrupted warfarin therapy with interrupted dabigatran (held 12–24 hours prior) show comparably low bleeding rates without any statistically significant difference.[46,47] These series were too small to demonstrate any difference in thromboembolic risk.

In addition to interrupted dabigatran, one series explored the possibility of uninterrupted dabigatran, showing bleeding complications in 1 of 48 (2.1%) of patients on uninterrupted dabigatran compared with 9 of 195 (4.6%) on uninterrupted warfarin ($P = .69$).[48] Nonetheless, recent surveys demonstrate that most implanting physicians do stop DOACs before device procedures.[49]

Rivaroxaban has been included in two studies: one with nine patients on uninterrupted therapy; and another with 83 patients on interrupted

therapy. In the nine patients who had uninterrupted rivaroxaban, there were five hematomas (56%), whereas in the 83 patients who had therapy interrupted 24 hours before the procedure there were only three hematomas (4%).[50,51]

Given the short half-life of most DOACs, the period of interruption for device implantation may be brief compared with that of warfarin. Despite this, the interruption could still pose some thromboembolic risk, and it is unknown if it is safe to continue DOAC therapy during device implantation. The ongoing BRUISE CONTROL-2 trial is a randomized controlled trial enrolling patients taking dabigatran, rivaroxaban, or apixaban with a plan to undergo cardiac rhythm device surgery. Patients are randomized to DOAC interruption or continuation, with a primary outcome of hematoma formation and secondary outcomes of other bleeding events and thromboembolic compilations.[52] This study may help to shed some light onto the perioperative role of DOAC therapy.

ANTIPLATELET AGENTS

Although anticoagulation with VKA, DOACs, and heparin has been extensively studied in cardiac rhythm device surgery, antiplatelet agents and their effect on bleeding are also important to consider. Following the advent of drug-eluting stents in the early to mid-2000s, an increasing number of patients now use dual antiplatelet therapy (DAPT) with aspirin and ADP/P2Y12 inhibitors for longer periods. Given frequent comorbidities in this population, this period of time often overlaps with an indication for either a PPM or ICD. In 2004, Weigand and colleagues[6] first considered the effect of antiplatelet agents in their large review of 3164 device implantations. Aspirin (ASA) therapy alone was common, seen in 40%, and was not associated with any increased risk of hematoma when compared with control subject (3.1% vs 2.5%; $P = $ NS). Combined therapy (ASA plus P2Y12 inhibitor) was still uncommon, with only 23 patients in the study, but five of these patients (22%) developed a hematoma following their CIED procedure.

Later observational series went on to highlight the bleeding risk of DAPT. Kutinsky and colleagues[5] prospectively evaluated 935 patients, of whom 100 were on uninterrupted ASA and clopidogrel at the time of surgery. Of the 100 patients with DAPT, 22 (22%) developed hematomas, compared with 9% of the study population as a whole or 5% of those not on any antiplatelet or anticoagulant therapy. In the group of patients who previously were on clopidogrel but had it stopped before the procedure, all hematomas developed in patients who had stopped clopidogrel within 4 days of the procedure (4 of 38). Tompkins and colleagues[12] echoed these results in reporting on a larger retrospective study of 1388 patients, of whom 139 were on DAPT. Compared with 255 patients not on any antiplatelet or anticoagulant agents, the bleeding risk of DAPT-treated patients was significantly higher (7.2% vs 1.6%; $P = .004$), although not as great as the bleeding risk associated with perioperative heparin in this study (14.3% vs 1.6%; $P<.0001$). A meta-analysis examining the antiplatelet effect on pocket hematomas found comparable results, with a 4.9% bleeding rate with DAPT compared with a 1.7% rate on no therapy (OR, 5.0; 95% confidence interval, 3.0–8.3).[31]

Several other points about antiplatelet therapy differ from full OAC. The timing of postoperative hematomas with DAPT seemed to be quicker, with most hematomas developing within 2 days as opposed to more evenly distributed within the first week.[53] Also, when ASA was evaluated by itself without DAPT, most observational studies found a slight but statistically insignificant increased risk of hematoma associated with its use.[54–56]

The consequences of DAPT interruption are also distinctly different from that of anticoagulation. Although anticoagulation interruption is associated with venous or arterial thromboembolism, the actual percentage of events is low. This percentage may be higher than fractionated annual averages, but is still less than 1% for 1 week of interruption of OAC.[17] In contrast, the risk of thrombosis when DAPT is interrupted after the recent placement of a coronary stent is high, and consequences can be drastic. The mortality of stent thrombosis as a consequence of DAPT cessation is significant: between 9% and 45%.[57] The rate of stent thrombosis after DAPT cessation is 29%, and typically occurs within 5 to 10 days.[58,59] There also is the hypercoagulable state that exists during surgery, which compounds the risk of stent thrombosis, resulting in high mortality rates when surgery is performed within 2 to 3 months of stenting.[60,61] Thus, when device surgery is performed after recent coronary stenting, it is typically preferable to continue DAPT therapy during the procedure. When device surgery is elective, physicians should consider delaying therapy until DAPT is no longer indicated.

SUMMARY

Implantable cardiac rhythm devices are common and growing in usage. With the increase in burden of diseases, such as congestive heart failure, the demand will only grow. Being able to implant these devices in the safest manner possible by minimizing perioperative risk is increasingly important. Consensus-based paradigms, such as perioperative bridging, can persist for decades without solid data to support their practice. The BRUISE CONTROL trial was pivotal in shifting practice patterns, and although novel, was based on years of observational data with similar conclusions. Nonetheless, further research is needed to establish the best approach for low-VTE-risk patients, and a better understanding of the role of DOAC therapy around the time of device implantation.

REFERENCES

1. Mond HG, Proclemer A. The 11th world survey of cardiac pacing and implantable cardioverter-defibrillators: calendar year 2009. A World Society of Arrhythmia's project. Pacing Clin Electrophysiol 2011;34(8):1013–27.
2. Greenspon AJ, Hart RG, Dawson D, et al. Predictors of stroke in patients paced for sick sinus syndrome. J Am Coll Cardiol 2004;43(9):1617–22.
3. Bardy GH, Lee KL, Mark DB, et al. Amiodarone or an implantable cardioverter-defibrillator for congestive heart failure. N Engl J Med 2005;352(3):225–37.
4. Raad D, Irani J, Akl EG, et al. Implantable electrophysiologic cardiac device infections: a risk factor analysis. Eur J Clin Microbiol Infect Dis 2012;31(11):3015–21.
5. Kutinsky IB, Jarandilla R, Jewett M, et al. Risk of hematoma complications after device implant in the clopidogrel era. Circ Arrhythm Electrophysiol 2010;3(4):312–8.
6. Wiegand UK, LeJeune D, Boguschewski F, et al. Pocket hematoma after pacemaker or implantable cardioverter defibrillator surgery: influence of patient morbidity, operation strategy, and perioperative antiplatelet/anticoagulation therapy. Chest 2004;126(4):1177–86.
7. Klug D, Balde M, Pavin D, et al. Risk factors related to infections of implanted pacemakers and cardioverter-defibrillators: results of a large prospective study. Circulation 2007;116(12):1349–55.
8. Reynolds MR, Cohen DJ, Kugelmass AD, et al. The frequency and incremental cost of major complications among Medicare beneficiaries receiving implantable cardioverter-defibrillators. J Am Coll Cardiol 2006;47(12):2493–7.
9. Sohail MR, Henrikson CA, Braid-Forbes MJ, et al. Mortality and cost associated with cardiovascular implantable electronic device infections. Arch Intern Med 2011;171(20):1821–8.
10. Birnie DH, Healey JS, Wells GA, et al. Pacemaker or defibrillator surgery without interruption of anticoagulation. N Engl J Med 2013;368(22):2084–93.

11. Tolosana JM, Berne P, Mont L, et al. Preparation for pacemaker or implantable cardiac defibrillator implants in patients with high risk of thrombo-embolic events: oral anticoagulation or bridging with intravenous heparin? A prospective randomized trial. Eur Heart J 2009;30(15):1880–4.

12. Tompkins C, Cheng A, Dalal D, et al. Dual antiplatelet therapy and heparin "bridging" significantly increase the risk of bleeding complications after pacemaker or implantable cardioverter-defibrillator device implantation. J Am Coll Cardiol 2010; 55(21):2376–82.

13. Cheng A, Nazarian S, Brinker JA, et al. Continuation of warfarin during pacemaker or implantable cardioverter-defibrillator implantation: a randomized clinical trial. Heart Rhythm 2011;8(4):536–40.

14. Ahmed I, Gertner E, Nelson WB, et al. Continuing warfarin therapy is superior to interrupting warfarin with or without bridging anticoagulation therapy in patients undergoing pacemaker and defibrillator implantation. Heart Rhythm 2010;7(6):745–9.

15. Feng L, Li Y, Li J, et al. Oral anticoagulation continuation compared with heparin bridging therapy among high risk patients undergoing implantation of cardiac rhythm devices: a meta-analysis. Thromb Haemost 2012;108(6):1124–31.

16. Gage BF, Waterman AD, Shannon W, et al. Validation of clinical classification schemes for predicting stroke: results from the National Registry of Atrial Fibrillation. JAMA 2001;285(22):2864–70.

17. Garcia DA, Regan S, Henault LE, et al. Risk of thromboembolism with short-term interruption of warfarin therapy. Arch Intern Med 2008;168(1):63–9.

18. Chen S, Liu J, Pan W, et al. Thromboembolic events during the perioperative period in patients undergoing permanent pacemaker implantation. Clin Cardiol 2012;35(2):83–7.

19. Douketis JD, Spyropoulos AC, Spencer FA, et al. Perioperative management of antithrombotic therapy: antithrombotic therapy and prevention of thrombosis, 9th ed: American College of Chest Physicians evidence-based clinical practice guidelines. Chest 2012;141(2 Suppl):e326S–50S.

20. Goldstein DJ, Losquadro W, Spotnitz HM. Outpatient pacemaker procedures in orally anticoagulated patients. Pacing Clin Electrophysiol 1998;21(9): 1730–4.

21. al-Khadra AS. Implantation of pacemakers and implantable cardioverter defibrillators in orally anticoagulated patients. Pacing Clin Electrophysiol 2003;26(1 Pt 2):511–4.

22. Michaud GF, Pelosi F Jr, Noble MD, et al. A randomized trial comparing heparin initiation 6 h or 24 h after pacemaker or defibrillator implantation. J Am Coll Cardiol 2000;35(7):1915–8.

23. Tischenko A, Gula LJ, Yee R, et al. Implantation of cardiac rhythm devices without interruption of oral anticoagulation compared with perioperative bridging with low-molecular weight heparin. Am Heart J 2009;158(2):252–6.

24. Ghanbari H, Feldman D, Schmidt M, et al. Cardiac resynchronization therapy device implantation in patients with therapeutic international normalized ratios. Pacing Clin Electrophysiol 2010;33(4):400–6.

25. Giudici MC, Paul DL, Bontu P, et al. Pacemaker and implantable cardioverter defibrillator implantation without reversal of warfarin therapy. Pacing Clin Electrophysiol 2004;27(3):358–60.

26. Cano O, Munoz B, Tejada D, et al. Evaluation of a new standardized protocol for the perioperative management of chronically anticoagulated patients receiving implantable cardiac arrhythmia devices. Heart Rhythm 2012;9(3):361–7.

27. Li HK, Chen FC, Rea RF, et al. No increased bleeding events with continuation of oral anticoagulation therapy for patients undergoing cardiac device procedure. Pacing Clin Electrophysiol 2011; 34(7):868–74.

28. Marquie C, De Geeter G, Klug D, et al. Post-operative use of heparin increases morbidity of pacemaker implantation. Europace 2006;8(4):283–7.

29. Robinson M, Healey JS, Eikelboom J, et al. Postoperative low-molecular-weight heparin bridging is associated with an increase in wound hematoma following surgery for pacemakers and implantable defibrillators. Pacing Clin Electrophysiol 2009; 32(3):378–82.

30. Ghanbari H, Phard WS, Al-Ameri H, et al. Meta-analysis of safety and efficacy of uninterrupted warfarin compared to heparin-based bridging therapy during implantation of cardiac rhythm devices. Am J Cardiol 2012;110(10):1482–8.

31. Bernard ML, Shotwell M, Nietert PJ, et al. Meta-analysis of bleeding complications associated with cardiac rhythm device implantation. Circ Arrhythm Electrophysiol 2012;5(3):468–74.

32. Chow V, Ranasinghe I, Lau J, et al. Peri-procedural anticoagulation and the incidence of haematoma formation after permanent pacemaker implantation in the elderly. Heart Lung Circ 2010;19(12):706–12.

33. Hammerstingl C, Omran H. Perioperative bridging of chronic oral anticoagulation in patients undergoing pacemaker implantation: a study in 200 patients. Europace 2011;13(9):1304–10.

34. Proietti R, Porto I, Levi M, et al. Risk of pocket hematoma in patients on chronic anticoagulation with warfarin undergoing electrophysiological device implantation: a comparison of different peri-operative management strategies. Eur Rev Med Pharmacol Sci 2015;19(8):1461–79.

35. Airaksinen KE, Korkeila P, Lund J, et al. Safety of pacemaker and implantable cardioverter-defibrillator implantation during uninterrupted warfarin treatment: the FinPAC study. Int J Cardiol 2013;168(4):3679–82.

36. Douketis JD, Spyropoulos AC, Kaatz S, et al. Periop-erative bridging anticoagulation in patients with atrial fibrillation. N Engl J Med 2015;373(9):823–33.

37. Rechenmacher SJ, Fang JC. Bridging anticoagula-tion: primum non nocere. J Am Coll Cardiol 2015; 66(12):1392–403.

38. Raunso J, Selmer C, Olesen JB, et al. Increased short-term risk of thrombo-embolism or death after interruption of warfarin treatment in patients with atrial fibrillation. Eur Heart J 2012;33(15):1886–92.

39. Cano O, Andres A, Jimenez R, et al. Systematic im-plantation of pacemaker/ICDs under active oral anti-coagulation irrespective of patient's individual preoperative thromboembolic risk. Pacing Clin Elec-trophysiol 2015;38(6):723–30.

40. Staerk L, Fosbol EL, Gadsboll K, et al. Non-vitamin K antagonist oral anticoagulation usage according to age among patients with atrial fibrillation: temporal trends 2011-2015 in Denmark. Sci Rep 2016;6: 31477.

41. Connolly SJ, Ezekowitz MD, Yusuf S, et al. Dabiga-tran versus warfarin in patients with atrial fibrillation. N Engl J Med 2009;361(12):1139–51.

42. Morin DP, Bernard ML, Madias C, et al. The state of the art: atrial fibrillation epidemiology, prevention, and treatment. Mayo Clin Proc 2016;91(12): 1778–810.

43. Rogers PA, Bernard ML, Madias C, et al. Current evidence-based understanding of epidemiology, prevention, and treatment of atrial fibrillation. Curr Probl Cardiol, in press.

44. Healey JS, Eikelboom J, Douketis J, et al. Periproce-dural bleeding and thromboembolic events with da-bigatran compared with warfarin: results from the Randomized Evaluation of Long-Term Anticoagula-tion Therapy (RE-LY) randomized trial. Circulation 2012;126(3):343–8.

45. Rowley CP, Bernard ML, Brabham WW, et al. Safety of continuous anticoagulation with dabigatran dur-ing implantation of cardiac rhythm devices. Am J Cardiol 2013;111(8):1165–8.

46. Madan S, Muthusamy P, Mowers KL, et al. Safety of anticoagulation with uninterrupted warfarin vs. inter-rupted dabigatran in patients requiring an implant-able cardiac device. Cardiovasc Diagn Ther 2016; 6(1):3–9.

47. Kosiuk J, Koutalas E, Doering M, et al. Comparison of dabigatran and uninterrupted warfarin in patients with atrial fibrillation undergoing cardiac rhythm de-vice implantations. Case-control study. Circ J 2014; 78(10):2402–7.

48. Jennings JM, Robichaux R, McElderry HT, et al. Car-diovascular implantable electronic device implanta-tion with uninterrupted dabigatran: comparison to uninterrupted warfarin. J Cardiovasc Electrophysiol 2013;24(10):1125–9.

49. Nascimento T, Birnie DH, Healey JS, et al. Managing novel oral anticoagulants in patients with atrial fibril-lation undergoing device surgery: Canadian survey. Can J Cardiol 2014;30(2):231–6.

50. Melton BL, Howard PA, Goerdt A, et al. Association of uninterrupted oral anticoagulation during cardiac device implantation with pocket hematoma. Hosp Pharm 2015;50(9):761–6.

51. Kosiuk J, Koutalas E, Doering M, et al. Treatment with novel oral anticoagulants in a real-world cohort of patients undergoing cardiac rhythm device im-plantations. Europace 2014;16(7):1028–32.

52. Essebag V, Healey JS, Ayala-Paredes F, et al. Strat-egy of continued vs interrupted novel oral anticoag-ulant at time of device surgery in patients with moderate to high risk of arterial thromboembolic events: the BRUISE CONTROL-2 trial. Am Heart J 2016;173:102–7.

53. Cano O, Osca J, Sancho-Tello MJ, et al. Morbidity associated with three different antiplatelet regimens in patients undergoing implantation of cardiac rhythm management devices. Europace 2011; 13(3):395–401.

54. Boule S, Marquie C, Vanesson-Bricout C, et al. Clo-pidogrel increases bleeding complications in pa-tients undergoing heart rhythm device procedures. Pacing Clin Electrophysiol 2012;35(5):605–11.

55. Thal S, Moukabary T, Boyella R, et al. The relation-ship between warfarin, aspirin, and clopidogrel continuation in the peri-procedural period and the incidence of hematoma formation after device im-plantation. Pacing Clin Electrophysiol 2010;33(4): 385–8.

56. Dai Y, Chen KP, Hua W, et al. Dual antiplatelet ther-apy increases pocket hematoma complications in Chinese patients with pacemaker implantation. J Geriatr Cardiol 2015;12(4):383–7.

57. Abualsaud AO, Eisenberg MJ. Perioperative man-agement of patients with drug-eluting stents. JACC Cardiovasc Interv 2010;3(2):131–42.

58. Iakovou I, Schmidt T, Bonizzoni E, et al. Incidence, predictors, and outcome of thrombosis after suc-cessful implantation of drug-eluting stents. JAMA 2005;293(17):2126–30.

59. Eisenberg MJ, Richard PR, Libersan D, et al. Safety of short-term discontinuation of antiplatelet therapy in patients with drug-eluting stents. Circulation 2009;119(12):1634–42.

60. Wilson SH, Fasseas P, Orford JL, et al. Clinical outcome of patients undergoing non-cardiac sur-gery in the two months following coronary stenting. J Am Coll Cardiol 2003;42(2):234–40.

61. Kaluza GL, Joseph J, Lee JR, et al. Catastrophic outcomes of noncardiac surgery soon after coro-nary stenting. J Am Coll Cardiol 2000;35(5): 1288–94.

Implantable Loop Recorders for Cryptogenic Stroke (Plus Real-World Atrial Fibrillation Detection Rate with Implantable Loop Recorders)

Dan L. Musat, MD, Nicolle Milstein, BS, Suneet Mittal, MD*

KEYWORDS

- Cryptogenic stroke • Implantable loop recorder • Atrial fibrillation

KEY POINTS

- Cryptogenic stroke (CS) represents a significant percentage of ischemic strokes and is associated with significant morbidity and high risk of recurrence.
- Undetected atrial fibrillation (AF) is an important consideration in these patients.
- Tools for electrocardiographic monitoring range from the 12-lead electrocardiogram (ECG) to implantable loop recorders (ILRs).
- Given the mantra, "the more you look, the more you shall find," ILRs have become an important tool for long-term ECG monitoring in patients with CS.
- A major unresolved issue is what duration of AF indicates that the CS patient is at high risk for recurrent stroke and thus would benefit from initiation of anticoagulation.

A stroke occurs in approximately 800,000 people each year in the United States; it can be a devastating diagnosis, associated with high morbidity and mortality, and results in a significant impact on society and the health care system.[1,2] The standard evaluation of a patient presenting with stroke includes a comprehensive physical examination (with emphasis on the blood pressure and heart rate, pattern and location of neurologic deficit, and physical signs of hyperlipidemia or vasculitis), basic hematologic tests, assessment of the cardiac rhythm (electrocardiography [ECG] and inpatient telemetry), and cardiac (transthoracic and transesophageal echocardiography) and neurologic (head computed tomography, head MRI and magnetic resonance angiography, and carotid ultrasound) imaging. Additional tests can also be performed as clinically indicated (**Fig. 1**). Despite these efforts, a definitive cause for stroke cannot be identified in 10% to 40% of patients[1,3,4]; these patients are considered to have suffered a cryptogenic stroke (CS).

Approximately a third of patients with CS suffer another event within 10 years; thus, it is critical to identify a definite cause and initiate treatment accordingly.[3,5] A strong consideration in these patients is cardioembolism, either because of a paradoxic embolism or from within the left atrial appendage, left ventricle, or aorta. There has been great interest in the association between

Disclosure Statement: None (D.L. Musat and N. Milstein). Consultant to Abbott, Boston Scientific, and Medtronic (S. Mittal).
Valley Health System and Snyder Center for Comprehensive Atrial Fibrillation, 223 N. Van Dien Avenue, Ridgewood, NJ 07450, USA
* Corresponding author.
E-mail address: mittsu@valleyhealth.com

Card Electrophysiol Clin 10 (2018) 111–118
https://doi.org/10.1016/j.ccep.2017.11.011
1877-9182/18/© 2017 Elsevier Inc. All rights reserved.

cardiacEP.theclinics.com

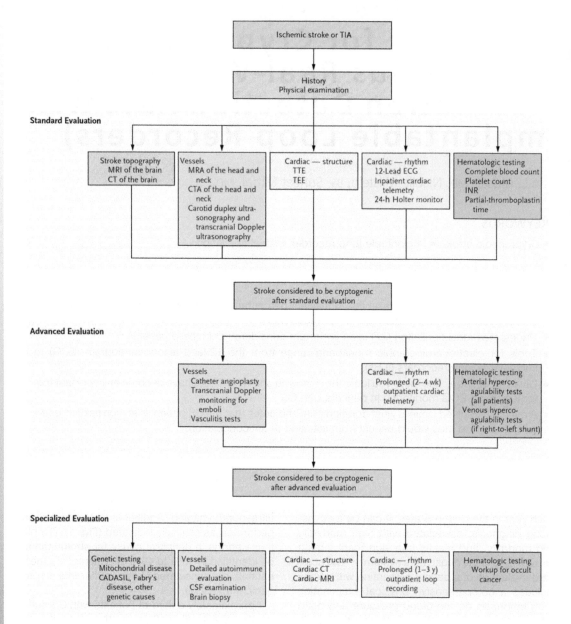

Fig. 1. Algorithm for the identification and diagnostic evaluation of patients with cryptogenic ischemic stroke or transient ischemic attack (TIA). CADASIL, cerebral autosomal-dominant arteriopathy with subcortical infarcts and leukoencephalopathy; CSF, cerebrospinal fluid; CT, computed tomography; CTA, computed tomographic angiography; INR, international normalized ratio; MRA, magnetic resonance angiography; TEE, transesophageal echocardiography; TTE, transthoracic echocardiography. (*Reproduced from* Saver JL. Clinical practice. Cryptogenic stroke. N Engl J Med 2016;374(21):2068; with permission.)

the presence of a patent foramen ovale and CS and the role of patent foramen ovale closure as a strategy to mitigate against recurrent stroke. However, only one randomized trial has suggested a benefit and a recent meta-analysis showed the benefit of patent foramen ovale closure to be only marginal.[6,7] Similarly, empiric anticoagulation was considered a possible solution. However, in

patients with CS, empiric treatment with warfarin was not superior to aspirin alone in preventing recurrent stroke, but was associated with a significant increase in bleeding events.[8] For these reasons, current guidelines do not recommend empiric anticoagulation in patients with CS.

Because the benefit of anticoagulation is well established in patients with atrial fibrillation (AF), and because AF is a known cause of stroke,[1] there has been great interest in ascertaining whether AF is present in patients presenting with stroke. A meta-analysis of 50 studies of 11,658 patients presenting with stroke found that 7.7% of these patients had AF on their admission ECG.[9] The same meta-analysis reported that in-hospital ECG monitoring (serial ECGs, continuous ECG monitoring, or Holter monitoring) identified an additional 5.1% of patients with AF. Posthospital discharge ECG monitoring for an additional 1 to 7 days identified another 10.7% of patients with AF. Finally, extended ECG monitoring using either external ECG monitors or implantable loop recorders (ILRs) found AF in 16.9% of patients (**Fig. 2**). Using this sequential approach to ECG monitoring, AF was ultimately diagnosed in approximately a quarter of all patients presenting with stroke.[9]

A central theme of ECG monitoring in patients in whom AF is being sought is that "the more you look, the more you shall find." Two recent randomized clinical trials have shown the value of extended ECG monitoring for the diagnosis of AF in patients with CS. The first was the EMBRACE trial,[10] which randomized 572 patients 55 years of age and older who had either a CS (62.9%) or transient ischemic attack (TIA; 37.1%) within the prior 6 months to undergo either another 24-hour Holter monitor or a 30-day autotriggered loop recorder. The mean time from event to randomization was 75.1 ± 38.6 days. AF lasting greater than or equal to 30 seconds was detected in 16.1% of the loop recorder group, as compared with a detection rate of only 3.2% in the Holter monitoring group (P<.001). Similarly, AF lasting greater than or equal to 2.5 minutes was detected in 9.9% of the loop recorder group, as compared with a detection rate of only 2.5% in the Holter monitoring group (P<.001). This translated into a much higher likelihood that a patient in the loop recorder group would have been prescribed anticoagulation (18.6% vs 11.1% in the Holter group; P = .01). Importantly, the diagnosis of AF increased with each week of monitoring (**Fig. 3**).

Ambulatory external ECG monitoring is not feasible for longer than 30 days. First, patients have a difficult time tolerating the leads and associated inconvenience of the ECG monitoring equipment. In the EMBRACE trial, in the patients randomized to the loop recorder arm, only 82% could complete more than a 3-week monitoring period.[10] Second, current payment guidelines only permit up to 30 days of monitoring. Yet, if the detection of AF increases as patients are monitored for 2 weeks instead of 1 week, 3 weeks instead of 2 weeks, and 4 weeks instead of 3 weeks, it seems even longer-term monitoring would be clinically useful. ILRs are currently the only available modality for longer-term ECG monitoring.

The first-generation ILRs, without a specific capability to detect AF, had a low yield in patients with CS.[11] The first ILR capable of detecting AF

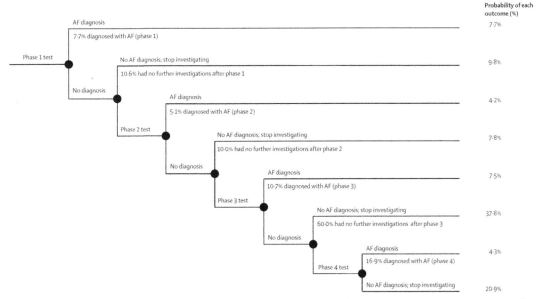

Fig. 2. Schematic of sequential cardiac monitoring model. (*Reproduced from* Sposato LA, Cipriano LE, Saposnik G, et al. Diagnosis of atrial fibrillation after stroke and transient ischaemic attack: a systematic review and meta-analysis. Lancet Neurol 2015;14(4):383; with permission.)

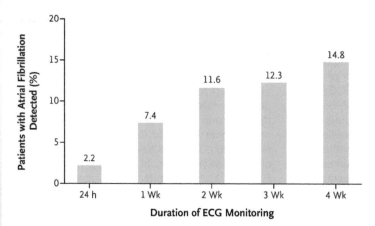

Fig. 3. Incremental yield of prolonged ECG monitoring for the detection of atrial fibrillation in patients with cryptogenic stroke or transient ischemic attack. (*Reproduced from* Gladstone DJ, Spring M, Dorian P, et al. Atrial fibrillation in patients with cryptogenic stroke. N Engl J Med 2014;370(26): 2473; with permission.)

was the REVEAL XT (Medtronic, Minneapolis, MN), and currently several other ILR types have been developed and miniaturized with the capability of AF detection. However, the experience in patients with CS has been mainly with the REVEAL devices. Different small series have reported a high incidence of AF detection rates of 16% to 36% (**Fig. 4**).[9] In these series, the ILRs were implanted 8 to 174 days after the stroke and the first AF episode was detected at a median of 48 to 153 days after implant. Most AF episodes were paroxysmal and asymptomatic.[12–17]

The role of the ILR was then explored in a second randomized ECG monitoring trial, called CRYSTAL-AF.[18] This trial enrolled 441 patients 40 years of age and older within 90 days of a CS or TIA. Patients were randomized to receive an ILR (REVEAL XT), which was implanted at a mean of 38 ± 27 days after index event, or conventional follow-up. By 6 months, AF was detected in significantly more ILR patients (8.9% vs 1.4%; P<.001); this continued at 12 months (12.4% vs 2.0%; P<.001). By 3 years of follow-up, 30% of patients in the ILR group had been found to have at

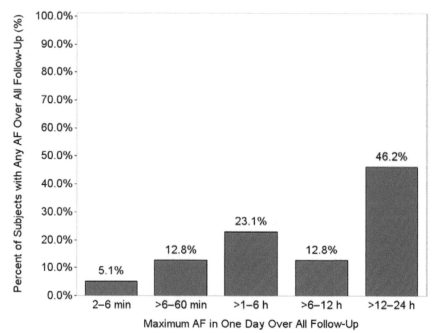

Fig. 4. Proportion of patients diagnosed with poststroke atrial fibrillation. (*From* Brachmann J, Morillo CA, Sanna T, et al. Uncovering atrial fibrillation beyond short-term monitoring in cryptogenic stroke patients: three-year results from the cryptogenic stroke and underlying atrial fibrillation trial. Circ Arrhythm Electrophysiol 2016;9(1):e003333; with permission.)

least one episode of AF greater than or equal to 2 minutes. Overall, the median time to first detection of AF was 8.4 months; in 81% of patients, the first AF episode was asymptomatic.[19] The median value for the maximum time in AF in a single day (maximal burden) was 10.5 hours (quartiles, 2.9–23.8 hours; **Fig. 5**). The duration of AF episodes increased over time; nearly 45% of patients in whom the AF was initially short (<1 hour) subsequently had at least one AF episode greater than 1 hour.[19]

Using the Medtronic Discovery Link database, Ziegler and colleagues[20] have subsequently reported the real-world incidence of AF in 1247 patients with CS implanted with second-generation ILR (REVEAL LINQ, Medtronic). During a median follow-up of 182 days, 1521 AF episodes were detected in 147 patients; the AF detection rates at 1 and 6 months post-ILR implant were 4.6% and 12.2%, respectively. The median time to AF detection was 58 days (interquartile range, 11–101 days) and the median duration of longest AF episode was 3.4 hours (interquartile range, 0.4–11.8 hours). At least one AF episode greater than 1 hour was detected in 71% of patients, greater than 6 hours in 37% of patients, and greater than 24 hours in 12% of patients. The median time to detection of nearly 2 months again illustrates the limitation of using ambulatory external ECG monitoring for AF detection in this patient population. Recent data also suggest that use of ILRs in patients with CS is a cost-effective strategy for AF detection.[21]

Having established that there is a direct relationship between duration of monitoring and detection of AF in patients with CS, and that ILRs are the only

feasible way of monitoring for AF for a long period of time (ie, several years), attention needs to be turned to several unresolved issues in this patient population. The first question is what to do with the patient who presents with stroke, the cause of which remains cryptogenic following initial evaluation. Should patients first undergo 30 days of ambulatory external ECG monitoring, with ILRs reserved for those with no AF detected during this period, or should these patients simply receive an ILR before hospital discharge? In the EMBRACE and CRYSTAL-AF trials, ECG monitoring did not occur for several weeks following the index TIA or stroke. Thus, the answer to this question remains unresolved.

Second, what duration of AF detected during follow-up should trigger initiation of anticoagulation? The reason for this dilemma is the relationship between the burden/duration of subclinical AF and the risk for stroke remains undefined. The duration of AF implicated to increase the risk of thromboembolic events has ranged from 5 minutes as seen in a substudy of the MOST trial,[22] 6 minutes in the ASSERT trial,[23] 1 hour in the pooled analysis of the SOS-AF project,[24] 5.5 hours in the TRENDS trial,[25] to 24 hours in the AT500 Registry.[26] To compound matters is the observation that there is no temporal relationship between the episode of AF and stroke, with more than half the patients having no AF episodes detected in the 30 days before stroke.[27] However, if short episodes of AF increase the risk of stroke, then ECG monitoring using ILRs makes sense because it can automatically capture ECG data over a long period of time without requiring participation of the patient.

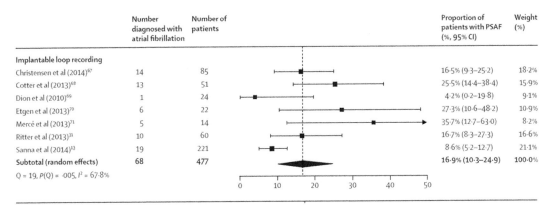

Fig. 5. Distribution of maximum atrial fibrillation burden in 1 day at different thresholds and throughout the study (36-month follow-up). CI, confidence interval; PSAF, poststroke atrial fibrillation. (*Reproduced from* Brachmann J, Morillo CA, Sanna T, et al. Uncovering atrial fibrillation beyond short-term monitoring in cryptogenic stroke patients: three-year results from the cryptogenic stroke and underlying atrial fibrillation trial. Circ Arrhythm Electrophysiol 2016;9(1):e003333; with permission.)

However, if predictive information is provided only by longer episodes, other technologies may be more feasible (especially from a convenience, patient acceptance, and cost-effectiveness standpoint). As an example, the Kardia Mobile (AliveCor, Mountain View, CA) is a low cost, patient-initiated, event monitor, which in conjunction with a smartphone can capture a high-resolution 30-second ECG. Furthermore, the device runs a Food and Drug Administration–approved AF detection algorithm to help the patient recognize whether they are having AF. By checking their ECG once or twice a day, a patient could easily ensure the absence of a longer episode of AF and potentially ensure they are at low risk for recurrent stroke. Even more appealing is the impending availability of the Kardia band, which is coupled with an Apple iWatch. The watch can alert the patient when the heart rate profile suggests an AF episode; the patient can then initiate acquisition of an ECG to confirm the diagnosis. Ultimately, the ideal system is a nonintrusive, external, ECG monitoring device (eg, ring, necklace, bracelet, tattoo, article of clothing) that is worn for long periods of time, has a robust algorithm for AF detection, and alerts the patient when it seems that AF is present. The availability of such a device could eliminate the need for implantable ECG recorders.

A third question is how do the various ILRs compare and how good are they for AF detection? Different manufacturers use different methods for AF detection and there are differences in options for device programming. Most of the commercial performance data are available for the Medtronic LINQ ILR. The AF detection algorithm in this device looks for patterns in a Lorenz plot of the differences in the RR intervals. An AF evidence score is computed every 2 minutes; the evidence score is compared against a threshold to detect AF. In addition, a P-wave evidence score is incorporated and subtracted from the AF evidence score before comparing with the threshold; the aim is to reduce false-positive detections of AF.[28,29] The incorporation of a P-wave evidence score results in a 46% relative reduction in inappropriately detected episodes of AF at the expense of only a less than 2% reduction in the total number of true AF episodes that were detected appropriately. Furthermore, the positive predictive value (PPV) increased to 72%, 83%, 90%, 93%, and 95% and the duration for detection increased from 2 minutes to 6, 10, 20, 30, and 60 minutes, respectively.[28]

The performance of the ILR improves as the duration of AF episode improves. The best PPV was observed when AF episodes lasted greater than 1 hour. Shorter episodes require a lot of time and effort for adjudication; false-positive detections occur because of noise, oversensing or undersensing, atrial or ventricular ectopy, and sinus arrhythmia. (These causes tend to be sporadic in nature and generally do not persist, unlike true AF, over a long period of time.) However, performance is also intrinsically linked to the type of population undergoing monitoring. As an example, in a recent study, 1106 patients with CS underwent Reveal LINQ ILR implantation; in the first 90 days of implant, 2807 episodes of device-detected AF (episodes ≥2 minutes) were identified.[30] Only 720 of these episodes were ultimately deemed to truly represent AF, yielding a PPV of only 26%. This is not entirely surprising because in a CS population, the incidence rate of AF is low yet the ILR is programmed to favor high sensitivity to ensure that any true episode of AF is not missed.

The workload is reduced dramatically by changing the ECG storage parameters on the device. For example, if the ILR is programmed to store ECGs only for episodes greater than or equal to 10 minutes (as opposed to all episodes ≥2 minutes), the number of AF episodes needing review decreases to 990 (relative reduction of 65%); the greatest reduction in workload occurs when the ILR is programmed to record an ECG only for the longest observed episode of AF. In this instance, the number of AF episodes needing review would decrease to 418 (relative reduction of 85%). Given the implications for workload, it is critical that one understand whether isolated short episodes, which would be missed by this type of programming approach, have predictive value in patients with CS.

A final question is whether the role of empiric anticoagulation should be reconsidered in the era of novel oral anticoagulants. The answer to this question will emerge from the results of two large ongoing prospective trials. The RESPECT ESUS (Dabigatran Etexilate for Secondary Stroke Prevention in Patients with Embolic Stroke of Undetermined Source; NCT02239120) trial is comparing dabigatran with aspirin in 6000 patients (≥60 years of age and one additional risk factor for stroke) with a nonlacunar CS; the primary outcome is time to first recurrent stroke (ischemic or hemorrhagic) over a 3-year follow-up.[5,31] The NAVIGATE ESUS (Rivaroxaban vs Aspirin in Secondary Prevention of Stroke and Prevention of Systemic Embolism in Patients With Recent Embolic Stroke of Undetermined Source; NCT02313909) trial is comparing rivaroxaban with aspirin in patients 50 years of age and older. The primary end point is time to recurrent stroke (ischemic or hemorrhagic) or systemic embolism and first occurrence of major bleeding over a 3-year follow-up.[5,32] Should these trials demonstrate superiority to empiric treatment with a novel oral anticoagulant, the strategy of long-term ECG monitoring to detect AF before initiation of anticoagulation would need to be re-evaluated.

If ILRs are ultimately deemed to be necessary for AF detection in patients with CS, several technological improvements will be necessary to optimize clinical utility of these devices. The first is the need for near 100% of successful data transmission from the device to a central World Wide Web server, from where the physician can adjudicate the stored ECG information. Unfortunately, available data suggest that automatic connectivity and data transfer are far from perfect. Over a 6-month period, automatic daily connectivity occurred in only 79% of 112 patients with a LINQ ILR; in a third of the patients, connectivity was lost for greater than 48 hours.[33] One solution to this problem is to involve the patient in this process. Toward this end, the Confirm RX (St. Jude Medical, Minneapolis, MN) ILR was recently approved for use in Europe and the United States; the ILR pairs with a patient's own smartphone and informs the patient when data did or did not transfer. The second is the need to develop processes to triage the incoming data to prevent major data deluge. The third is the creation of remote monitoring systems capable of helping clinicians quickly triage hundreds or thousands of patients who may be undergoing monitoring in a practice. The last is a method to integrate device-related information with clinical information, which is necessary to help manage the patient.

In summary, AF is detected in a high percentage of patients diagnosed with CS. The likelihood of AF detection progressively increases with the duration of ECG monitoring. By 3 years, nearly 30% of patients with CS will have an ILR-detected episode of AF. Future studies will establish the causative link between device-detected AF and stroke, the relationship between duration and burden of AF and stroke, and whether detection of AF is even necessary before anticoagulation is initiated in patients with CS. The answers to these questions need to be coupled with improvements in ILR technology and the recognition that patient participation and engagement are ultimately necessary to achieve the best outcomes in this patient population.

REFERENCES

1. Benjamin EJ, Blaha MJ, Chiuve SE, et al. Heart disease and stroke statistics-2017 update: a report from the American Heart Association. Circulation 2017;135(10):e146–603.

2. Krishnamurthi RV, Moran AE, Feigin VL, et al. Stroke prevalence, mortality and disability-adjusted life years in adults aged 20-64 years in 1990-2013: data from the global burden of disease 2013 study. Neuroepidemiology 2015;45(3):190–202.

3. Li L, Yiin GS, Geraghty OC, et al. Incidence, outcome, risk factors, and long-term prognosis of cryptogenic transient ischaemic attack and ischaemic stroke: a population-based study. Lancet Neurol 2015;14(9):903–13.

4. Saver JL. Clinical practice. Cryptogenic stroke. N Engl J Med 2016;374(21):2065–74.

5. Yaghi S, Bernstein RA, Passman R, et al. Cryptogenic stroke: research and practice. Circ Res 2017;120(3):527–40.

6. Rengifo-Moreno P, Palacios IF, Junpaparp P, et al. Patent foramen ovale transcatheter closure vs. medical therapy on recurrent vascular events: a systematic review and meta-analysis of randomized controlled trials. Eur Heart J 2013;34(43):3342–52.

7. Carroll JD, Saver JL, Thaler DE, et al. Closure of patent foramen ovale versus medical therapy after cryptogenic stroke. N Engl J Med 2013;368(12):1092–100.

8. Mohr JP, Thompson JL, Lazar RM, et al. A comparison of warfarin and aspirin for the prevention of recurrent ischemic stroke. N Engl J Med 2001;345(20):1444–51.

9. Sposato LA, Cipriano LE, Saposnik G, et al. Diagnosis of atrial fibrillation after stroke and transient ischaemic attack: a systematic review and meta-analysis. Lancet Neurol 2015;14(4):377–87.

10. Gladstone DJ, Spring M, Dorian P, et al. Atrial fibrillation in patients with cryptogenic stroke. N Engl J Med 2014;370(26):2467–77.

11. Dion F, Saudeau D, Bonnaud I, et al. Unexpected low prevalence of atrial fibrillation in cryptogenic ischemic stroke: a prospective study. J Interv Card Electrophysiol 2010;28(2):101–7.

12. Cotter PE, Martin PJ, Ring L, et al. Incidence of atrial fibrillation detected by implantable loop recorders in unexplained stroke. Neurology 2013;80(17):1546–50.

13. Jorfida M, Antolini M, Cerrato E, et al. Cryptogenic ischemic stroke and prevalence of asymptomatic atrial fibrillation: a prospective study. J Cardiovasc Med (Hagerstown) 2016;17(12):863–9.

14. Ritter MA, Kochhäuser S, Duning T, et al. Occult atrial fibrillation in cryptogenic stroke: detection by 7-day electrocardiogram versus implantable cardiac monitors. Stroke 2013;44(5):1449–52.

15. Rojo-Martinez E, Sandin-Fuentes M, Calleja-Sanz AI, et al. High performance of an implantable Holter monitor in the detection of concealed paroxysmal atrial fibrillation in patients with cryptogenic stroke

and a suspected embolic mechanism. Rev Neurol 2013;57(6):251–7 [in Spanish].

16. Etgen T, Hochreiter M, Mundel M, et al. Insertable cardiac event recorder in detection of atrial fibrillation after cryptogenic stroke: an audit report. Stroke 2013;44(7):2007–9.

17. Merce J, Garcia M, Ustrell X, et al. Implantable loop recorder: a new tool in the diagnosis of cryptogenic stroke. Rev Esp Cardiol (Engl Ed) 2013;66(8):665–6.

18. Sanna T, Diener H-C, Passman RS, et al. Cryptogenic stroke and underlying atrial fibrillation. N Engl J Med 2014;370(26):2478–86.

19. Brachmann J, Morillo CA, Sanna T, et al. Uncovering atrial fibrillation beyond short-term monitoring in cryptogenic stroke patients: three-year results from the cryptogenic stroke and underlying atrial fibrillation trial. Circ Arrhythm Electrophysiol 2016;9(1): e003333.

20. Ziegler PD, Rogers JD, Ferreira SW, et al. Real-world experience with insertable cardiac monitors to find atrial fibrillation in cryptogenic stroke. Cerebrovasc Dis 2015;40(3–4):175–81.

21. Diamantopoulos A, Sawyer LM, Lip GY, et al. Cost-effectiveness of an insertable cardiac monitor to detect atrial fibrillation in patients with cryptogenic stroke. Int J Stroke 2016;11(3):302–12.

22. Glotzer TV, Hellkamp AS, Zimmerman J, et al. Atrial high rate episodes detected by pacemaker diagnostics predict death and stroke: report of the Atrial Diagnostics Ancillary Study of the MOde Selection Trial (MOST). Circulation 2003;107(12):1614–9.

23. Healey JS, Connolly SJ, Gold MR, et al. Subclinical atrial fibrillation and the risk of stroke. N Engl J Med 2012;366(2):120–9.

24. Boriani G, Tukkie R, Manolis AS, et al. Atrial antitachycardia pacing and managed ventricular pacing in bradycardia patients with paroxysmal or persistent atrial tachyarrhythmias: the MINERVA randomized multicentre international trial. Eur Heart J 2014;35(35):2352–62.

25. Glotzer TV, Daoud EG, Wyse DG, et al. The relationship between daily atrial tachyarrhythmia burden from implantable device diagnostics and stroke risk: the TRENDS study. Circ Arrhythm Electrophysiol 2009;2(5):474–80.

26. Capucci A, Santini M, Padeletti L, et al. Monitored atrial fibrillation duration predicts arterial embolic events in patients suffering from bradycardia and atrial fibrillation implanted with antitachycardia pacemakers. J Am Coll Cardiol 2005;46(10): 1913–20.

27. Daoud EG, Glotzer TV, Wyse DG, et al. Temporal relationship of atrial tachyarrhythmias, cerebrovascular events, and systemic emboli based on stored device data: a subgroup analysis of TRENDS. Heart Rhythm 2011;8(9):1416–23.

28. Purerfellner H, Pokushalov E, Sarkar S, et al. P-wave evidence as a method for improving algorithm to detect atrial fibrillation in insertable cardiac monitors. Heart Rhythm 2014;11(9):1575–83.

29. Sanders P, Purerfellner H, Pokushalov E, et al. Performance of a new atrial fibrillation detection algorithm in a miniaturized insertable cardiac monitor: results from the reveal LINQ usability study. Heart Rhythm 2016;13(7):1425–30.

30. Mittal S, Rogers J, Sarkar S, et al. Real-world performance of an enhanced atrial fibrillation detection algorithm in an insertable cardiac monitor. Heart Rhythm 2016;13(8):1624–30.

31. Dabigatran etexilate for secondary stroke prevention in patients with embolic stroke of undetermined source (RE-SPECT ESUS). Secondary dabigatran etexilate for secondary stroke prevention in patients with embolic stroke of undetermined source (RE-SPECT ESUS). Available at: https://clinicaltrials.gov/ct2/show/NCT02239120. Accessed June 1, 2017.

32. Rivaroxaban versus aspirin in secondary prevention of stroke and prevention of systemic embolism in patients with recent embolic stroke of undetermined source (ESUS) (NAVIGATE ESUS). Secondary rivaroxaban versus aspirin in secondary prevention of stroke and prevention of systemic embolism in patients with recent embolic stroke of undetermined source (ESUS) (NAVIGATE ESUS). Available at: https://clinicaltrials.gov/ct2/show/NCT02313909. Accessed June 1, 2017.

33. Musat DL, Deihl S, Preminger MW, et al. Understanding Automatic connectivity limitations in patients undergoing long-term ECG monitoring with an implantable cardiac monitor. Heart Rhythm 2017;14(5):S245.

Implantable Cardioverter Defibrillator Implantation with or Without Defibrillation Testing

Stephen Duffett, MD, FRCPC, Imane El Hajjaji, MD,
Jaimie Manlucu, MD, FRCPC, Raymond Yee, MD, FRCPC, FHRS*

KEYWORDS

- Implantable cardioverter-defibrillator • Defibrillation testing • Defibrillation threshold testing
- Defibrillation safety margin

KEY POINTS

- DFT is performed by assessing ICD shock efficacy for induced VF and is performed in several ways.
- DFT was routinely performed at initial ICD implant with early devices, with ICD system revision performed for inadequate test results.
- Large randomized trials have failed to demonstrate clinical benefit of routinely performing DFT at implant.
- DFT still has a role in specific clinical scenarios and remains current standard of care during subcutaneous ICD implants.

INTRODUCTION

The practice of testing an implantable cardioverter-defibrillator (ICD) postimplant to assess for defibrillation efficacy, otherwise known as defibrillation testing (DFT), dates to the beginning of the technology when it was considered essential to ensure device efficacy at the time of implantation for this new therapy. It was considered standard of practice for many years and remains so for many centers. DFT can also be performed on chronic follow-up, especially at device replacement. When DFT results are poor, modification of the ICD system is required and options range from altering shock pathway configuration, lead repositioning, removal or addition of a superior vena cava (SVC) coil or subcutaneous electrode, or the use of an ICD with higher shock output. It has been reported that extensive modifications requiring multiple lead positions are required in 2.2% of patients.[1] After modification, acceptable DFT results are obtainable in virtually all patients.[2]

The premise underlying DFT is that defibrillation efficacy assessed under controlled conditions in the electrophysiology laboratory predicts shock efficacy for spontaneous ventricular fibrillation (VF), and that patients with high DF energy requirements are at increased risk for death from failed ICD therapy in the ambulatory setting. It assumes that VF induced in the laboratory is similar to spontaneous VF in the ambulatory setting. However, DFT also carries real risks, and lack of clear evidence that DFT impacts hard clinical outcomes has led many to question the need for DFT and some to abandon testing altogether. This article summarizes the arguments and data for and

Disclosures: Consulting for Medtronic, Inc (J. Manlucu).
Heart Rhythm Program, Department of Medicine, Western University, PO Box 5339, 339 Windermere Road, London, Ontario N6A 5A5, Canada
* Corresponding author.
E-mail address: ryee@uwo.ca

Card Electrophysiol Clin 10 (2018) 119–125
https://doi.org/10.1016/j.ccep.2017.11.012

cardiacEP.theclinics.com

against DFT so that the reader can decide if or when DFT is appropriate.

Before proceeding, one word of clarification is worthwhile to avoid confusion. The acronym "DFT" has historically been used to mean defibrillation threshold, one specific method of assessing defibrillation efficacy and the measured value derived. For the purposes of this discussion, DFT is used to describe the general approach to assessing DF efficacy.

METHODS OF DEFIBRILLATION TESTING

To understand the benefits and risks of DFT, an understanding of how DFT is performed is needed. DFT is performed at the time of ICD implantation or as a stand-alone outpatient procedure with the patient under intravenous sedation or general anesthesia.[3] There are two basic approaches to evaluating DF efficacy. The first approach involves VF induction followed by shock delivery. Sustained VF is induced by rapid ventricular stimulation at rates up to 50 Hz or by critically timed low-energy shocks delivered within the vulnerable period of ventricular repolarization. Once VF is induced, a single DF test shock is delivered, followed by a rescue transthoracic shock from the external defibrillator, if necessary. In some centers, two ICD test shocks are delivered before any rescue transthoracic shock. After an intervening recovery period, the VF induction–defibrillation cycle is repeated. The number of VF inductions and DF shock values tested is dictated

by the specific test protocol and there are several in use (**Fig. 1**). In the safety margin test protocol, the shock strength tested is usually 10 J lower than the maximum energy output of the implanted ICD and must be successful on two occasions to be considered to have passed implant testing.[4,5] The defibrillation threshold test method involves determining the lowest delivered energy that successfully defibrillates, recognizing that the term "threshold" is misleading because DF is a probabilistic phenomenon. Thus, for any given patient, there exists an S-shaped dose response curve that describes the relationship between shock strength and defibrillation success.[2] For example, if a 15-J shock is unsuccessful but 20-J shock is successful, the DF threshold is said to be 20 J but the probability of success at that shock output is not 100%. The test shock energy value tested with each VF episode induced is successively decreased (step-down protocol) until the test shock fails, successively increased (step-up protocol) until the test shock successfully defibrillates, or a combination of the two methods (down-up or binary protocol). The DF threshold value obtained with the step-down method correlates with a probability of 70% to 80% success.[6] Adequate defibrillation threshold is believed to be a value that is at least 10 J lower than the maximum energy output of the implanted ICD.

The second approach for estimating DF efficacy of an ICD system involves determining the upper limit of vulnerability, which has been shown to correlate with DF threshold.[7] It is based on the

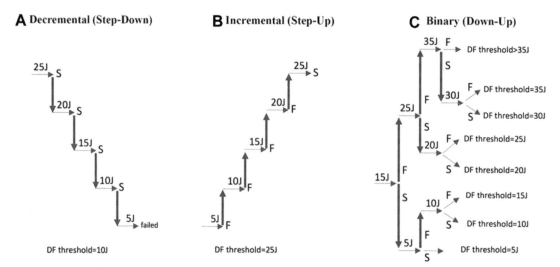

Fig. 1. Three methods of defibrillation threshold testing. (*A*) Starting shock output is high with decreasing shock output until a failed shock occurs (decremental). (*B*) Starting shock output is low with increasing shock output until a successful shock occurs (incremental). (*C*) Shock output is increased or decreased from previous value in response to a success or failure, until the lowest successful shock output is determined (binary). DF, defibrillation; F, failed shock; J, joules; S, successful shock.

principle that test shocks of intermediate strength delivered during baseline rhythm and timed to the vulnerable period induce VF. Shocks above the upper limit of vulnerability value fail to induce VF.[8] The test protocol involves delivering test shocks of decreasing strength until VF is finally induced. The advantage of this method is that VF is induced only once during DFT.

DFT does come with some risk, and when balancing that risk, it is important to understand the magnitude of benefit during routine ICD insertion. DFT was originally evaluated in old studies, when ICD generator and lead technology was in its infancy, and occasionally required the use of epicardial patches.[9] Initially, the energy required for successful defibrillation was high, but has steadily decreased over the years with improvements in technology.[10] As a consequence, the use of DFT during routine transvenous ICD implantation has decreased as confidence in the technology has grown. However, DFT testing continues to be recommended in certain situations with conventional ICDs and for subcutaneous ICD (S-ICD) implantation, where the technology is new.[11] Careful patient selection is important to minimize risk, while still providing patients with some assurance that their defibrillator will function properly when they need it most.

DETERMINANTS OF DEFIBRILLATION TESTING RESULTS

DFT results are heterogeneous in the ICD population and there has been interest in identifying clinical risk factors that predict DFT results. One study by Hodgson and colleagues[12] in 2002 assessed 34 clinical parameters, including standard data from echocardiography and radiologic investigations. Multivariate analysis demonstrated that only left ventricular mass was an independent predictor of high DF threshold values, but this only accounted for approximately 5% of variability in measurements. Another study, by Russo and colleagues[13] in 2005, identified reduced ejection fraction (relative risk, 0.981) and amiodarone use (relative risk, 3.347) as risk factors for inadequate DFT results leading to system modification. This study also suggested that younger age and absence of coronary disease were risk factors for high threshold values. In contrast, Val-Mejias and Oza[14] reported little variability in DF threshold values irrespective of left ventricular dysfunction or clinical indication (primary vs secondary).

A recent study by Shih and colleagues[15] on 1642 patients identified five patient factors associated with high DF values. These risk factors were used to develop a risk score, EF-SAGA (ejection fraction <20%, secondary prevention indication, age <60 years, gender [male], and amiodarone use). Patients with a low EF-SAGA score (only one risk factor) had a 0.4% probability of poor DFT result. The incidence of poor DFT result increased to 8.9% in patients with four or five of these risk factors. Of the patients with high DFT values, subcutaneous leads were implanted with resultant lowering of DFT values in 32 of 38 patients (84%). The authors concluded that DFT could be abandoned as a routine procedure in patients with ejection fraction less than 20% and no other risk factors were present.

In one single-center study of implants from 2005 to 2012, the incidence of high DF energy requirements was 13%.[16] In most this was adequately addressed by change in lead position, replacement of the generator with one of higher delivered energy capacity, or a change in shock vector. The impact of dual-coil versus single-coil ICDs leads on DF efficacy is discussed elsewhere in this issue.

CLINICAL VALUE OF DEFIBRILLATION TESTING

DFT is based on several premises. First is that the ventricular tachyarrhythmia induced during testing is the same as VF that would occur spontaneously. Second, shock efficacy in the laboratory reflects that which would occur in the ambulatory setting. Third, patients who fail DFT or have high DF energy requirements have a poorer prognosis. Knowing this is important to appreciating the limitations and concerns about DFT.

DFT assesses an implanted ICD system's ability to adequately detect VF and the efficacy of shocks to terminate it. Both functions require intact leads that are properly connected to the generator. Careful scrutiny of sensing, pacing threshold, and pathway impedance values during routine interrogations can identify most lead integrity issues (conductor wire fracture or insulation breaches), as can delivering low-energy test shocks in sinus rhythm. However, there are rare case reports of concealed lead fracture where high impedance values could only be exposed by high output shocks delivered during DFT.[17] Lead failures secondary to the conductor wire externalization have also been discovered through DFT for the Riata lead.[18]

For an intact ICD system to detect VF, however, sensed right ventricular electrograms (VEGM) must be of sufficient amplitude and rate. Typically, VEGMs are measured during baseline rhythm (sinus rhythm or atrial fibrillation) and values of 5 to 7 mV or greater are believed sufficient to allow for VEGM amplitude decrease and variability of nearly 50% to 70% during VF.[2] For baseline VEGM values less than 5 mV, many recommend performing DFT to directly assess sensing during induced VF. However, Ruetz and colleagues did a retrospective study and reported no correlation between VEGM amplitude in sinus rhythm and undersensing during VF. Even sinus VEGM amplitudes below 3 mV were adequately sensed, suggesting that the sinus rhythm VEGM amplitude that might provoke CF testing in modern ICD's can be reduced to values less than 3 mV in most cases.[19] The other important VEGM parameter is the VEGM rate during VF. In most cases of VF, the right ventricular VEGM rate is consistent with rapid ventricular activation in the left ventricle but there are rare reported cases of dissimilar right and left ventricular rhythms.[20] This rare phenomenon is virtually impossible to identify without DFT.

For advocates of DFT, the results translate into clinical decisions. Where DFT identifies patients with low DFT energy requirements, programming the ICD initial shock energy to submaximal values can increase battery longevity and decrease charge times.[2] Charge times were a significant issue with early generation devices but this concern has receded with modern ICD technology.[21] In addition, high-energy electrical shocks may cause structural damage to myocardial cells, resulting in postshock mechanical dysfunction and potentially lead to patient morbidity and mortality.[22,23] However, the clinical benefits of careful ICD shock output titration have not been adequately studied.

In contrast, patients with high DF output requirements at initial implantation were considered at higher risk of death from failed ICD therapy, especially in the early years when there was uncertainty about the reliability of ICD technology. Subsequent improvements in ICD technology, including the use of a biphasic waveform, have increased confidence in defibrillation efficacy and caused many to re-evaluate the relevance of continued DFT. A retrospective analysis by Pires and Johnson in 2006 noted that more than 75% of their patient cohort had some form of DFT.[24] Russo and colleagues[25] reported in 2013 that DFT was not performed in up to 29% of patients. In a recent study by Leshem and colleagues,[26] the use of DFT during implant was 11.2%. This study was a prospective study of 6343 consecutive ICD implants between July 2010 and March of 2015. A significant drop in DFT was noted during the period of the study, with initial DFT testing rates dropping from 31% down to 2% near the end of the study. The Canadian Registry of ICD Implant Testing Procedures (CREDIT) study reported that DFT was not performed in up to one-third of ICD implants.[1] Meanwhile, the European SAFE-ICD registry reported that only 39% of 2150

consecutive patients from 2008 to 2011 underwent DFT.[27] The central issue is whether there remains clinical value in performing DFT in the current era of modern ICD technology.

There have been two well designed randomized clinical trials addressing the question of the impact of DFT on hard clinical outcomes. The Shockless Implant Evaluation (SIMPLE) trial was a single-blind, multicenter trial that randomly assigned 2500 patients to DFT (n = 1253) versus no DFT (n = 1247) at the time of ICD implantation.[28] This was a noninferiority trial powered for a primary composite outcome of arrhythmic death or failed appropriate shock. After a mean follow-up of 3.1 years, the primary end point occurred in fewer patients in the no DFT group than the DFT group (90 [7%] vs 104 patients [8%]; $P_{\text{non-inferiority}}$<.0001). The rate of pre-specified adverse events in the two groups was similar. Thus, although DFT was reasonably safe, it did not seem to offer incremental clinical benefit.

The slightly smaller NORDIC ICD Study was also a noninferiority trial that randomized 1077 patients to DFT versus no DFT at the time of initial ICD implantation.[29] The primary end point was mean first shock efficacy for all true ventricular tachycardia (VT) and fibrillation episodes. During follow-up, ICDs were programmed to deliver maximum shock output (40 J) irrespective of the DFT result. In SIMPLE, maximum shock output of ICDs was specified at 31 J because not all implanted ICDs were capable of 41-J shocks. After a median follow-up of 22.8 months, first shock efficacy in the no DFT group was 3% better but certainly noninferior to the DFT group (97.1% vs 94.1%; $P_{\text{non-inferiority}}$<.001). Serious adverse events within 30 days of implant were reported in 94 DFT patients compared with 74 no DFT patients (17.6% vs 13.9%; P = .095).

The large European prospective observational study, SAFE-ICD, demonstrated similar results in real-world practice with low event rates irrespective of peri-implant testing or not.[27] The overall mortality at 2-year follow-up in DFT patients was 12.9% compared with 14.6% in no DFT patients (P = .29), with no difference in the rate of sudden cardiac death or failed shocks between the two groups.

One explanation for these results is that the mortality benefit of an ICD is small, but significant, when amortized over a longer time horizon. However, the chance that arrhythmic death will occur in the infrequent patient with failed DFT is so unlikely that a statistical difference is difficult to demonstrate. This was evaluated using a mathematical model that assessed efficacy of DFT on a hypothetical patient cohort over a 5-year period.[30] The study found the impact of DFT to be limited, with confidence intervals that included no benefit of DFT.

It is important to consider the potential risks and disadvantages of DFT rate in clinical practice. Serious associated risks include stroke and systemic embolism, myocardial infarction, heart failure, and nonelective supported ventilation, in addition to ICD implantation risks, such as pneumothorax, pericarditis/tamponade, device infection, and death.

A large Canadian study encompassing 19,067 ICD implant patients from 2000 to 2006 reported 0.016% incidence of death related to the DFT (three cases), stroke rate of 0.026% (five cases), and prolonged resuscitation in 0.14% (27 cases).[31] Two patients had poor outcomes following prolonged resuscitation, with one having serious neurologic deficits and the other requiring cardiac transplantation for hemodynamic collapse. Prolonged hypotension requiring the use of vasopressors or inotropes related to DFT has been reported to occur in up to 3% of cases.[1] In a recent systematic review of the major DFT clinical trials, Phan and colleagues[32] found that the complication rate was generally low with a 30-day mortality rate of 0% to 0.6% for no DFT and 0% to 0.9% for DFT. Although no significant difference was identified, there was a clear trend in favor of not performing DFT.

Any ICD implant strategy that includes DFT as part of the routine practice needs to be flexible and/or mitigate these risks in high-risk individuals. Although clinical and procedural factors may indicate those at higher risk of having high DFT values at the time of implant, their predictive value is modest at best and does not seem to translate to clinically important outcomes. A composite score that encompasses each of the risk factors evaluated may provide a more predictive model that could classify those at higher risk of a failed initial shock during intraoperative testing. However, the question remains as to whether there is any meaningful benefit to identifying these patients, given that the chance of failing multiple high-energy shocks in modern devices is exceedingly rare. For patients who have high DFT values only identified at follow-up, the additional risks associated with reoperation need to be considered.[33]

One specific patient group worth discussing are those at increased risk for stroke. The presence of concomitant atrial fibrillation must be considered before DFT testing. If there is a history of ongoing atrial fibrillation or inadequate preimplant anticoagulation, transesophageal echocardiography may be required to rule out intracardiac thrombus before DFT.

In addition to the complications listed, additional disadvantages of routine testing include increased cost and procedure time. In the CREDIT study, DFT was associated with an $844 incremental cost compared with no DFT.[1] Increased cost was attributed to professional fees secondary to the need for more support staff, the cost of complications, and increased length of hospital stay. DFT increased procedure time by an average of 102 ± 45 minutes in one study.[34]

DFT evaluates an ICD system's likely response to VF but not to VT. Although many arrhythmia episodes may fall in the VF therapy zone, fast monomorphic VT commonly occurs and is effectively treated with antitachycardia pacing in many instances. The PainFREE study found that fast VT episodes with cycle lengths of 240 to 320 ms accounted for 40% of episodes during follow-up, whereas true VF accounted for only 3% of the episodes.[35] The shock energy required to terminate VT may differ significantly from that needed for VF, and patients failing DFT may still have most clinically encountered ventricular tachyarrhythmias treated successfully.

SPECIFIC SITUATIONS THAT WARRANT CONSIDERATION OF DEFIBRILLATION TESTING

DFT during routine implant has steadily declined in recent years but there are specific situations where DFT remains relevant. Nonstandard site (eg, right-sided or abdominal) ICD implants and some cases of device upgrades or generator replacements have been associated with significantly higher shock output.[13,16,27,36]

DFT is currently standard of practice during S-ICD insertion.[37] Vector testing is performed before planned S-ICD to assess for appropriate QRS and T-wave amplitude from the skin surface. An additional consideration for the S-ICD is the potential for concomitant use of a transvenous pacemaker, because the S-ICD is limited to short duration postshock transcutaneous pacing, but does not provide chronic pacing support.[11] DFT is useful to exclude adverse device interactions.

Occasionally, electrogram oversensing or undersensing in ICD systems can raise concerns about adequate arrhythmia detection. It may be reasonable to perform DFT to ensure an appropriate response to VF, especially if adjustment in ICD settings is required.

In the population receiving cardiac resynchronization defibrillators (CRT-D), poorer ventricular function and functional class are often present and have been associated with high DFT values at the time of implant. DFT is higher risk in this population with severe heart failure. Testing is delayed safely to several months postimplant if needed to lessen the hemodynamic consequence.[38,39] A CRT-focused study in 2010 failed to show clinical benefit of routine DFT during CRT-D implant long-term follow-up.[40] In the setting of CRT, routine DFT is not supported by evidence but can be safely delayed to 2 months if needed.

SUMMARY

DFT assesses the critical functions of an ICD under controlled conditions at ICD implantation or on follow-up. However, risks and lack of evidence demonstrating clinical benefit has caused many to be more selective in performing DFT. To be clear, DFT is safe but no benefit has been shown for DFT on mortality or first-shock efficacy in large randomized-controlled trials. DFT is associated with an increased procedural time and cost. Some clinical and procedural factors identify those at risk of poor DFT response at the time of implant, but the ability of these factors to sufficiently predict DFT outcome is modest at best. DFT remains standard of practice following implantation of S-ICDs. Selective application of DFT to specific patient situations that raise concerns about ICD efficacy is warranted. Physicians should remain familiar with the process of DFT and situations where it remains relevant.

REFERENCES

1. Healey JS, Dorian P, Mitchell LB, et al. Canadian registry of ICD implant testing procedures (CREDIT): current practice, risks, and costs of intraoperative defibrillation testing. J Cardiovasc Electrophysiol 2010;21(2):177–82.

2. Russo AM, Chung MK. Is defibrillation testing necessary? Cardiol Clin 2014;32(2):211–24.

3. Al Fagih A, Al Shurafa H, Al Ghamdi S, et al. Safe and effective use of conscious sedation for defibrillation threshold testing during ICD implantation. J Saudi Heart Assoc 2010;22(4):209–13.

4. Leong-Sit P, Gula LJ, Diamantouros P, et al. Effect of defibrillation testing on management during implantable cardioverter-defibrillator implantation. Am Heart J 2006;152(6):1104–8.

5. Marchlinski FE, Flores B, Miller JM, et al. Relation of the intraoperative defibrillation threshold to successful postoperative defibrillation with an automatic implantable cardioverter defibrillator. Am J Cardiol 1988;62(7):393–8.

6. Hani Kanj M, Wilkoff BL. Implantable cardioverter defibrillators. In: Zipes DP, Jalife J, editors. Cardiac electrophysiology: from cell to bedside. 6th edition. Philadelphia: Elsevier/Saunders; 2014. p. 1139–50.

7. Birgersdotter-Green U, Undesser K, Fujimura O, et al. Correlation of acute and chronic defibrillation threshold with upper limit of vulnerability determined in normal sinus rhythm. J Interv Card Electrophysiol 1999;3(2):155–61.

8. Lesigne C, Levy B, Saumont R, et al. An energy-time analysis of ventricular fibrillation and defibrillation thresholds with internal electrodes. Med Biol Eng 1976;14(6):617–22.

9. Pinski SL, Vanerio G, Castle LW, et al. Patients with a high defibrillation threshold: clinical characteristics, management, and outcome. Am Heart J 1991; 122(1 Pt 1):89–95.

10. Gan T, Cao X, Yu Z, et al. Intraoperative defibrillation threshold testing and postoperative long-term efficacy of cardioverter-defibrillator implantation. Exp Ther Med 2013;5(1):323–7.

11. Bardy GH, Smith WM, Hood MA, et al. An entirely subcutaneous implantable cardioverter–defibrillator. N Engl J Med 2010;363(1):36–44.

12. Hodgson DM, Olsovsky MR, Shorofsky SR, et al. Clinical predictors of defibrillation thresholds with an active pectoral pulse generator lead system. Pacing Clin Electrophysiol 2002;25(4 Pt 1):408–13.

13. Russo AM, Sauer W, Gerstenfeld EP, et al. Defibrillation threshold testing: is it really necessary at the time of implantable cardioverter-defibrillator insertion? Heart Rhythm 2005;2(5):456–61.

14. Val-Mejias JE, Oza A. Does defibrillation threshold increase as left ventricular ejection fraction decreases? Europace 2010;12(3):385–8.

15. Shih MJ, Kakodkar SA, Kaid Y, et al. Reassessing risk factors for high defibrillation threshold: the EF-SAGA risk score and implications for device testing. Pacing Clin Electrophysiol 2016;39(5): 483–9.

16. Keyser A, Hilker MK, Ucer E, et al. Significance of intraoperative testing in right-sided implantable cardioverter-defibrillators. J Cardiothorac Surg 2013;8:77.

17. Bun SS, Duytschaever M, Tavernier R. Defibrillation testing can reveal 'concealed' lead fracture. Europace 2013;15(1):54.

18. Shah P, Singh G, Chandra S, et al. Failure to deliver therapy by a riata lead with internal wire externalization and normal electrical parameters during routine interrogation. J Cardiovasc Electrophysiol 2013; 24(1):94–6.

19. Ruetz LL, Koehler JL, Brown ML, et al. Sinus rhythm R-wave amplitude as a predictor of ventricular fibrillation undersensing in patients with implantable cardioverter-defibrillator. Heart Rhythm 2015;12(12): 2411–8.

20. Barold SS, Kucher A, Nägele H, et al. Dissimilar ventricular rhythms: implications for ICD therapy. Heart Rhythm 2013;10(4):510–6.

21. Mann DE, Kelly PA, Robertson AD, et al. Significant differences in charge times among currently available implantable cardioverter defibrillators. Pacing Clin Electrophysiol 1999;22(6 Pt 1):903–7.

22. Jones JL, Proskauer CC, Paull WK, et al. Ultrastructural injury to chick myocardial cells in vitro following 'electric countershock'. Circ Res 1980;46(3):387–94.

23. Mitchell LB, Pineda EA, Titus JL, et al. Sudden death in patients with implantable cardioverter defibrillators: the importance of post-shock electromechanical dissociation. J Am Coll Cardiol 2002;39(8):1323–8.

24. Pires LA, Johnson KM. Intraoperative testing of the implantable cardioverter-defibrillator: how much is enough? J Cardiovasc Electrophysiol 2006;17:140–5.

25. Russo AM, Wang Y, Al-Khatib SM, et al. Patient, physician, and procedural factors influencing the use of defibrillation testing during initial implantable cardioverter defibrillator insertion: findings from the NCDR®. Pacing Clin Electrophysiol 2013;36(12):1522–31.

26. Leshem E, Suleiman M, Laish-Farkash A, et al, Israeli Working Group of Pacing and Electrophysiology. Contemporary rates and outcomes of single- vs. dual-coil implantable cardioverter defibrillator lead implantation: data from the Israeli ICD Registry. Europace 2017;19(9):1485–92.

27. Brignole M, Occhetta E, Bongiorni MG, et al. Clinical evaluation of defibrillation testing in an unselected population of 2,120 consecutive patients undergoing first implantable cardioverter-defibrillator implant. J Am Coll Cardiol 2012;60(11):981–7.

28. Healey JS, Hohnloser SH, Glikson M, et al. Cardioverter defibrillator implantation without induction of ventricular fibrillation: a single-blind, non-inferiority, randomised controlled trial (SIMPLE). Lancet 2015;385(9970):785–91.

29. Bänsch D, Bonnemeier H, Brandt J, et al. Intra-operative defibrillation testing and clinical shock efficacy in patients with implantable cardioverter-defibrillators: the NORDIC ICD randomized clinical trial. Eur Heart J 2015;36(37):2500–7.

30. Gula LJ, Massel D, Krahn AD, et al. Is defibrillation testing still necessary? A decision analysis and Markov model. J Cardiovasc Electrophysiol 2008;19(4):400–5.

31. Birnie D, Tung S, Simpson C, et al. Complications associated with defibrillation threshold testing: the Canadian experience. Heart Rhythm 2008;5(3):387–90.

32. Phan K, Ha H, Kabunga P, et al. Systematic review of defibrillation threshold testing at de novo implantation. Clrc Arrhythm Electrophysiol 2016;9(4):e003439.

33. Viskin S, Rosso R. The top 10 reasons to avoid defibrillation threshold testing during ICD implantation. Heart Rhythm 2008;5(3):391–3.

34. Gold MR, Higgins S, Klein R, et al. Efficacy and temporal stability of reduced safety margins for ventricular defibrillation: primary results from the Low Energy Safety Study (LESS). Circulation 2002;105(17):2043–8.

35. Wathen MS, Sweeney MO, DeGroot PJ, et al. Shock reduction using antitachycardia pacing for spontaneous rapid ventricular tachycardia in patients with coronary artery disease. Circulation 2001;104(7):796–801.

36. Gasparini M, Galimberti P, Ceriotti C. The values of defibrillation testing at implantable cardioverter defibrillator implantation: 'and then there were none'. Curr Opin Cardiol 2012;27(1):8–12.

37. Bennett M, Parkash R, Nery P, et al. Canadian Cardiovascular Society/Canadian Heart Rhythm Society 2016 implantable cardioverter-defibrillator guidelines. Can J Cardiol 2017;33(2):174–88.

38. Gasparini M, Galimberti P, Regoli F, et al. Delayed defibrillation testing in patients implanted with biventricular ICD (CRT-D): a reliable and safe approach. J Cardiovasc Electrophysiol 2005;16(12):1279–83.

39. Bianchi S, Ricci RP, Biscione F, et al. Primary prevention implantation of cardioverter defibrillator without defibrillation threshold testing: 2-year follow-up. Pacing Clin Electrophysiol 2009;32(5):573–8.

40. Michowitz Y, Lellouche N, Contractor T, et al. Defibrillation threshold testing fails to show clinical benefit during long-term follow-up of patients undergoing cardiac resynchronization therapy defibrillator implantation. Europace 2011;13(5):683–8.

Lead Management and Lead Extraction

Charles J. Love, MD, FHRS, CCDS

KEYWORDS

- Cardiac implantable electronic devices • Lead extraction • Pacing complications

KEY POINTS

- Management of patients with cardiac implantable electronic devices (CIEDs) has become complex given the complications that can occur with implanted lead systems.
- Clinical problems such as infection, lead failure, and occluded vessels create situations that demand intervention to remove leads.
- Due to adhesions that occur in the venous system and at the endomyocardial attachment site, simple traction to remove a lead is often not sufficient, and is in many cases dangerous.
- Infection is, with few exceptions, a mandatory reason to remove the entire CIED system.
- Tools and techniques are now available that enable a skilled operator with a well trained team to extract leads with a great deal of efficacy and safety.

Lead extraction has become an indispensable procedure to manage patients with cardiac implantable electronic devices (CIED). Since the first implanted pacemaker in 1958 resulted in a lead fracture (2 hours after the implant), the weak link in any CIED system remains the lead. Although lead failure is not uncommon, it does not in itself represent an urgent cause for removal. The most compelling cause is infection. This article will provide an overview of lead extraction and what is now called lead management.

INDICATIONS FOR EXTRACTION

The current indications for lead extraction are listed in **Box 1**. Infection of any part of the CIED system is recognized as being the most noncontroversial reason to extract leads. This is true whether the infection is in the device pocket (other than a superficial cellulitis), or if it is intravascular with endocarditis. Failure to extract leads in an infected system almost always results in a failure to cure (at best), or severe sepsis and death. Delay in complete system removal is associated with worse patient outcomes and increased mortality.[1–4] Beyond infection, Class I indications are somewhat less common or compelling. Occlusions of the vasculature preventing placement of new leads, or a need to perform a vasculature intervention that would require placing a stent that would cover and incarcerate existing leads has become a more common reason for need to extract leads.

With the advent of MRI conditionally safe CIED systems, there are several conditions that must be present in order to proceed with an MRI in keeping with the labeling requirements. Having leads that are not attached to the pacemaker or defibrillator, leads that are fractured, or leads that are not themselves labeled as MRI conditionally safe would result in a non-MRI conditionally safe system. Although some medical centers are willing to do scans on patients with these noncompliant systems, most do not do so. By extracting superfluous leads rather than abandoning them, patients have the option of getting a needed MRI scan at most imaging centers.

Accumulation of leads in the vasculature can create future problems for a patient. Factors that have been shown to increase the difficulty and risk of extraction include longer dwell time and

Johns Hopkins Hospital, 600 North Wolfe Street/Carnegie 592B, Baltimore, MD 21287, USA
E-mail address: clove14@jhmi.edu

Card Electrophysiol Clin 10 (2018) 127–136
https://doi.org/10.1016/j.ccep.2017.11.013
1877-9182/18/© 2017 Elsevier Inc. All rights reserved.

Box 1
Lead management recommendations

- Class I indications (strong)

  - Careful consideration with the patient on the decision on whether to abandon or remove a lead is recommended before starting the procedure. The risks and benefits of each course of action should be discussed, and any decision should take the patient's preference, comorbidities, future vascular access, and available programming options into account.

  - If antibiotics are going to be prescribed, drawing at least 2 sets of blood cultures before starting antibiotic therapy is recommended for all patients with suspected CIED infection to improve the precision and minimize the duration of antibiotic therapy.

  - Gram stain and culture of generator pocket tissue and the explanted lead(s) are recommended at the time of CIED removal to improve the precision and minimize the duration of antibiotic therapy.

  - Preprocedural transesophageal echocardiography is recommended for patients with suspected systemic CIED infection to evaluate the absence or size, character, and potential embolic risk of identified vegetations.

  - Evaluation by physicians with specific expertise in CIED infection and lead extraction is recommended for patients with documented CIED infection.

  - A complete course of antibiotics based on identification and in vitro susceptibility testing results after CIED removal is recommended for all patients with definite CIED system infection.

  - Complete device and lead removal is recommended for all patients with definite CIED system infection.

  - Complete removal of epicardial leads and patches is recommended for all patients with confirmed infected fluid (purulence) surrounding the intrathoracic portion of the lead.

  - Complete device and lead removal is recommended for all patients with valvular endocarditis without definite involvement of the lead(s) and/or device.

  - Complete device and lead removal is recommended for patients with persistent or recurrent bacteremia or fungemia, despite appropriate antibiotic therapy and no other identifiable source for relapse or continued infection.

  - Careful consideration of the implications of other implanted devices and hardware is recommended when deciding on the appropriateness of CIED removal and for planning treatment strategy and goals.

  - Lead removal is recommended for patients with clinically significant thromboembolic events attributable to thrombus on a lead or a lead fragment that cannot be treated by other means.

  - Lead removal is recommended for patients with superior vena cava stenosis or occlusion that prevents implantation of a necessary lead.

  - Lead removal is recommended for patients with planned stent deployment in a vein already containing a transvenous lead, to avoid entrapment of the lead.

  - Lead removal as part of a comprehensive plan for maintaining patency is recommended for patients with superior vena cava stenosis or occlusion with limiting symptoms.

  - Lead removal is recommended for patients with life-threatening arrhythmias secondary to retained leads.

  - Extraction programs and operator-specific information on volume, clinical success rates, and complication rates for lead removal and extraction should be available and discussed with the patient prior to any lead removal procedure.

- Class IIa Indications (moderate)

  - Lead abandonment or removal can be a useful treatment strategy if a lead becomes clinically unnecessary or nonfunctional.

  - Transesophageal echocardiography can be useful for patients with CIED pocket infection with and without positive blood cultures to evaluate the absence or size, character, and potential embolic risk of identified vegetations.

  - Evaluation by physicians with specific expertise in CIED infection and lead extraction can be useful for patients with suspected CIED infection.

- o Device and/or lead removal can be useful for patients with severe chronic pain at the device or lead insertion site or believed to be secondary to the device, which causes significant patient discomfort, is not manageable by medical or surgical techniques, and for which there is no acceptable alternative.
- o Lead removal can be useful for patients with ipsilateral venous occlusion preventing access to the venous circulation for required placement of an additional lead.
- o Lead removal can be useful for patients with a CIED location that interferes with the treatment of a malignancy.
- o Lead removal can be useful for patients if a CIED implantation would require more than 4 leads on 1 side or more than 5 leads through the SVC.
- o Lead removal can be useful for patients with an abandoned lead that interferes with the operation of a CIED system.
- Class IIb indications (weak)
  - o Additional imaging may be considered to facilitate the diagnosis of CIED pocket or lead infection when it cannot be confirmed by other methods.
  - o Lead removal may be considered for patients with leads that because of their design or their failure pose a potential future threat to the patient if left in place.
  - o Lead removal may be considered for patients to facilitate access to MRI.
  - o Lead removal may be considered in the setting of normally functioning nonrecalled pacing or defibrillation leads for selected patients after a shared decision-making process.

Data from Kusumoto FM, Schoenfeld MH, Wilkoff BL, et al. 2017 HRS expert consensus statement on cardiac implantable electronic device lead management and extraction. Presented at Asian Pacific Heart Rhythm Meeting. Yokohama (Japan), 2017; with permission.

more leads in place. Thus, it is felt by many physicians that if a lead may need to be removed, that doing so sooner will result in a higher degree of procedural success and a lower risk to the patient.[5,6]

FACILITY REQUIREMENTS

When a lead extraction is to be performed, having a qualified and experienced physician is certainly a key requirement. However, there are several additional requirements needed to achieve success and safety. Having a trained and competent team of professionals working together is key to the success of an extraction program (**Box 2**). All team members must know their role in the extraction procedure, as well as when a complication occurs. Most members of the team will be in the operating room at the time of the procedure. If not, they should be immediately available to assist at any time during the procedure.

When a problem occurs during an extraction (eg, hypotension, SVC tear, or cardiac perforation), there is often little time between the recognition that help is needed until the patient's condition becomes irreversible. All personnel must be in the operating room, or immediately available to come to the operating room to lend their expertise. In most cases, there is no time to bring someone in from outside of the institution or to move the patient to another venue.

This raises the question of where in the facility these procedures should be performed. My preference is that procedures be done in a hybrid operating room. This is really nothing more than a surgical suite capable of managing open heart procedures that also has a high-quality fluoroscopy system that can be moved out of the way. Alternatively, an electrophysiology (EP) laboratory that has a fluoroscopy system that can be moved out of the way and that also has room for all of the equipment to perform open heart procedures provides an equivalent venue. Such rooms provide the excellent fluoroscopy needed to perform lead extraction procedures (allowing for visualization of small lead conductors and parts), as well as all items needed to perform an immediate surgical rescue of a patient.

Optimally, the institution will provide support for a lead extraction program. This will allow for the purchase of the needed equipment and supplies to perform extraction procedures. More importantly, it will provide for a culture of cooperation and mutual support between all parties involved. For noncardiac surgeons performing lead extraction, it is necessary to have the support of one's cardiac surgical colleagues. This can be challenging, as in most institutions the surgeon is not being clinically productive while on standby during the extraction. Depending on the employment model, there are several options that are used to remedy this situation. These include

1. The institution provides virtual RVUs or payment to the standby surgeon.
2. The institution assigns the physician to that role as part of his or her employment model.

3. The surgeon operates with the extractor as a cosurgeon, both receiving a portion of the revenue collected.
4. The surgeon and extractor alternate billing 1 case to the next.
5. The surgeon is working in a clinic, office or other operating room, but is available to leave that venue to be at the extraction in short order.

Options 1 to 4 have the advantage of allowing the cardiac surgeon to be in the operating room during the extraction procedure. Option 5 is only viable if the surgeon can be immediately available to the operating room where the extraction is taking place.

PREPARATION FOR THE EXTRACTION PROCEDURE
Evaluation of the Cardiac Implantable Electronic Device System

It is important to know exactly what lies beneath the surface when attempting to extract a lead. Once the decision is made to proceed with an extraction, it is important to know

- What device is present, and what is the condition of the device?
  - Recalls or alerts
  - Battery condition
  - Need for device change because of the condition of the patient (upgrade or downgrade)
  - Connector type (IS-1, LV-1, DF-1, DF-4, or other special connections)
  - Presence of adapters
- What lead(s) is/are present?
  - All leads should be identified as to manufacturer, model, and implant date
  - Presence of fractures or visible loss of integrity
  - Presence of special connectors or adapters being used
  - Recall or reliability issues on any of the leads
  - Special construction issues impacting extraction (such as Riata leads)
  - Unique lead characteristics such as fragility and lack of isodiametric design
  - High risk leads (noncovered or nonbackfilled shock coils, StarFix active fixation leads)

Evaluation of the Patient

Knowledge of the patient is important to all phases of management. Management of anticoagulation and antiplatelet medications can be particularly challenging. So-called bridging of oral anticoagulants with heparin products was common in the past. However, given the plethora of data regarding increased complication rates with bridging therapy, this strategy has fallen out of favor in most clinical situations. Management should be individualized for each patient, and will depend on many factors including recent coronary or vascular stent implants, mechanical heart valves, and patients at high risk of thrombosis or thromboembolic events. Initial evaluation should include

- A full history and physical examination
- Laboratory work
  - Chest radiograph
  - Echocardiogram
  - Complete blood cell count
  - Coagulation studies
  - Type and cross-match (includes screening for any unusual antibodies)
  - Blood and wound cultures (when indicated)
  - Other imaging studies as indicated (may include gated cardiac computed tomography [CT] or positron emission tomography [PET] imaging)

Preparation of the Operating Room

The operating room should be checked to assure that all equipment is present and fully functional. It is useful to have an extraction cart that can be stocked with all devices and equipment that may be needed during an extraction procedure (**Box 3**). Duplicates of most items should be on hand, as well as multiple sizes of each item when available. It is helpful to have an individual assigned to ensure that the cart remains stocked, and that the items that may be required are present in the operating room.

In addition to having the previously mentioned equipment and supplies available, it is critical that all personnel involved or likely to be involved in the operation have an opportunity to discuss the plan. It is equally important that everyone knows their individual role in the event of a complication. Some institutions practice emergency response by having a drill with a simulated emergency. This is especially important when a center has a relatively low volume of lead extraction, or when new personnel are hired. Having an organized response can save time and increase the odds of a successful outcome for the patient.

Preparation of the Patient

Once the patient enters the operating room, the focus is on preparation of the patient for the procedure as well as for potential complications.

Box 3
Procedure room requirements

- Extraction cart contents
  - Locking stylets and/or lead locking devices
  - Long, heavy suture ties
  - Extraction sheaths
    - Mechanical
    - Laser
    - Cutting
  - Snares
  - Femoral workstation
- Sternotomy/thoracotomy tray with working sternal saw
- Cardiac bypass pump
- Working external defibrillator/external pacemaker
- Temporary pacing lead and working temporary pacemaker
- Fluoroscopy unit that is operational
- TEE machine
- SVC occlusion balloon
- Cross-matched blood (at least 2 units, but 4 are preferable)
- All items needed for new implant if one is to be performed

In most circumstances, the patient should be prepped as if undergoing an open heart procedure. This will include

- Intravenous access in the upper body
- Large bore femoral intravenous access (extremely important in the case of an SVC tear)
- General anesthesia with endotracheal intubation
- Full torso preparation and draping (from above the clavicles to upper thigh)
- Placement of adhesive defibrillator/external pacing pads
- Placement of a long, stiff guidewire from femoral vein to above the SVC origin (for placement of an SVC occlusion balloon in the case of an SVC tear)
- Placement of a temporary transvenous pacing electrode (as needed)
- Programming of the implanted device (if present) to appropriate mode and deactivation of shock therapies as appropriate

Lead Extraction Procedure

Once the patent is prepped, draped, under anesthesia, and stable, it is time to begin the operation. When intact leads are present that can be accessed in the pectoral area, the first task is to open the pocket and to free the leads from all of the adhesive tissues. If an infection is present, it is critical that all foreign material be identified, dissected free, and removed. Tissue specimens should be sent for culture, as they have been shown to enhance the yield for finding the culprit organism(s).[7] Removal of all (or as much as possible) of the infected tissues is helpful to expedite the healing process. Once the leads are dissected free down to the insertion into the venous system, they are prepared with locking stylets. Any lead being retained will typically have a standard stylet placed into it to help stabilize it and reduce the risk of it from being damaged during the removal of the targeted leads. When leads have a central lumen, each lead that is going to be removed has the connector pin cut off and the inner conductor coil exposed (note: some leads are lumenless, in which case no locking stylet is used; also, some leads tend to pull apart easily when the connector pin is cut off, and therefore some operators will leave the connector in place). Because most leads lack sufficient tensile strength to survive the extraction process, a locking stylet is placed into the lumen of the central coil and advanced to the tip of the lead. It is then locked into place (**Fig. 1**). The purpose of this stylet is twofold. First, it locks either into the tip of the lead, or along the length of the lead, serving to strengthen the lead and prevent it from uncoiling when traction is applied. Second, it adds stiffness to the lead,

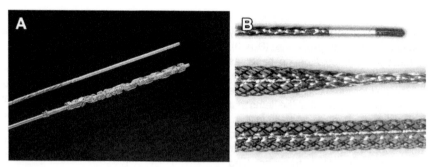

Fig. 1. Locking stylets. (*A*) Cook medical locking stylet. (*B*) Spectranetics lead locking device (LLD). ([*A*] Permission for use granted by Cook Medical, Bloomington, Indiana; [*B*] Reproduced with the permission of Koninklijke Philips N.V. and its subsidiary, The Spectranetics Corporation. All rights reserved.)

helping to provide a rail over which the extraction sheath can follow. Should a lead not have a lumen, or if a locking stylet cannot be inserted, a lead extender can be used to clamp onto the exposed end of the lead and thus provide a suitable working length over which an extraction sheath may be placed (**Fig. 2**).

Once the stylet is locked, and all leads either have been prepared or stabilized, a suture is tied over the end of the targeted lead to compress the lead components and to provide traction on the outer insulation. The latter is important to prevent the insulation from bunching up in front of the sheath (so called snow-plowing of the insulation), which could prevent advancement of the sheath. For some leads, especially those with multiple conductor cables (such as the St. Jude Riata lead), placement of a compression device, such as the Cook Medical One Tie, is helpful (**Fig. 3**). This is a loop of metal wire that is wrapped around the distal end of the lead and twisted to compress and hold in place all of the inner components of the lead. Some extractors tie onto each of the cable components of a lead (when present) to prevent prolapsing of the cables ahead of the sheath. It is important that all targeted leads be prepared before application of an extraction sheath, as it is common that leads adjacent to a lead over which a sheath is being used can become damaged to the point that placement of a locking stylet is not possible.

At this point, a sheath is passed over the lead passing through binding sites and releasing adhesions, and advanced close to the tip of the lead (**Fig. 4**). Then, the lead is pulled into the sheath (traction) while the sheath localizes the stress on the myocardium (countertraction). The lead tip releases from the myocardium and is retracted into the sheath. If a new implant is being performed, the lead is removed from the sheath without removing the sheath from the venous system, and a guidewire may be placed through it to maintain venous access. Otherwise, the sheath and lead are removed from the venous system. Placement of an absorbable hemostatic suture around the sheath before it is removed is useful to minimize bleeding. In essence, all sheaths perform the same function, passing over the lead, releasing adhesions, and providing countertraction. The main difference is what is at the cutting end of the sheath. This may be tapered polypropylene, fiberoptics through which laser energy is delivered, or a rotating metal cutting surface (**Fig. 5**). No one tool works in all situations. For example, a laser sheath is flexible and excellent in ablating soft tissue binding sites, and one

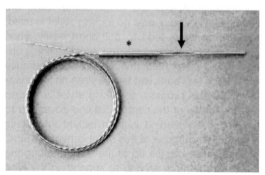

Fig. 2. Bulldog lead extender. (Permission for use granted by Cook Medical, Bloomington, Indiana.)

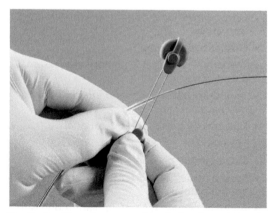

Fig. 3. OneTie coil compression device. (Permission for use granted by Cook Medical, Bloomington, Indiana.)

procedure. Sheaths come in several internal luminal diameters. A sheath must be sized to accommodate the lead body and components (eg, anode ring, tines, coils), suture tie, compression device (if used), and allow space for fibrous material that remains fixed to the lead body. It is often necessary to upsize during a procedure if forward progress is halted.

Some leads are not accessible from the superior veins, or they may break during an extraction procedure. To remove a lead fragment, and in some cases as a primary approach to extraction, it is necessary to proceed from a femoral route. If the lead to be removed is attached to a device, the pocket must be opened and the lead prepared to the point where the connector is cut off. If the lead is severed or has prolapsed into the vasculature, then it is not necessary to enter the pocket unless an infection is present or there is another reason to do so.

The femoral vein is accessed, and a 16F long Teflon sheath is advanced over a guidewire to the right atrium. The lead is then snared or grasped using any one of several devices and pulled into the sheath. The sheath may be advanced over the lead to provide countertraction if needed. Unfortunately, the typical femoral sheath is not very capable of cutting through adhesions, and the powered sheaths are not long enough (in most cases) to be used from the femoral approach (**Fig. 6**).

A disadvantage of the femoral approach is that it is much more challenging to maintain venous access to place a new lead from the pocket. However,

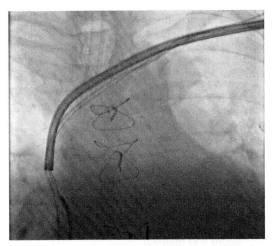

Fig. 4. Frame from fluoroscopy showing extraction sheath tracking down the lead on the way to the heart, passing through binding sites to free the lead from the vein wall.

does not need to use as much forward pressure to advance it under most conditions. However, laser energy does not pass through calcified adhesions well, whereas mechanical sheaths and rotating metal sheaths are more effective in this scenario. It is also common to use different sheaths during different phases of an extraction. Some will use a short, stiff mechanical sheath to bore through the tough tissues under the clavicle, then switch to a laser or other more flexible mechanical sheath for the remainder of the

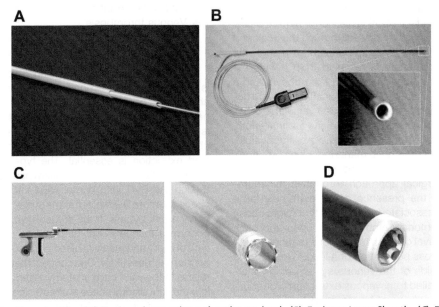

Fig. 5. Extraction sheaths. (*A*) Basic polypropylene sheaths on lead. (*B*) Excimer Laser Sheath. (*C*) EvolutionRL rotating cutting sheath. (*D*) TightRail mechanical cutting sheath. ([*B*] Reproduced with the permission of Koninklijke Philips N.V. and its subsidiary, The Spectranetics Corporation. All rights reserved; [*C*] Permission for use granted by Cook Medical, Bloomington, Indiana; [*D*] Reproduced with the permission of Koninklijke Philips N.V. and its subsidiary, The Spectranetics Corporation. All rights reserved.)

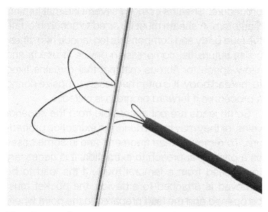

Fig. 6. Needle's Eye snare and femoral extraction sheath.

it can be accomplished if there is still lead in the pocket area. Once the lead is prepared and the connector cut off, a 0.014-inch guidewire is placed into the lumen of the lead. As the lead is pulled down through the femoral vein while the other end is maintained at the pectoral venous entry site, the guidewire follows the lead into the inferior vena cava, and can then be used from the pectoral site to reaccess the central circulation.

In many cases, when removing a lead from the superior approach, the lead will pull free from the myocardium before the sheath has advanced beyond an occluded part of the venous system. Should this occur, a useful technique that can maintain access to the circulation involves snaring the free end of the lead in the atrium from the femoral approach, and maintaining traction on it from below to allow the sheath to dissect through the occluded area from above. Once the sheath is through the occlusion, the snare is released from below; the lead pulled through the sheath from above, and a guidewire placed through the sheath to provide access through the newly expanded vein lumen.

Certain circumstances may make a transvenous approach to extraction inadvisable or impossible. These cases are best managed using an open heart approach via sternotomy, or a minimally invasive surgical approach through a minithoracotomy. In the presence of an extremely large vegetation associated with a lead that might cause a major pulmonary embolism, an open approach allows removal of the mass. Other situations would involve a gross perforation of a lead, a lead that is clearly outside of the venous system or myocardium, or a failed transvenous extraction procedure when the lead(s) must be removed.

Complications

Even in the best of hands, complications resulting from an extraction may occur. Many of these are

related to the anatomy of the patient, and the adhesion of the lead to the thin wall of the superior vena cava. Many factors have been related to the risk of complications occurring during a procedure.[8] The most important ones are

- Duration of lead implant
- Female sex
- Number of implanted leads extracted
- Small body surface area (BSA)
- Female gender (possibly also related to small BSA)
- Presence of calcification in the venous system
- History of a CVA
- Advanced heart failure
- Renal dysfunction (especially end-stage renal failure and dialysis)
- Presence of a dual coil ICD lead
- Infection as an indication for extraction
- Diabetes mellitus
- Anemia
- Lack of operator experience

Major complications include

- Death
- Superior vena cava tear
- Pericardial tamponade
- Cardiac avulsion
- Pulmonary embolism
- Hemothorax
- Cardiac arrest
- Tricuspid valve damage
- AV fistula formation
- Venous thrombosis
- Paradoxic embolism (in the presence of a patent foramen ovale or atrial septal defect)

Because complications are going to occur, the key is to be prepared to respond quickly to minimize the chance of a poor outcome. Having availability of all necessary equipment and personnel to affect a repair is important, but having a surgeon who is knowledgeable of the unique types of injuries associated with lead extraction is essential. The types of injuries such as long tears from the inominate vein down though the SVC with hemorrhage into the pleural space are more like major trauma surgery than a coronary artery bypass. If the surgeon who is going to perform a rescue is not prepared to manage this type of injury and massive bleeding, rescue of the patient is much less likely. One concept that is important relates to the vena cava anatomy. Although bleeding into the right pleural space is often a sign of SVC tear, typically half of the SVC is intrapericardial. Thus, it should also be noted that one can encounter hemothorax and/or pericardial tamponade with an SVC tear, depending on whether the defect occurs above and/or below the pericardial reflection.

Recently, a new device has been made available to help control hemorrhage when an SVC tear occurs. This is known as the Bridge Balloon. The Bridge Balloon is a large, compliant balloon that occludes the SVC from the inominate veins to the atrium. When an SVC tear occurs, the balloon is advanced over a prepositioned guidewire and inflated, thus occluding the SVC (**Fig. 7**). This typically takes no more than 1 minute to deploy. In the animal laboratory, blood pressure was maintained via flow from the IVC to the heart, the azygous vein, and other collateral vessels. Having the SVC occluded allows more time for a surgeon to open the chest and make a repair. In addition, the inflated balloon allows better visualization of the anatomy by slowing the torrent of blood that is usually encountered upon opening the mediastinum.

When a drop in blood pressure occurs, a decision must be made quickly as to the cause. Having a transesophageal echocardiography (TEE) probe in place during sheath advancement can help the operator make a diagnosis as to the cause of the hypotension. A growing pericardial effusion suggests either an SVC tear below the pericardial refection, or a myocardial tear. An empty ventricle suggests massive blood loss, most often into the pleural space. Often, vagal reflexes are activated during the extraction process, and these are generally benign, with restoration of a normal blood pressure when the procedure is paused. A critical point to understand is that if an SVC tear occurs with bleeding into the pleural space, much of the fluids and medications that are given will not be channeled into the heart, but will end up in the pleural space. It is for this reason that having a large femoral catheter in place, and using that access as the primary port during and SVC tear, is so important.

Vegetations are frequently found in the setting of endocarditis. Most vegetations are sheared off by the extraction sheath and either remain in the heart or embolize to the lungs. These typically do not cause a significant problem, although occasionally a patient may experience hemodynamic instability due to the embolic event itself, or because of the release of necrotic material, toxins, and debris from the infected material as it is avulsed from the lead. In most cases, these events are transient. However, as noted previously, large vegetations can pose a substantial threat of major pulmonary embolism should they break free. When the size of a vegetation approaches the size of a mainstem pulmonary artery (or even the size of the pulmonic valve), there should be consideration of an open heart approach. One alternative that is being used more frequently with variable success is the AngioVac system. This consists of a large cannula that is placed into the femoral vein and advanced to the right atrium. The other end is attached to a bypass pump, and one attempts to suck in the vegetation. Although this sounds enticing, in practice many of the vegetations are well organized or even calcified and will not fit into the suction sheath. Finally, when a vegetation is present in a patient who has a patent foramen ovale or atrial septal defect, a paradoxic embolism is possible.

It is important to consider whether a patient needs a new system prior to replacing a CIED. In my experience and in some studies, many patients no longer need a new CIED. This may be because their ventricle has recovered function, or it may be that the original indication was questionable. If an infection is not present, a new system can be implanted as part of the extraction procedure. However, if an infection is present, one should wait until the bacteremia has cleared (usually 5 days of negative blood cultures), or in the case of a nonsystemic infection, a 3-day waiting period is recommended to minimize the risk of seeding the new implant.[1] In the case of endocarditis, some patients may benefit from a leadless pacemaker, subcutaneous ICD

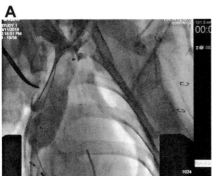 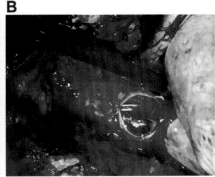

Fig. 7. BridgeTM superior vena cava occlusion balloon. (*A*) Fluoroscopic frame of balloon inflated in the SVC of a swine. (*B*) Balloon inflated in the SVC of a swine showing occlusion of the vessel with minimal blood flow, thereby maintaining hemostasis. (*Courtesy of* the Spectranetics Corporation, Colorado Springs, CO; with permission.)

(nontransvenous lead system), or an epicardial system. This is especially important for patients that have recurrent bacteremia, such as intravenous drug users, hemodialysis patients, and patients with little or no venous access available. It is strongly advised that a collaboration with the infectious disease consultant be developed, and that the infectious disease consultant be consulted on cases of CIED infection.

In the case of an infected device pocket, management of the local infected tissues is important. If all of the necrotic and infected material is able to be removed, primary closure with a closed drainage system is optimal. If complete debridement is not possible, partial pocket closure with packing to the base of the pocket and daily packing changes is one option. If the pocket is on the larger side, a WoundVac system may be used to accelerate healing.

SUMMARY

Lead extraction and management have become indispensable to the management of patients with CIED systems. The increasing incidence of CIED infection and failure of both recalled and good lead systems are the main drivers of the need to extract. Although the risk of a major adverse event during the procedure in experienced hands is around 1.2% with a mortality rate of 0.2%, this is not the risk to the individual. Consideration of an individual's unique situation for each patient given the risk profile of that patient is necessary to have an appropriate discussion with the patient. Only then can the risk of the extraction versus the risk of lead abandonment be truly evaluated and applied to that patient. With that being said, in experienced hands at a high-volume center, lead extraction can be performed in most cases with minimal risk and excellent results.

REFERENCES

1. Baddour LM, Epstein AE, Erickson CC, et al. Update on cardiovascular implantable electronic device infections and their management: a scientific statement from the American Heart Association. Circulation 2010;121:458–77.

2. Deharo JC, Quatre A, Mancini J, et al. Long-term outcomes following infection of cardiac implantable electronic devices: a prospective matched cohort study. Heart 2012;98:724–31.

3. Viganego F, O'Donoghue S, Eldadah Z, et al. Effect of early diagnosis and treatment with percutaneous lead extraction on survival in patients with cardiac device infections. Am J Cardiol 2012;109:1466–71.

4. Le KY, Sohail MR, Friedman PA, et al. Mayo Cardiovascular Infections Study Group. Impact of timing of device removal on mortality in patients with cardiovascular implantable electronic device infections. Heart Rhythm 2011;8:1678–85.

5. Wilkoff BL, Love CJ, Byrd CL, et al, Heart Rhythm Society, American Heart Association. Transvenous lead extraction: Heart Rhythm Society expert consensus on facilities, training, indications, and patient management: this document was endorsed by the American Heart Association (AHA). Heart Rhythm 2009;6: 1085–104.

6. Abu-El-Haija B, Bhave PD, Campbell DN, et al. Venous stenosis after transvenous lead placement: a study of outcomes and risk factors in 212 consecutive patients. J Am Heart Assoc 2015;4:e001878.

7. Dy Chua J, Abdul-Karim A, Mawhorter S, et al. The role of swab and tissue culture in the diagnosis of implantable cardiac device infection. Pacing Clin Electrophysiol 2005;28:1276–81.

8. Kusumoto FM, Schoenfeld MH, Wilkoff BL, et al. 2017 HRS expert consensus statement on cardiac implantable electronic device lead management and extraction. Heart Rhythm 2017;14(12):e503–48.

When Is It Safe Not to Reimplant an Implantable Cardioverter Defibrillator at the Time of Battery Depletion?

Sana M. Al-Khatib, MD, MHS*, Daniel J. Friedman, MD,
Gillian D. Sanders, PhD

KEYWORDS

- Sudden cardiac death • Implantable cardioverter defibrillator • Cardiac resynchronization therapy
- Left ventricular ejection fraction recovery

KEY POINTS

- Available data suggest that up to 45% of recipients of primary prevention implantable cardioverter defibrillators (ICDs) have significant improvement in their left ventricular function during follow-up. Although prospective data on the outcomes of patients with a primary prevention ICD and substantial improvement in left ventricular function are scarce, such patients appear to be at a low risk of ventricular arrhythmias.
- Prospective data are limited on the outcomes of patients with a cardiac resynchronization therapy defibrillator (CRT-D) who have significant improvement in their left ventricular function; however, the cumulative evidence from retrospective studies suggests that the risk of future ventricular arrhythmias is low in patients with a primary prevention indication whose LV ejection fraction (LVEF) improves to at least 45% with cardiac resynchronization therapy (CRT).
- It is not known when it is safe to not reimplant an ICD in patients with a primary prevention ICD with or without CRT.
- Until more data are available, the 2 situations in which it may be safe not to reimplant an ICD are: (1) patients with a primary prevention ICD who have significant improvement in LV function (LVEF ≥45%), no prior ICD therapies, and no bradycardia pacing indication, and (2) patients with a primary prevention CRT-D who have an improvement of the LVEF to at least 45% with CRT. If ICD replacement is forgone, it may be important to periodically assess the LVEF to look for worsening to less than or equal to 35%, at which point replacement of the ICD may be appropriate.
- Randomized clinical trials are needed on ICD replacement versus no replacement and on CRT-D versus CRT-P at the time of battery depletion.

Several randomized clinical trials have demonstrated the efficacy of the implantable cardioverter defibrillator (ICD) in reducing sudden cardiac death and all-cause mortality in survivors of cardiac arrest, patients with sustained ventricular tachycardia and structural heart disease, and patients with significant systolic dysfunction.[1–7] This robust evidence of the survival benefit of ICDs

---

Disclosures: Dr S.M. Al-Khatib reports nothing to disclose. Dr D.J. Friedman has received modest research grants from Boston Scientific, significant research grants from the National Cardiovascular Data Registry, modest educational grants from St. Jude Medical and Boston Scientific, and salary support from the NIH T-32 training grant HL069749. Dr G.D. Sanders reports nothing to disclose.
Duke Clinical Research Institute, Duke University Medical Center, 2400 Pratt Street, Durham, NC 27705, USA
* Corresponding author.
E-mail address: sana.alkhatib@duke.edu

Card Electrophysiol Clin 10 (2018) 137–144
https://doi.org/10.1016/j.ccep.2017.11.014
1877-9182/18/© 2017 Elsevier Inc. All rights reserved.

has not only informed professional guidelines,[8] but it has transformed clinical practice with about 100,000 new ICDs being implanted in patients in the United States annually.[9] The continued use of primary prevention ICDs in clinical practice has been further supported by analyses of the National Cardiovascular Data Registry ICD Registry.[10,11]

Current guidelines provide recommendations regarding when to implant a primary prevention or a secondary prevention ICD in a given patient.[8] However, guidance on when it is safe not to replace an ICD is missing from these guidelines. In fact, this issue was identified by the most recent guidelines that were published in 2012 as a gap in knowledge in need of further research. Specifically, the guidelines state that: "Indicators should be identified that provide direction about when it is safe to not replace an ICD that has reached the end of its effective battery life."[8]

The appropriate use criteria document generated by the Heart Rhythm Society (HRS) and the American College of Cardiology (ACC) also reflects the current uncertainty regarding the best treatment strategy for older patients whose ICD reaches end of life in the setting of an improved left ventricular ejection fraction (LVEF) and no prior ICD shocks for life-threatening arrhythmias. The document states that among patients with improved heart function and no prior ICD shocks, generator replacement may be "at times an appropriate option."[12] This recommendation was supported mainly by expert opinion and not by high-quality studies. This article will review guideline recommendations regarding ICDs, summarize published data on the outcomes of patients with primary prevention ICDs with or without cardiac resynchronization therapy (CRT) who have improvement in the left ventricular (LV) function, provide some guidance regarding situations in which it may be safe to not replace an ICD, and identify gaps in the existing evidence on this topic that should be addressed by future research.

CURRENT INDICATIONS FOR IMPLANTABLE CARDIOVERTER DEFIBRILLATORS

The most recent guideline document on device-based therapy of cardiac rhythm abnormalities lists several class I indications for the ICD[8]:

1. Survivors of cardiac arrest caused by ventricular fibrillation or hemodynamically unstable sustained ventricular tachycardia (VT) after evaluation to define the cause of the event and to exclude any completely reversible causes
2. Patients with structural heart disease and spontaneous sustained VT, whether hemodynamically stable or unstable
3. Patients with syncope of undetermined origin with clinically relevant, hemodynamically significant sustained VT or ventricular fibrillation induced at electrophysiological study
4. Patients with LV dysfunction due to prior myocardial infarction (MI), at least 40 days after MI, LVEF no more than 35%, New York Heart Association (NYHA) class II or III
5. Patients with nonischemic cardiomyopathy and LVEF of no more than 35%, NYHA class II or III
6. Patients with LV dysfunction caused by prior MI who are at least 40 days post-MI, have an LVEF less than or equal to 30%, and are in NYHA functional class I.
7. Patients with nonsustained VT caused by prior MI, LVEF less than or equal to 40%, and inducible ventricular fibrillation or sustained VT at electrophysiological study[8]

Multiple class IIa indications for ICDs are also listed in the guideline document. These class IIa indications involve milder presentations of class I scenarios such as unexplained syncope with significant systolic dysfunction caused by nonischemic cardiomyopathy or sustained VT in patients with normal or near-normal ventricular function.[8] All recommendations on ICDs stipulate that patients be on optimal medical therapy and have a reasonable expectation of survival for more than 1 year.[8] As stated previously, the guidelines do not offer any guidance on when not to reimplant an ICD.

DATA ON IMPLANTABLE CARDIOVERTER DEFIBRILLATORS

During an ICD generator's typical lifetime of approximately 7 to 10 years, about 65% of patients do not receive ICD shocks, and up to 45% of patients have a substantial improvement in their LVEF to greater than 35%, such that they would no longer meet accepted indications for a new ICD.[13,14] In a study of 195 patients, 50 (25.6%) had 10% improvement in LVEF, reaching a median LVEF during follow-up of 41% (25th, 75th percentiles 37%, 49%, respectively).[15] Studies have shown that LVEF improvement is associated with a significant long-term reduction in heart failure hospitalizations, ICD shocks, and death.[13,16–18] Among patients with ICDs, among the strongest predictors of ICD shocks is a prior heart failure hospitalization.[19] The close correlation between the LVEF, worsening heart failure, and the risk of ventricular arrhythmias has raised questions about the benefits of ICD in patients with substantial improvement in the LVEF.[20,21]

However, a few retrospective studies with relatively small sample sizes have shown a nontrivial rate of appropriate ICD shocks even in patients with significant LVEF improvement.[22–24] In a secondary analysis of the Defibrillators in Non-Ischemic Cardiomyopathy Treatment Evaluation (DEFINITE), patients whose LVEF improved had lower mortality risk compared with patients whose LVEF decreased, but appropriate shocks did not significantly correlate with LVEF improvement during follow-up.[22] Another study of 91 patients with primary prevention ICDs found that at generator replacement, 25 patients (27%) had improved LVEF. During a mean follow-up of 6 years, 9 patients (36%) with improved LVEF versus 19 (29%) with unchanged LVEF had appropriate ICD shocks.[23] In an analysis of 154 primary prevention ICD patients needing replacement because of battery depletion, 114 (74%) patients had not received appropriate ICD therapy. Following ICD generator replacement, the 3-year incidence of appropriate therapy in these patients was 14%; however, this study did not include information on the incidence of LVEF improvement.[24] In a similar study, 275 of 403 patients (68%) needing a primary prevention ICD replacement had not received appropriate therapy from the initial device. After ICD generator replacement, the 3-year risk of appropriate ICD therapy was 13.7%, but no information on follow-up LVEF was provided.[25] So, based on these data, it seems appropriate to replace the ICD in patients with a primary prevention ICD who continue to meet the guideline recommendations at the time of device replacement.

Given the conflicting data on the outcomes of ICD patients with an improved LVEF and the paucity of data from prospective studies on the best management practices, it is not known whether ICD generator replacement should be performed in patients who no longer meet current indications for an ICD (due to an improved LVEF to >35% and in the absence of prior ICD shocks).[20,26] This uncertainty is amplified in patients 65 years of age and older in whom the burden of comorbid diseases and competing modes of death reduce ICD benefit.[26,27] Although many studies have defined the risks associated with ICD generator replacement,[28,29] there are currently no studies that have examined whether this invasive procedure leads to any benefit among these lower-risk patients.

The critical importance of understanding the best care strategy for individuals who no longer meet current indications for an ICD (due to an improved LVEF >35% and absence of prior ICD shocks) has been emphasized by patients, care partners, physicians, and professional organizations. In early 2015, as part of its prioritization process, the Patient Centered Outcomes Research Institute (PCORI) tasked the Duke University Evidence Synthesis Group (ESG) to work with diverse stakeholders to identify and prioritize the future research most needed by patients and other decision makers on the topic of ICDs in older patients. The results identified clinical effectiveness and safety of ICD replacements in older patients who have not had an appropriate shock or those with improved LVEF as a key research priority for PCORI.[26]

ICD generator replacement is associated with a nontrivial risk of complications; within 6 months after the procedure, the risk of major complications is 4%, and the risk of minor complications is 7.4%.[28] Major complications associated with ICD generator replacement include lead dislodgement or damage, device infection requiring removal of the entire ICD system, significant bleeding requiring ICD pocket evacuation, and prolonged hospitalization.[28] Minor complications include nerve injury, minor bleeding, skin infection, and pain. The risk of device infection is particularly troubling, as it does not only appear to be increasing, but it generally requires removal of the whole ICD system. In a study of the National Hospital Discharge Survey database from 1996 through 2006, the risk of device infection was noted to have increased from 2004 to 2006 by 57%.[30] Factors that could account for this rise in device infection included an increase in the rate of comorbid illnesses like end-organ failure and diabetes mellitus and an increase in the use of CRT devices.[30] Removal of the entire ICD system (generator and leads) is associated with substantial risks including cardiac perforation with or without tamponade, vascular damage, and even death.[31,32]

Therefore, until more data become available, the algorithm in **Fig. 1** can be used to make decisions regarding ICD generator replacements.

In reviewing this algorithm, it is important to note that the LVEF measurement is subjective with interobserver variability and intraobserver variability that approach 5% to 8%, so it may be better to use a cutoff for the improved LVEF at battery depletion of greater than 40% or greater than 45% to allow for that variability. Also, although the annual risk of receiving ICD therapy among patients with LVEF improvement is relatively small, low- to moderate-quality studies have shown that over 5 years, greater than 10% (sometimes >20%) of patients end up receiving appropriate therapy. This information should be considered and shared with the patient during clinical decision making. Finally, if ICD replacement is forgone, it may be important to obtain periodic follow-up assessments of the LVEF to look for worsening of no more than 35%, at which point replacement of the ICD may be appropriate.

DATA ON CARDIAC RESYNCHRONIZATION THERAPY-DEFIBRILLATOR

CRT has become one of the mainstay therapies in patients with heart failure with a reduced LVEF (≤35%) who have a wide QRS and symptomatic heart failure despite optimal medical therapy.[8] Many studies have shown that this therapy improves patients' survival, quality of life, and functional status, and reduces heart failure hospitalization.[33–37] CRT devices are either pacemakers (CRT-P) or defibrillators (CRT-D). Both types of devices resynchronize the heart through biventricular pacing; CRT-D can also deliver high-energy shocks

or antitachycardia pacing to terminate life-threatening ventricular arrhythmias. Patients who receive a primary prevention CRT-D as their initial device may have significant improvement in their LVEF due to CRT and as such their risk of ventricular arrhythmias may decrease substantially. In such patients, when the battery reaches end of life, it is not known whether a CRT-P may suffice. The HRS/ACC Appropriate Use Criteria document considered these types of scenarios and determined that it may be appropriate to replace a CRT-D with a CRT-P device in patients who received a CRT-D device when the LVEF is no more than 35% and the LVEF at end of battery life is at least 36%.[12]

A few studies have reported on the risk of appropriate ICD shocks from CRT-Ds in patients with an improved LVEF. In a landmark analysis of 270 patients with post-CRT-D LVEF assessment and no ICD therapy within 1 year of device implantation, the 2-year risk of appropriate ICD therapy was 3.0%, 2.1%, and 1.5% for post-CRT-D LVEF of 45%, 50%, and 55%, respectively. This study concluded that when the LVEF near normalizes to at least 45%, the incidence of ICD therapies for ventricular arrhythmias decreases appreciably.[38] In another study of 270 patients, the

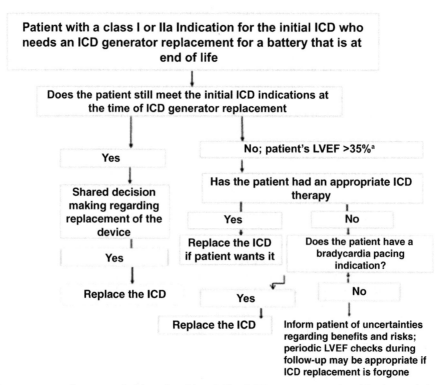

Fig. 1. ICD generator replacement decision algorithm. [a] The LVEF measurement is subjective and the variability may be up to 8%, so it may be better to use a cutoff of 40% or 45% to allow for that variability.

LVEF improved to greater than 35% in 21% of patients during a follow-up period of 12 months. Patients with an LVEF improvement to greater than 35% received fewer ICD therapies during follow-up than those who did not (23 vs 38%; P value 0.03). Limiting the analysis to patients with a primary prevention ICD showed that the rate of ICD therapies was 31% in patients with no LVEF improvement versus 6% in patients with an LVEF improvement to greater than 35%.[39]

Another study reported on the risk of appropriate ICD shocks in 110 patients with CRT-D who had an absolute increase in the LVEF of at least 10%, a decrease in LV end-systolic volume of at least 30%, or a decrease in LV end-diastolic volume of at least 20%. They found these 3 groups of patients received ICD shocks (3-year risk: 64% vs 82% for LVEF ≥10%; 63% vs 92% for end-systolic volume ≥30%; and 62% vs 94% for end-diastolic volume ≥20%; all P<.001) during a mean follow-up duration of 25 months. However, this study was limited by the relatively small sample size and short follow-up.[40] In another study of 142 patients with a primary prevention CRT-D and a baseline LVEF less than 35%, 42 patients had an improvement in the LVEF to greater than 35% over a median follow-up of 3 years. None of these 42

patients had appropriate ICD therapies during follow-up.[41]

A secondary analysis of the Multicenter Automatic Defibrillator Implantation Trial With Cardiac Resynchronization Therapy (MADIT-CRT) focused on 752 patients who survived and had echocardiographic data at enrollment and at 12 months. During an average follow-up period of 2.2 years, 7.3% patients had LVEF normalization. The risk of ventricular arrhythmias was significantly lower in patients with LVEF greater than 50% (hazard ratio [HR], 0.24; 95% confidence interval [CI], 0.07-0.82; P = .023) and LVEF of 36% to 50% (HR, 0.44; 95% CI, 0.28–0.68; P<.001). Because the risk of inappropriate ICD therapy was nontrivial, the authors concluded that patients with LVEF improvement could be considered for downgrade from CRT-D to CRT-P when the battery reaches end of life if no ventricular arrhythmias had occurred.[42]

Finally, a meta-analysis was conducted to determine the association between LVEF recovery following CRT and the risk of appropriate ICD therapy.[43] Six retrospective cohort studies were included (n = 1740). The risk of appropriate ICD therapy was significantly lower in patients with post-CRT LVEF of at least 35% (5.5/100 person-years) than in patients with post-CRT LVEF less

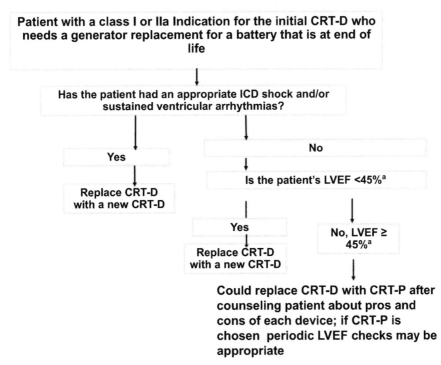

Fig. 2. CRT-D generator replacement decision algorithm. [a] LVEF cutoff of 45% was used based on data from Chatterjee et al.[43] (*Data from* Chatterjee NA, Roka A, Lubitz SA, et al. Reduced appropriate implantable cardioverter-defibrillator therapy after cardiac resynchronization therapy-induced left ventricular function recovery: a meta-analysis and systematic review. Eur Heart J 2015;36(41):2780–9.)

than 35% (incidence rate difference −6.5/100 person-years, 95% CI: −8.8 to −4.2, P = .001). Focusing the analysis on patients with a post-CRT LVEF of at least 45% showed a lower risk of ICD therapy (2.3/100 person-years) compared with patients without such recovery (−5.8/100 person-years, 95% CI: −7.6–24.0, P = .001). Patients with a primary prevention ICD had low rates of ICD therapy (0.4–0.8/100-person years) irrespective of LVEF recovery. The investigators concluded that LVEF recovery post-CRT is associated with significantly reduced appropriate ICD therapy, and this risk is lowest in patients with improvement of LVEF to at least 45% and those with a primary prevention ndication.[43]

Based on the aforementioned studies, it is not known how to best manage patients with a CRT-D device with no prior ICD therapies who have significant improvement in the LVEF at the time of battery depletion. Therefore, randomized clinical trials of CRT-P versus CRT-D, especially at the time of device replacement, are needed. Until such trials are completed, the algorithm in **Fig. 2** can be used to make decisions regarding CRT-D generator replacements.

SUMMARY

Many patients with a primary prevention ICD or a CRT-D have significant improvement in their LV function during follow-up. Patients with an ICD and improved LVEF to greater than 45% appear to be at a low risk of ventricular arrhythmias; however, there are no data from prospective studies on whether it is safe to not replace the ICD in such patients. In patients with a CRT-D who have significant improvement in their LV function, evidence from retrospective studies suggests that the risk of future ventricular arrhythmias is low in patients with a primary prevention indication whose LVEF improves to at least 45% with CRT. However, there are no data on whether replacing the CRT-D with a CRT-P in such patients is safe. It is noteworthy that the absolute LVEF value during follow-up may not be enough in assessing the risk of ventricular arrhythmias; it is possible that the magnitude of improvement is more important than whether the LVEF is less than or greater than 35%. Future studies should look at the predictive power of the LVEF as a continuous variable. In addition, future randomized clinical trials should compare the outcomes of ICD replacement versus not replacing and CRT-D versus CRT-P at the time of battery depletion. Until data from clinical trials are available to guide clinical recommendations, shared decision making is essential taking into account the uncertainties in the data and the known pros and cons of replacing versus not replacing the ICD.

REFERENCES

1. Moss AJ, Hall WJ, Cannom DS, et al. Improved survival with an implanted defibrillator in patients with coronary disease at high risk for ventricular arrhythmia. Multicenter automatic defibrillator implantation trial investigators. N Engl J Med 1996; 335(26):1933–40.

2. Antiarrhythmics versus Implantable Defibrillators (AVID) investigators. A comparison of antiarrhythmic-drug therapy with implantable defibrillators in patients resuscitated from near-fatal ventricular arrhythmias. N Engl J Med 1997;337(22):1576–83.

3. Buxton AE, Lee KL, Fisher JD, et al. A randomized study of the prevention of sudden death in patients with coronary artery disease. Multicenter unsustained tachycardia trial investigators. N Engl J Med 1999;341(25):1882–90.

4. Connolly SJ, Hallstrom AP, Cappato R, et al. Meta-analysis of the implantable cardioverter defibrillator secondary prevention trials. AVID, CASH and CIDS studies. Antiarrhythmics vs implantable defibrillator study. Cardiac arrest study Hamburg. Canadian implantable defibrillator study. Eur Heart J 2000; 21(24):2071–8.

5. Moss AJ, Zareba W, Hall WJ, et al. Prophylactic implantation of a defibrillator in patients with myocardial infarction and reduced ejection fraction. N Engl J Med 2002;346(12):877–83.

6. Kadish A, Dyer A, Daubert JP, et al. Prophylactic defibrillator implantation in patients with nonischemic dilated cardiomyopathy. N Engl J Med 2004; 350(21):2151–8.

7. Bardy GH, Lee KL, Mark DB, et al. Amiodarone or an implantable cardioverter-defibrillator for congestive heart failure. N Engl J Med 2005; 352(3):225–37.

8. Epstein AE, DiMarco JP, Ellenbogen KA, et al. 2012 ACCF/AHA/HRS focused update incorporated into the ACCF/AHA/HRS 2008 guidelines for device-based therapy of cardiac rhythm abnormalities: a report of the American College of Cardiology Foundation/American Heart Association Task Force on Practice Guidelines and the Heart Rhythm Society. Circulation 2013;127(3):e283–352.

9. Kremers MS, Hammill SC, Berul CI, et al. The national ICD registry report: version 2.1 including leads and pediatrics for years 2010 and 2011. Heart Rhythm 2013;10(4):e59–65.

10. Al-Khatib SM, Hellkamp A, Bardy GH, et al. Survival of patients receiving a primary prevention ICD in clinical practice versus clinical trials. JAMA 2013; 309:55–62.

11. Al-Khatib SM, Hellkamp AS, Fonarow GC, et al. Association between prophylactic implantable cardioverter defibrillators and survival in patients with left ventricular ejection fraction between 30% and 35%. JAMA 2014;311:2209–15.

12. Russo AM, Stainback RF, Bailey SR, et al. ACCF/HRS/AHA/ASE/HFSA/SCAI/SCCT/SCMR 2013 appropriate use criteria for implantable cardioverter-defibrillators and cardiac resynchronization therapy: a report of the American College of Cardiology Foundation appropriate use criteria task force, Heart Rhythm Society, American Heart Association, American Society of Echocardiography, Heart Failure Society of America, Society for Cardiovascular Angiography and Interventions, Society of Cardiovascular Computed Tomography, and Society for Cardiovascular Magnetic Resonance. Heart Rhythm 2013; 10(4):e11–58.

13. Kini V, Soufi MK, Deo R, et al. Appropriateness of primary prevention implantable cardioverter-defibrillators at the time of generator replacement: are indications still met? J Am Coll Cardiol 2014;63(22):2388–94.

14. Adabag S, Patton KK, Buxton AE, et al. Association of implantable cardioverter defibrillators with survival in patients with and without improved ejection fraction: secondary analysis of the sudden cardiac death in heart failure trial. JAMA Cardiol 2017;2(7): 767–74.

15. Friedman DJ, Overton R, Shaw L, et al. The role of baseline versus long-term follow-up ejection fraction in predicting adverse events among primary prevention implantable cardioverter defibrillator recipients. J Am Coll Cardiol 2017;69(11):741.

16. Kalogeropoulos AP, Fonarow GC, Georgiopoulou V, et al. Characteristics and outcomes of adult outpatients with heart failure and improved or recovered ejection fraction. JAMA Cardiol 2016;1(5):510–8.

17. Madhavan M, Waks JW, Friedman PA, et al. Outcomes after implantable cardioverter-defibrillator generator replacement for primary prevention of sudden cardiac death. Circ Arrhythm Electrophysiol 2016;9(3):e003283.

18. Zhang Y, Guallar E, Blasco-Colmenares E, et al. Changes in follow-up left ventricular ejection fraction associated with outcomes in primary prevention implantable cardioverter-defibrillator and cardiac resynchronization therapy device recipients. J Am Coll Cardiol 2015;66(5):524–31.

19. Singh JP, Hall WJ, McNitt S, et al. Factors influencing appropriate firing of the implanted defibrillator for ventricular tachycardia/fibrillation: findings from the Multicenter Automatic Defibrillator Implantation Trial II (MADIT-II). J Am Coll Cardiol 2005; 46(9):1712–20.

20. Merchant FM, Quest T, Leon AR, et al. Implantable cardioverter-defibrillators at end of battery life:

21. Kramer DB, Buxton AE, Zimetbaum PJ. Time for a change–a new approach to ICD replacement. N Engl J Med 2012;366(4):291–3.

22. Schliamser JE, Kadish AH, Subacius H, et al. DEFINITE Investigators (2013) Significance of follow-up left ventricular ejection fraction measurements in the Defibrillators in Non-Ischemic Cardiomyopathy Treatment Evaluation trial (DEFINITE). Heart Rhythm 2013;10:838–46.

23. Naksuk N, Saab A, Li JM, et al. Incidence of appropriate shock in implantable cardioverter-defibrillator patients with improved ejection fraction. J Card Fail 2013;19:426–30.

24. Van Welsenes GH, Van Rees JB, Thijssen J, et al. Primary prevention implantable cardioverter defibrillator recipients: the need for defibrillator back-up after an event-free first battery service-life. J Cardiovasc Electrophysiol 2011;22:1346–50.

25. Yap SC, Schaer BA, Bhagwandien RE, et al. Evaluation of the need of elective implantable cardioverter-defibrillator generator replacement in primary prevention patients without prior appropriate ICD therapy. Heart 2014;100:1188–92.

26. Al-Khatib SM, Gierisch JM, Crowley MJ, et al. Future research prioritization: implantable cardioverter-defibrillator therapy in older patients. J Gen Intern Med 2015;30(12):1812–20.

27. Steinberg BA, Al-Khatib SM, Edwards R, et al. Outcomes of implantable cardioverter-defibrillator use in patients with comorbidities: results from a combined analysis of 4 randomized clinical trials. JACC Heart Fail 2014;2(6):623–9.

28. Poole JE, Gleva MJ, Mela T, et al. Complication rates associated with pacemaker or implantable cardioverter-defibrillator generator replacements and upgrade procedures: results from the REPLACE registry. Circulation 2010;122(16):1553–61.

29. Prutkin JM, Reynolds MR, Bao H, et al. Rates of and factors associated with infection in 200 909 Medicare implantable cardioverter-defibrillator implants: results from the National Cardiovascular Data Registry. Circulation 2014;130(13):1037–43.

30. Voigt A, Shalaby A, Saba S. Continued rise in rates of cardiovascular implantable electronic device infections in the United States: temporal trends and causative insights. Pacing Clin Electrophysiol 2010;33(4):414–9.

31. Wazni O, Epstein LM, Carrillo RG, et al. Lead extraction in the contemporary setting: the LExICon study: an observational retrospective study of consecutive laser lead extractions. J Am Coll Cardiol 2010;55(6): 579–86.

32. Wilkoff BL, Love CJ, Byrd CL, et al. Transvenous lead extraction: Heart Rhythm Society expert consensus on facilities, training, indications, and

patient management: this document was endorsed by the American Heart Association (AHA). Heart Rhythm 2009;6(7):1085–104.

33. Bristow MR, Saxon LA, Boehmer J, et al. Cardiac-resynchronization therapy with or without an implantable defibrillator in advanced chronic heart failure. N Engl J Med 2004;350(21):2140–50.

34. Cleland JG, Daubert JC, Erdmann E, et al. The effect of cardiac resynchronization on morbidity and mortality in heart failure. N Engl J Med 2005;352: 1539–49.

35. Linde C, Abraham WT, Gold MR, et al. Randomized trial of cardiac resynchronization in mildly symptomatic heart failure patients and in asymptomatic patients with left ventricular dysfunction and previous heart failure symptoms. J Am Coll Cardiol 2008; 52(23):1834–43.

36. Moss AJ, Hall WJ, Cannom DS, et al. Cardiac-resynchronization therapy for the prevention of heart failure events. N Engl J Med 2009;361(14):1329–38.

37. Tang AS, Wells GA, Talajic M, et al. Cardiac-resynchronization therapy for mild-to-moderate heart failure. N Engl J Med 2010;363(25):2385–95.

38. Manfredi JA, Al-Khatib SM, Shaw LK, et al. Association between left ventricular ejection fraction post-cardiac resynchronization treatment and subsequent ICD therapy for sustained ventricular tachyarrhythmias. Circ Arrhythm Electrophysiol 2013;6:257–64.

39. Schaer BA, Osswald S, Di Valentino M, et al. Close connection between improvement in left ventricular function by cardiac resynchronization therapy and the incidence of arrhythmias in cardiac resynchronization therapy-defibrillator patients. Eur J Heart Fail 2010;12:1325–32.

40. Steffel J, Milosevic G, Hurlimann A, et al. Characteristics and long-term outcome of echocardiographic super-responders to cardiac resynchronization therapy: 'real world' experience from a single tertiary care centre. Heart 2011;97:1668–74.

41. Van Boven N, Bogaard K, Ruiter J, et al. Functional response to cardiac resynchronization therapy is associated with improved clinical outcome and absence of appropriate shocks. J Cardiovasc Electrophysiol 2013;24:316–22.

42. Ruwald MH, Solomon SD, Foster E, et al. Left ventricular ejection fraction normalization in cardiac resynchronization therapy and risk of ventricular arrhythmias and clinical outcomes: results from the Multicenter Automatic Defibrillator Implantation Trial with Cardiac Resynchronization Therapy (MADIT-CRT) trial. Circulation 2014;130:2278–86.

43. Chatterjee NA, Roka A, Lubitz SA, et al. Reduced appropriate implantable cardioverter-defibrillator therapy after cardiac resynchronization therapy-induced left ventricular function recovery: a meta-analysis and systematic review. Eur Heart J 2015; 36(41):2780–9.

Important Parameters for Implantable Cardioverter Defibrillator Selection

Nath Zungsontiporn, MD, Michael Loguidice, MD,
James Daniels, MD*

KEYWORDS

- ICD • Implantable cardioverter defibrillator • Single-chamber • Dual-chamber • DF-1 • DF-4

KEY POINTS

- Several important parameters relating to device characteristics, patient attributes, and comorbidities should be considered when selecting the appropriate implantable cardioverter defibrillator (ICD) for each patient.
- Single-chamber ICDs are appropriate for most primary and secondary prevention patients without a pacing indication.
- The need for atrial or A-V sequential pacing is the only well-established indication for dual-chamber ICD implantation.

INTRODUCTION

The efficacy of implantable cardioverter defibrillators (ICDs) in reducing the risk of sudden cardiac death (SCD) has been well established by several clinical trials in both patients with previous ventricular tachycardia (VT) and fibrillation (VF) (secondary prevention)[1] and those at higher risk of developing such arrhythmias (primary prevention).[2–5]

However, there are several important parameters that should be considered when selecting the appropriate ICD for each patient. This review aims to examine some of these issues. Other articles in this issue will specifically address the issues surrounding the choice between transvenous and subcutaneous ICDs (S-ICD), and between single- and dual-coil leads.

SINGLE- VERSUS DUAL-CHAMBER IMPLANTABLE CARDIOVERTER DEFIBRILLATOR

The single-chamber ICD has a single lead in the right ventricle (RV). The dual-chamber ICD has a lead in the right atrium in addition to the lead in the RV. These devices are able to deliver antitachycardia pacing (ATP) as well as a high-energy electrical shock for the treatment of VT and VF. In addition, ICDs can also deliver pacing to treat bradycardia if needed. Most of the randomized controlled trials that established the efficacy of ICDs for primary and secondary prevention of SCD used single-chamber ICDs.[6]

In addition to atrial or A-V sequential pacing capability, the dual-chamber ICD has the additional potential advantages of providing enhanced

None of the authors has any potential financial conflict of interest related to this article.

Division of Cardiology, Department of Internal Medicine, University of Texas Southwestern Medical Center, 5323 Harry Hines Boulevard, Dallas, TX 75390, USA

* Corresponding author. Division of Cardiology, University of Texas Southwestern Medical Center, 5323 Harry Hines Boulevard, Suite HP8.110, Dallas, TX 75390-9047.

E-mail address: James.Daniels@UTSouthwestern.edu

Card Electrophysiol Clin 10 (2018) 145–152
https://doi.org/10.1016/j.ccep.2017.11.015

arrhythmia discrimination, monitoring for atrial arrhythmias, and delivering atrial ATP to treat such arrhythmias. There also are potential drawbacks to dual-chamber ICDs, including increased device-related complications, increased RV pacing, and increased cost.

Arrhythmia Discrimination

Because ICDs determine the need to deliver therapy (ATP and/or shocks) largely by the rate or cycle length of the tachycardia, a single-chamber ICD can have difficulty differentiating between VT and supraventricular tachycardia (SVT) based solely on rate. During ventricular arrhythmias (VA), the ventricular rate is often faster than the atrial rate, whereas, during some SVTs, the atrial rate is faster than the ventricular rate. Therefore, because the ICD is able to sense the atrial electrogram, 1 potential advantage of the dual-chamber ICD over the single-chamber device is enhanced arrhythmia discrimination (beyond the available single-chamber rhythm discriminators) and a reduction in inappropriate shocks.

Several randomized controlled trials have sought to determine if dual-chamber ICDs improve arrhythmia discrimination. Several trials that included predominantly a secondary prevention population conducted in the 1990s to early 2000s did not demonstrate a difference in the number of SVTs misclassified as VT, inappropriate ICD therapies, or in mortality and arrhythmogenic morbidity.[7–9] Limitations of these trials include relatively small sample sizes (each with N ≤100) and noncontemporary device programming.

Subsequent studies in predominantly secondary prevention patients without a pacing indication suggested some benefits of dual-chamber ICDs. The Detect Supraventricular Tachycardia Study randomly assigned 400 participants who received a dual-chamber ICD (75% secondary prevention) to a single- or dual-chamber detection algorithm. This study used more contemporary rhythm discrimination algorithms, including morphologic criteria. However, the investigators used a VT detection rate no faster than 150 bpm, which is very low compared with current practice. This study demonstrated significant reduction in the number of SVT episodes inappropriately classified as VT in the dual-chamber arm (30.9%) compared with the single-chamber detection arm (39.5%) with an odds ratio (OR) of inappropriate detection of 0.53 ($P = .03$). The odds of inappropriate therapy delivery (ATP or shock) were also decreased by 46% ($P = .02$).[10] However, no difference in the number of arrhythmia-related hospitalizations or additional clinic visits was seen.

The Dual chamber and Atrial Tachyarrhythmias Adverse events Study (DATAS) trial randomized 334 participants with an ICD indication (88% secondary prevention) to dual-chamber ICDs, single-chamber ICDs, or dual-chamber ICDs programmed as a single-chamber ICD. This study showed 33% lower composite score rate of clinically significant adverse events (all-cause mortality, invasive intervention due to cardiovascular causes, hospitalizations >24 hours for cardiovascular causes, 2 or more episodes of inappropriate shocks, and sustained symptomatic atrial tachyarrhythmias lasting >48 hours) in the dual-chamber ICD group.[11] This study is limited by nonstandardized device programming and the use of combined outcome.

The 2 most recent studies focused on primary prevention patients and reported conflicting results. The Optimal Anti-Tachycardia Therapy in Implantable Cardioverter-Defibrillator Patients Without Pacing Indications (OPTION) trial randomized 453 participants with an ICD indication (75% primary prevention) who received a dual-chamber ICD to dual-chamber or single-chamber device programming. The devices in both groups were programmed with lower VT detection rate of 170/min. The single-chamber programming group used onset, stability, and long cycle search discrimination criteria (but no morphologic criteria), whereas the dual-chamber group used a proprietary dual-chamber rhythm discrimination algorithm that included ventricular rate stability, rate-onset analysis, atrioventricular association analysis, long cycle search, and determination of the chamber of origin in the case of 1:1 tachycardia. Of note, the investigators did not specify the duration that was required to diagnose an arrhythmia episode. This study demonstrated a significantly longer time to first inappropriate shock in the dual-chamber ICD group compared with the single-chamber ICD group. At the end of 27-month study period, 10 patients in the dual-chamber setting group (4.3%) and 23 patients in the single-chamber setting group (10.3%) received at least 1 inappropriate shock ($P = .015$). Based on these results, the number of patients needed to treat with a dual-chamber ICD to prevent 1 patient from experiencing an inappropriate shock was 17.[12] The rate of death or cardiovascular hospitalization remained similar in both groups in this study.

The Reduction And Prevention of Tachyarrhythmias and Shocks Using Reduced Ventricular Pacing with Atrial Algorithms Study (the RAPTURE Study) randomized 100 participants receiving primary prevention ICD to dual-chamber or single-chamber devices. The devices in both groups were programmed to use high detection cutoff rates (>182 bpm) and to wait approximately 17 seconds before shocking ventricular tachyarrhythmias. Single-chamber devices in this study used an SVT-VT discrimination algorithm that included morphologic criteria, whereas dual-chamber devices use a proprietary algorithm that evaluated A and V rhythms as well as their relationship. There was no difference between groups in the number of patients receiving an inappropriate shock during 12-month follow-up period of this study.[13] However, the small sample size and short follow-up are limitations of this trial.

Detection of Atrial Arrhythmias

Another potential advantage of a dual-chamber ICD is enhanced detection of subclinical atrial tachycardia (AT)/atrial fibrillation (AF) episodes. In the RAPTURE study, the use of dual-chamber ICDs led to the detection of new AT/AF in 24% of patients compared with 0% with single-chamber devices after 1 year of follow-up.[13] These newly detected AT/AF episodes were predominantly asymptomatic. Although episodes of subclinical AT/AF have been associated with increased risk of stroke,[14,15] it remains unknown if treatment of such episodes would improve clinical outcomes.

Antitachycardia Pacing to Treat Atrial Arrhythmias

Certain dual-chamber ICDs have the ability to deliver atrial ATP and shocks, which has been reported to be effective in terminating atrial tachyarrhythmias in patients who have received an ICD.[16,17] However, most randomized controlled studies of atrial ATP in patients with dual-pacemakers did not show significant reduction of atrial arrhythmia burden.[18–20] Recently, a post hoc analysis of a randomized controlled trial that enrolled patients with nonpermanent AF with a dual-chamber pacing indication suggested that a new-generation atrial ATP algorithm in addition to RV pacing minimization was associated with a lower risk of progressing permanent AF compared with RV pacing minimization alone (hazard ratio [HR] 0.49, $P = .034$).[21] However, this study excluded patients who were ICD candidates.

Device-Related Complications

One concern regarding the use of dual-chamber ICDs is associated risk of complications. A study using the National Cardiovascular Data Registry (NCDR) ICD Registry reported increased odds of periprocedural complications (OR 1.40; $P<.001$) and in-hospital mortality (OR 1.45; $P<.001$) with

dual-chamber versus single-chamber ICD implantation after adjusting for demographics, medical comorbidities, diagnostic test data, and ICD indication.[6] Another study using the NCDR ICD registry linking to Centers for Medicare and Medicaid Services fee-for-service Medicare claims data reported higher risk of device-related complications up to 90 days after implantation with dual-chamber versus single-chamber ICD implantation but similar 1-year mortality and hospitalization outcomes in a propensity-matched cohort.[22] The additional intricacy of atrial lead implantation probably explains the observed increased risk of complication. However, the observational nature of these studies represents a major limitation.

Potential Increased Right Ventricle Pacing

Another concern regarding the utilization of dual-chamber ICDs in patients without pacing indication is raised by The Dual Chamber and VVI Implantable Defibrillator (DAVID) Trial.[23] This trial randomized 506 patients with left ventricular ejection fraction $\leq40\%$ who received a dual-chamber ICD to ventricular backup pacing at 40/min (VVI-40) or dual-chamber rate responsive pacing at 70/min (DDDR-70). The DDDR-70 group had more occurrences of death or hospitalization for new or worsened congestive heart failure compared with the VVI-40 group (relative hazard, 1.61; $P\leq.03$). These adverse events are likely due to the increased RV pacing noted in the dual-chamber ICD group of the DAVID trial. Studies that use pacing algorithms that minimize RV pacing, such as INTRINSIC RV study[24] and OPTION study,[12] demonstrated similar mortality and cardiovascular morbidities in patients who received single-chamber and dual-chamber ICDs.

In summary, the need for atrial or A-V sequential pacing is the only well-established indication for dual-chamber ICD implantation. Although the use of a dual-chamber ICD in patients without such a pacing indication may reduce the rate of inappropriate ICD shock, improvement in clinical outcomes such as hospitalization rate or mortality has yet to be demonstrated. Furthermore, it is not clear if enhanced detection of subclinical AT/AF by the dual-chamber ICD or using atrial ATP to treat such arrhythmias improves clinical outcomes either. Given the uncertain benefit as well as potential complications and increased cost, at this point in time, the use of a dual-chamber ICD cannot be routinely recommended in patients without a pacing indication. In exceptional circumstances, such as slow VTs with significant rate overlapping with SVT whereby inappropriate shocks cannot be adequately reduced with device programming, there may be a role for the dual-chamber ICD to enhance arrhythmia discrimination. However, the specific subgroups of patients in which the benefit of dual-chamber ICD therapy may outweigh the risk remain unknown and should be the focus of future studies.

IMPLANTABLE CARDIOVERTER DEFIBRILLATORS SYSTEM LONGEVITY

Once the decision to implant an ICD has been reached, it is critical to assess the potential duration that the patient will be exposed to ICD therapy. The durability of a particular ICD system should factor into the device selection decision for all patients, but this issue is especially important for younger patients, who are likely to have a defibrillator for decades. It is important to select a durable lead and a generator with long battery life to minimize the number of future generator changeouts, lead revisions, and lead extractions.

Lead Durability

Within the past decade, 2 smaller-caliber ICD leads (<8 French) were withdrawn from the market by the US Food and Drug Administration because of poor durability and lead failure.[25] The Medtronic Sprint Fidelis lead (Medtronic, Minneapolis, MN) was withdrawn in October 2007 because of a 17% failure rate at 5 years because of ineffective shocks and failure to pace caused by a fracture-prone pace-sense conductor.[25] The St. Jude Riata (St. Jude, Saint Paul, MN) lead had redundant conductors to prevent lead failure but was recalled in 2011 because of a higher rate of insulation failure.[26] Failure rates with the Riata lead have been reported as high as 12% to 13% over 54.8 ± 26.3 months of follow-up.[27]

A recent meta-analysis of 17 observational studies assessed the performance of 5 of the most used transvenous ICD (TV-ICD) lead families (Boston Scientific Endotak Reliance [Boston Scientific, Marlborough, MA], Medtronic Sprint Quattro [Medtronic, Minneapolis, MN], Medtronic Sprint Fidelis [Medtronic, Minneapolis, MN], St. Jude Riata [St. Jude, Saint Paul, MN], and St. Jude Durata [St. Jude, Saint Paul, MN]). In this study, 1265 lead failures (defined as externalization of conductors, insulation defect, fracture, or electrical malfunction) occurred over 136,509 lead-years observation (0.93/100 lead-years, 95% confidence interval 0.88–0.98). A higher lead failure rate was demonstrated with the Riata (1.0% per year increase) and Sprint Fidelis (>2.0% per year increase) leads compared with non-recalled leads. Comparisons between

the non-recalled lead families showed similarly low failure rates of the Durata, Endotak, and Quattro leads (0.45% vs 0.36% vs 0.29% incidence per year, respectively).[25] However, the shorter follow-up period of the Durata family lead (6716 lead-years) may obligate further evaluation.

Controversies remain regarding the durability of the Biotronik Linox ICD lead (Biotronik, Berlin, Germany). An estimated cumulative survival probability at 5 years after implant was reported to be 96.3% in a large registry-based study.[28] However, another registry-based study reported that Linox lead failed more frequently than the Durata lead (3.4% vs 0.4%, respectively; $P<.001$) over a median follow-up of 39 months.[29] A retrospective study also reported significantly higher failure rate of Linox lead (3.2% per year) than that of Endotak lead (0.61% per year) ($P = .049$). In this study, the failure rate of Linox lead was comparable to Sprint Fidelis lead (3.4% per year).[30]

Generator Longevity

A study evaluating a multicenter ICD registry between 1998 and 2005 demonstrated that at 5 years from implantation, 26% of the ICDs had not yet been replaced or explanted.[31] Multiple single-center, prospectively analyzed databases have shown that the ICD generator longevity is dependent on the manufacturer, percent of RV pacing, and type of device (VVI-ICD vs DDD-ICD).[32–35] In the late 1990s and early 2000s, Medtronic ICDs (Medtronic, Minneapolis, MN) seemed to have better battery longevity compared with other manufacturers.[32–35] In a large prospective study of 3436 patients in whom 4881 ICDs (44.2% VVI-ICDs, 27.4% DDD-ICDs, 26.3% cardiac resynchronization therapy–ICDs, 2.0% S-ICDs) were implanted from 1994 to 2014, the 6-year longevity of Medtronic ICDs implanted before 2006 was 64.1%, whereas the 6-year longevity of St. Jude Medical (St. Jude, Saint Paul, MN), Boston Scientific (Marlborough, MA), Sorin (Sorin Group, Milan, Italy), and Biotronik (Berlin, Germany) devices implanted during this period was 49.8%, 45.7%, 27.8%, and 10.5%, respectively.[36] For ICDs implanted after 2006, the same study showed that Boston Scientific ICDs displayed the highest 6-year longevity of 98%, whereas 6-year longevity of Sorin, Medtronic, St. Jude Medical, and Biotronik were 77.5%, 72.6%, 60.7%, and 42.1%, respectively.[36] The change in longevity seen in this study may be related to the incorporation of a higher-capacity Lithium Manganese battery into newer Boston Scientific devices, whereas other manufacturers usually use a lower-capacity Lithium Silver Vanadium battery. The overall longevity of the ICDs made by all manufacturers continues to improve over time and likely will continue to change with evolving technology.

A decrease in the percentage of ventricular pacing (VP) was reported to be associated with a decreased risk of generator replacement (HR 0.934 for 10% decrease in VP, P<.0001) in an analysis of a prospective database that included 980 patients (follow-up 58 ± 51 months) with 1502 ICDs.[35] Superior longevity of the single-chamber ICD (62.7% at 6 years after implantation) over the dual-chamber ICD (43.4% at 6 years after implantation) was also reported in the aforementioned prospective study.[36] In summary, the longevity of an ICD seems to be associated with the degree of RV pacing and the type of device implanted, which should be considered when trying to anticipate a generator's lifespan.

DF-1 VERSUS DF-4 IMPLANTABLE CARDIOVERTER DEFIBRILLATORS LEAD

The DF-1 ICD lead divides at the yoke into 1 pace/sense IS-1 low-voltage connector plug and 1 (in single-coil lead) or 2 (in dual-coil lead) DF-1 high-voltage connector plugs (**Fig. 1**). Each of these connector plugs needs to be inserted into a specific port on the device generator header. The proximal end of the DF-4 ICD lead has only 1 connector plug, incorporating up to 2 high-voltage terminals for the defibrillator coils and 2 pace/sense low-voltage terminals (see **Fig. 1**). The DF-4 system also places its seal rings, which

function to isolate the connecting interface between the lead and the header from outside body fluid and tissue, in the generator header instead of on the lead (as the DF-1 system does). This configuration ensures that the seal rings, which could wear down over time, get automatically replaced every time the generator is changed out. There is a concern that the high- and low-voltage terminals of the DF-4 system are located in close proximity and could potentially interfere with 1 another, especially during a high-voltage ICD shock. However, no difference in overall incidence of electrical lead failure between DF-1 and DF-4 connector was reported in an age- and sex-matched controlled study.[37]

This design of the DF-4 system results in smaller ICD header size, less pocket bulk, a simpler connecting process that potentially reduces the risk of terminal pin misconnection, and easier lead dissection and potentially less risk of lead damage during generator replacement. A trend toward shorter procedure time associated with the use of DF-4 system was also reported in an age- and sex-matched controlled study.[37]

A potential drawback of the DF-4 lead design includes less flexibility in lead modification. This issue could be important for patients who have a high defibrillation threshold (DFT) and need the addition of a subcutaneous coil. Such an addition would be easy with a DF-1 lead but requires a bulky adaptor for a DF-4 lead. Similarly, if the pace/sense component of a DF-4 lead

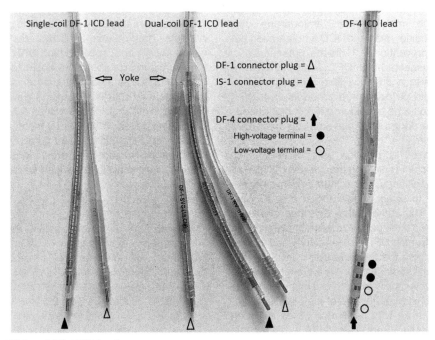

Fig. 1. The DF-1 and DF-4 ICD leads.

malfunctions, a pace/sense lead with an IS-1 lead cannot be easily added to the system.

PATIENT CHARACTERISTICS

There are several patient characteristics that factor into the type of ICD that is selected. These patient characteristics include the presence of certain comorbidities, the likelihood of an elevated DFT, as well as the age and size of the patient.

Certain comorbidities have been associated with higher risk of cardiac implantable electronic device (CIED) infection. In a recent meta-analysis, the most significant of these comorbidities include end-stage renal disease (OR = 8.73 [3.42–22.31]), history of previous device infection (OR = 7.84 [1.94–31.60]), corticosteroid drug use (OR = 3.44 [1.62–7.32]), renal insufficiency (OR = 3.02 [1.38–6.64]), chronic obstructive pulmonary disease (OR = 2.95 [1.78–4.90]), malignancy (OR = 2.23 [1.26–3.95]), diabetes mellitus (OR = 2.08 [1.62–2.67]), and congestive heart failure (OR = 1.65 [1.14–2.39]).[38] In patients with these conditions, the number of leads should be minimized. Although the overall rate of device infection of S-ICDs seems to be similar to TV-ICDs,[39,40] pocket infection associated with S-ICDs is generally easier to manage than endovascular infection associated with TV-ICDs. Thus, S-ICDs may be appropriate in patients at higher risk of CIED.

Certain patient characteristics are known to increase the risk for having high DFTs. These factors include left ventricular systolic dysfunction, younger age, male gender, amiodarone use, habitual cocaine use, and ICD implantation for secondary prevention.[41–43] In the presence of a known or suspected high DFT, a left pectoral implantation with a dual-coil lead and high-output device should be performed. In addition, a DF-1 ICD lead should be considered if a subcutaneous coil must be added to achieve an adequate DFT safety margin.

As discussed above, the patient's age is an important factor in selecting the specific ICD generator and lead or leads. For younger patients, the authors prefer to select a device that has a longer battery life. The authors also will often choose a single-coil lead if the patient does not have risk factors for an elevated DFT to make future lead extraction easier. Last, the S-ICD is also considered for young patients to preserve upper extremity vascular access; however, this is often offset by the large size and (current) short battery life of the S-ICD.

The size of an ICD generator varies between different manufacturers. This is not a major issue in general, but the size of the device relative to

patient's body size can be significant in smaller patients. In these cases, the authors generally try to use the most compact generator possible with the use the DF-4 lead. A potential drawback of a smaller generator size is often shorter battery longevity. With continuing advancement in ICD technology, the sizes of the ICDs made by all manufacturers continue to decrease with time.

SUMMARY

In conclusion, the choice of ICD to be implanted is often a result of a complex decision based on existing data while attempting to account for the relative importance of certain patient attributes and comorbidities along with each device's characteristics.

The authors' approach is to use single-chamber ICDs in almost all primary and secondary prevention patients without a pacing indication. They use device programming (eg, higher VT detection rate, prolonged detection duration, appropriate SVT-VT discriminators, routine use of antitachycardia pacing) to reduce the risk of inappropriate ICD shock. They use dual-chamber ICDs only in patients undergoing ICD implantation who require atrial or A-V sequential pacing, and they enable algorithms that minimize RV pacing in those patients requiring atrial pacing but with normal AV conduction. Because atrial lead sensing plays a pivotal role in dual-chamber SVT discrimination algorithms, the atrial lead should be carefully positioned to minimize far-field R-wave oversensing and ensure adequate P-wave amplitude.

The authors use DF-4 ICD leads in most of their patients. They reserve DF-1 systems for patients with a known or suspected high DFT. ICD system longevity and size should be optimized according to each individual patient characteristics. The authors' general rule is to use the device with the best longevity that is as small as feasible. Given continuing development of ICD technology, physicians who implant ICDs must be aware of current device specifications and projections in order to select the most optimal devices for each patient.

REFERENCES

1. Antiarrhythmics versus Implantable Defibrillators Investigators. A comparison of antiarrhythmic-drug therapy with implantable defibrillators in patients resuscitated from near-fatal ventricular arrhythmias. N Engl J Med 1997;337(22):1576–83.
2. Moss AJ, Hall WJ, Cannom DS, et al. Improved survival with an implanted defibrillator in patients with coronary disease at high risk for ventricular arrhythmia. Multicenter Automatic Defibrillator

Implantation Trial Investigators. N Engl J Med 1996; 335(26):1933–40.

3. Buxton AE, Lee KL, Fisher JD, et al. A randomized study of the prevention of sudden death in patients with coronary artery disease. Multicenter Unsustained Tachycardia Trial Investigators. N Engl J Med 1999;341(25):1882–90.

4. Moss AJ, Zareba W, Hall WJ, et al. Prophylactic implantation of a defibrillator in patients with myocardial infarction and reduced ejection fraction. N Engl J Med 2002;346(12):877–83.

5. Bardy GH, Lee KL, Mark DB, et al. Amiodarone or an implantable cardioverter-defibrillator for congestive heart failure. N Engl J Med 2005;352(3):225–37.

6. Dewland TA, Pellegrini CN, Wang Y, et al. Dual-chamber implantable cardioverter-defibrillator selection is associated with increased complication rates and mortality among patients enrolled in the NCDR implantable cardioverter-defibrillator registry. J Am Coll Cardiol 2011;58(10):1007–13.

7. Deisenhofer I, Kolb C, Ndrepepa G, et al. Do current dual chamber cardioverter defibrillators have advantages over conventional single chamber cardioverter defibrillators in reducing inappropriate therapies? A randomized, prospective study. J Cardiovasc Electrophysiol 2001;12(2):134–42.

8. Theuns DA, Klootwijk AP, Goedhart DM, et al. Prevention of inappropriate therapy in implantable cardioverter-defibrillators: results of a prospective, randomized study of tachyarrhythmia detection algorithms. J Am Coll Cardiol 2004;44(12):2362–7.

9. Kolb C, Deisenhofer I, Schmieder S, et al. Long-term follow-up of patients supplied with single-chamber or dual-chamber cardioverter defibrillators. Pacing Clin Electrophysiol 2006;29(9):946–52.

10. Friedman PA, McClelland RL, Bamlet WR, et al. Dual-chamber versus single-chamber detection enhancements for implantable defibrillator rhythm diagnosis: the detect supraventricular tachycardia study. Circulation 2006;113(25):2871–9.

11. Almendral J, Arribas F, Wolpert C, et al. Dual-chamber defibrillators reduce clinically significant adverse events compared with single-chamber devices: results from the DATAS (Dual chamber and Atrial Tachyarrhythmias Adverse events Study) trial. Europace 2008;10(5):528–35.

12. Kolb C, Sturmer M, Sick P, et al. Reduced risk for inappropriate implantable cardioverter-defibrillator shocks with dual-chamber therapy compared with single-chamber therapy: results of the randomized OPTION study. JACC Heart Fail 2014; 2(6):611–9.

13. Friedman PA, Bradley D, Koestler C, et al. A prospective randomized trial of single- or dual-chamber implantable cardioverter-defibrillators to minimize inappropriate shock risk in primary sudden

cardiac death prevention. Europace 2014;16(10): 1460–8.

14. Healey JS, Connolly SJ, Gold MR, et al. Subclinical atrial fibrillation and the risk of stroke. N Engl J Med 2012;366(2):120–9.

15. Swiryn S, Orlov MV, Benditt DG, et al. Clinical implications of brief device-detected atrial tachyarrhythmias in a cardiac rhythm management device population: results from the registry of atrial tachycardia and atrial fibrillation episodes. Circulation 2016;134(16):1130–40.

16. Ricci R, Pignalberi C, Disertori M, et al. Efficacy of a dual chamber defibrillator with atrial antitachycardia functions in treating spontaneous atrial tachyarrhythmias in patients with life-threatening ventricular tachyarrhythmias. Eur Heart J 2002; 23(18):1471–9.

17. Adler SW 2nd, Wolpert C, Warman EN, et al. Efficacy of pacing therapies for treating atrial tachyarrhythmias in patients with ventricular arrhythmias receiving a dual-chamber implantable cardioverter defibrillator. Circulation 2001;104(8):887–92.

18. Lee MA, Weachter R, Pollak S, et al. The effect of atrial pacing therapies on atrial tachyarrhythmia burden and frequency: results of a randomized trial in patients with bradycardia and atrial tachyarrhythmias. J Am Coll Cardiol 2003;41(11): 1926–32.

19. Mont L, Ruiz-Granell R, Martinez JG, et al. Impact of anti-tachycardia pacing on atrial fibrillation burden when added on top of preventive pacing algorithms: results of the prevention or termination (POT) trial. Europace 2008;10(1):28–34.

20. Gillis AM, Morck M, Exner DV, et al. Impact of atrial antitachycardia pacing and atrial pace prevention therapies on atrial fibrillation burden over long-term follow-up. Europace 2009;11(8):1041–7.

21. Boriani G, Tukkie R, Manolis AS, et al. Atrial antitachycardia pacing and managed ventricular pacing in bradycardia patients with paroxysmal or persistent atrial tachyarrhythmias: the MINERVA randomized multicentre international trial. Eur Heart J 2014;35(35):2352–62.

22. Peterson PN, Varosy PD, Heidenreich PA, et al. Association of single- vs dual-chamber ICDs with mortality, readmissions, and complications among patients receiving an ICD for primary prevention. JAMA 2013;309(19):2025–34.

23. Wilkoff BL, Cook JR, Epstein AE, et al. Dual-chamber pacing or ventricular backup pacing in patients with an implantable defibrillator: the dual chamber and VVI implantable defibrillator (DAVID) trial. JAMA 2002;288(24):3115–23.

24. Olshansky B, Day JD, Moore S, et al. Is dual-chamber programming inferior to single-chamber programming in an implantable cardioverter-defibrillator? Results of the INTRINSIC RV (Inhibition

of Unnecessary RV Pacing with AVSH in ICDs) study. Circulation 2007;115(1):9–16.

25. Providencia R, Kramer DB, Pimenta D, et al. Transvenous implantable cardioverter-defibrillator (ICD) lead performance: a meta-analysis of observational studies. J Am Heart Assoc 2015;4(11) [pii:e002418].

26. Hauser RG. Please leave the reliable ICD leads alone. Heart Rhythm 2013;10(4):562–3.

27. Fazal IA, Shepherd EJ, Tynan M, et al. Comparison of Sprint Fidelis and Riata defibrillator lead failure rates. Int J Cardiol 2013;168(2):848–52.

28. Good ED, Cakulev I, Orlov MV, et al. Long-term evaluation of Biotronik Linox and Linox(smart) implantable cardioverter defibrillator leads. J Cardiovasc Electrophysiol 2016;27(6):735–42.

29. Padfield GJ, Steinberg C, Karim SS, et al. Early failure of the Biotronik Linox implantable cardioverter defibrillator lead. J Cardiovasc Electrophysiol 2015;26(3):274–81.

30. Kawada S, Nishii N, Morimoto Y, et al. Comparison of longevity and clinical outcomes of implantable cardioverter-defibrillator leads among manufacturers. Heart Rhythm 2017;14(10):1496–503.

31. Hauser RG, Hayes DL, Epstein AE, et al. Multicenter experience with failed and recalled implantable cardioverter-defibrillator pulse generators. Heart Rhythm 2006;3(6):640–4.

32. Biffi M, Ziacchi M, Bertini M, et al. Longevity of implantable cardioverter-defibrillators: implications for clinical practice and health care systems. Europace 2008;10(11):1288–95.

33. Schaer BA, Koller MT, Sticherling C, et al. Longevity of implantable cardioverter-defibrillators, influencing factors, and comparison to industry-projected longevity. Heart Rhythm 2009;6(12):1737–43.

34. Thijssen J, Borleffs CJ, van Rees JB, et al. Implantable cardioverter-defibrillator longevity under clinical circumstances: an analysis according to device type, generation, and manufacturer. Heart Rhythm 2012;9(4):513–9.

35. Horlbeck FW, Mellert F, Kreuz J, et al. Real-world data on the lifespan of implantable cardioverter-defibrillators depending on manufacturers and the amount of ventricular pacing. J Cardiovasc Electrophysiol 2012;23(12):1336–42.

36. von Gunten S, Schaer BA, Yap SC, et al. Longevity of implantable cardioverter defibrillators: a comparison among manufacturers and over time. Europace 2016;18(5):710–7.

37. Forleo GB, Di Biase L, Mantica M, et al. First clinical experience with the new four-pole standard connector for high-voltage ICD leads. Early results of a multicenter comparison with conventional implant outcomes. J Interv Card Electrophysiol 2013;38(1):11–8.

38. Polyzos KA, Konstantelias AA, Falagas ME. Risk factors for cardiac implantable electronic device infection: a systematic review and meta-analysis. Europace 2015;17(5):767–77.

39. Chue CD, Kwok CS, Wong CW, et al. Efficacy and safety of the subcutaneous implantable cardioverter defibrillator: a systematic review. Heart 2017; 103(17):1315–22.

40. Brouwer TF, Yilmaz D, Lindeboom R, et al. Long-term clinical outcomes of subcutaneous versus transvenous implantable defibrillator therapy. J Am Coll Cardiol 2016;68(19):2047–55.

41. Shih MJ, Kakodkar SA, Kaid Y, et al. Reassessing risk factors for high defibrillation threshold: the EF-SAGA risk score and implications for device testing. Pacing Clin Electrophysiol 2016;39(5):483–9.

42. Al-Atia B, Vandenberk B, Voros G, et al. Predictors of a high defibrillation threshold test during routine ICD implantation. Acta Cardiol 2017. [Epub ahead of print].

43. Chen J, Naseem RH, Obel O, et al. Habitual cocaine use is associated with high defibrillation threshold during ICD implantation. J Cardiovasc Electrophysiol 2007;18(7):722–5.

Management of Device Infections

Khalid Aljabri, MD, Ann Garlitski, MD, Jonathan Weinstock, MD,
Christopher Madias, MD*

KEYWORDS

- Pacemaker • Defibrillator • Infection • Endocarditis

KEY POINTS

- The rate of cardiac implantable electronic device (CIED) infection has increased disproportionately to that of implantation.
- Device-related infections are most commonly due to perioperative contamination. Notably, early pocket re-exploration and upgrade procedures are at particularly high risk for infection.
- Risk factors for CIED infection include diabetes, heart failure, and renal disease.
- Confirmed infection of a CIED requires prompt removal of the entire system (generator and leads) in combination with antimicrobial therapy.
- An understanding of the risks of CIED infection and using preventive measures is critical for the implanting physician.

INTRODUCTION

Because of the expanding indications and longer life expectancy, implantations of cardiac implantable electronic devices (CIEDs) have increased dramatically over the past 2 decades. Infection represents a potential complication of CIED implantation that can have severe consequences. Although most infections are limited to the generator pocket, systemic infection and endocarditis associated with device implantation has been recognized since the early days of permanent pacemaker (PPM) placement and occurs in nearly 10% of device-related infections.[1] Such complex infections can be associated with substantial morbidity and mortality. The rate of CIED infection has increased disproportionately to that of implantation.[2,3] Here the authors provide a contemporary review of the pathogenesis, management, and prevention of CIED infection.

PATHOGENESIS AND MICROBIOLOGY

Device-related infections are most commonly due to perioperative contamination, either during initial implantation or at times of subsequent surgical manipulation (eg, generator replacement).[4] Infection can also occur because of a breach of the skin barrier in the setting of generator or lead erosion. A less common mechanism of CIED infection is the hematogenous spread of bacteria from another site with secondary involvement of the device components.[5]

Staphylococcal species are the predominant organisms isolated in large series of CIED infection, accounting for 60% to 80% of cases (**Fig. 1**).[1,6,7] Of these, *Staphylococcus aureus* and coagulase-negative staphylococci are the most frequent culpable isolated organisms. Gram-positive bacilli (*Corynebacterium* spp, *Propionibacterium* spp), *Pseudomonas* spp, and Enterobacteriaceae are less commonly involved in CIED infections. Polymicrobial involvement has been described. Rarely, fungi (*Candida* spp) or molds are identified as causative organisms.[7,8] A minority of patients will have negative cultures despite signs and symptoms of clinical infection, including some patients that demonstrate localized inflammation of the generator pocket or device erosion.[6]

Disclosure Statement: The authors have no disclosures.
The Cardiovascular Center, Tufts Medical Center, Tufts University School of Medicine, 800 Washington Street, Boston, MA 02111, USA
* Corresponding author. Tufts Medical Center, 800 Washington Street, Boston, MA 02111.
E-mail address: cmadias@tuftsmedicalcenter.org

Card Electrophysiol Clin 10 (2018) 153–162
https://doi.org/10.1016/j.ccep.2017.11.016
1877-9182/18/© 2017 Elsevier Inc. All rights reserved.

cardiacEP.theclinics.com

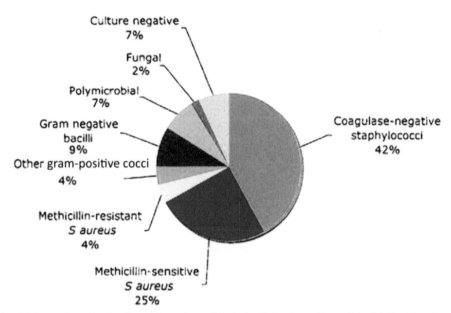

Fig. 1. Microbiology of cardiac implantable endocardial device infections. (*From* Sohail MR, Uslan DZ, Khan AH, et al. Management and outcome of permanent pacemaker and implantable cardioverter-defibrillator infections. J Am Coll Cardiol 2007;49(18):1853; with permission.)

EPIDEMIOLOGY (INCIDENCE AND RISK FACTORS)

It is difficult to accurately estimate the exact incidence of CIED infection because of the universal deficiencies in standardized registries and limitations associated with long-term surveillance. Reported incidence rates differ among observational studies because of the variation in definitions and follow-up duration. Infection risk after PPM implant is estimated to be 0.5% to 1.0% within the first 12 months.[9–11] Implantable cardioverter defibrillators (ICDs) carry a higher risk of infection than PPMs, although this higher risk might be partially explained by the fact that ICD patients are generally sicker and carry more comorbidities than PPM patients.[12] Infection risk also seems to increase in conjunction with the procedural complexity of the implanted CIED system.[13–16] In an analysis of device-related infections in the National Cardiovascular Data Registry (NCDR) ICD database, the infection rates were 1.4%, 1.5%, and 2.0% for single, dual, and biventricular ICDs, respectively.[16] CIED replacements and upgrades are associated with an even higher risk of infection than de novo implants.[10,16] In the NCDR, generator replacement had a higher rate of infection compared with initial implant (1.9% vs 1.6%; P<.001).[16] Reimplantation or device upgrade has been independently associated with infection in both ICD (odds ratio [OR] 1.354 [95% confidence interval [CI], 1.196–1.533; P<.0001]) and PPM patients (OR 2.79 [95% CI 2.38–3.28; P<.001]).[10,16]

The rate of CIED infection seems to be increasing.[17] It is thought that expanded indications for CIED implantation (ICD and biventricular devices) combined with an older and sicker patient population, in part, contributes to this increased rate. Multiple risk factors and comorbidities have been associated with CIED infections in several case series. These factors can be grouped into patient-, procedure-, or device-related factors (**Table 1**).[18] In a contemporary cohort of patients with CIED infection, 7 independent risk factors predicted infection: early pocket re-exploration, male sex, diabetes, upgrade procedure, heart failure, hypertension, and glomerular filtration rate less than 60 mL/min.[19] In a multicenter, French nationwide, prospective cohort study, secondary procedures, such as pulse generator replacements, were associated with an almost 2-fold risk of device infection as compared with de novo implants. Notably, early reinterventions for hematoma or lead dislodgment were the leading risk factors of infection in this cohort.[9]

CLINICAL PRESENTATION AND DIAGNOSIS

CIED infection can have varying presentation, ranging from isolated superficial infection to more complex deep infection (**Table 2**).[5] Uncomplicated pocket infections involve the subcutaneous pulse generator pocket and the extravascular portion of the transvenous leads. Typical pocket infection signs are local erythema, warmth, pain, and swelling. Less commonly, adherence of skin to the device with incipient or overt erosion of skin

Table 1
Risk factors associated with cardiac device-related infection

Patient-Related Factors	Procedure-Related Factors	Device-Related Factors
Age >60 y	Lack of antibiotic prophylaxis	Defibrillator (vs pacemaker)
Male sex	Device replacement/revision	Dual chamber (vs single chamber)
Chronic obstructive	Early reintervention	Biventricular device
pulmonary disease	Procedure duration	Abdominal pocket
Congestive heart failure	Operator experience	Epicardial leads
Diabetes	Postimplant hematoma	
Renal disease (dialysis)		
Steroid use		
Prior infection		
Presence of a central venous		
catheter		
Anticoagulant use		
Preoperative fever		

with draining sinus can be observed (**Fig. 2**). Any sign or symptom from the device pocket should raise suspicion of infection. Percutaneous aspiration of the device pocket is not recommended because of the lack of adequate diagnostic yield and the potential of introducing microorganisms into the pocket.[1,20] Early postimplantation inflammation can easily be misperceived as infection, as it is also characterized by isolated erythema of the pocket site; however, this entity occurs very early after device implantation (<7 days) and is usually secondary to local inflammatory skin reaction to disinfectants or wound dressings. Postimplantation inflammation should not be treated as an infection; however, close monitoring for signs of developing infection might be warranted.[21] Importantly, erosion through the skin barrier of any portion of the pulse generator or leads signifies definite infection.[20]

Complicated pocket infections and lead infections involve intravascular (or epicardial) portions of the device. CIED infections can be more difficult to diagnose, when there is absence of overt pocket involvement.[22] Isolated lead infections, including those with endocardial involvement, can have a subacute presentation with the most common symptoms related to systemic infection, including fevers, chills, sweats, malaise, and anorexia. The incidence of bacteremia or endocarditis associated with CIED infection has been reported between 0.06% and 0.6% per year or 1.14 per 1000 device.[13,23] Embolic phenomenon should raise the suspicion for lead or endocardial involvement.[21] Notably, CIED with concomitant valve infection was associated with high in-hospital mortality in the International Collaboration of Endocarditis-Prospective Cohort Study (OR 3.31, 95% CI, 1.71 – 6.39; P = .04).[23]

When CIED infection is suspected, at least 2 sets of blood cultures should be drawn before the initiation of antibiotics.[1] Positive blood cultures should bolster concern for complicated CIED infection, especially if staphylococcal species are isolated. Echocardiographic evaluation is indicated when CIED infection is suspected. Transthoracic echocardiography (TTE) can be limited in excluding the diagnosis of lead-related endocarditis. Transesophageal echocardiography (TEE) should be obtained in bacteremic patients, or in those in whom endocardial involvement might be suspected despite a nondiagnostic TTE.[1] TEE can visualize vegetation associated with device leads, as well as assessing for endocardial vegetation, abscess, or other cardiac complications.[24] Because of the proximity with device leads, the tricuspid valve is the most frequent site of endocardial involvement.[23] TEE has a sensitivity of more than 90% for diagnosis of endocarditis; however, the specificity is not 100% for lead-related endocarditis and false positives can occur.[24] Notably, thrombi and fibrous strands associated with device leads can be found in patients without clinical evidence of endocarditis. In fact, lead-associated masses can be commonly identified during TTE/TEE; when endocarditis is not the primary indication for obtaining the imaging, these findings are highly unlikely to represent an infectious process.[25]

Other imaging modalities can also aid in the diagnosis of CIED-associated endocarditis. PET using 18F-labeled fluorodeoxyglucose computed tomography (CT) can be useful in the diagnosis of endocarditis associated with CIED infections, particularly in bacteremic patients with nondiagnostic echocardiograms.[26] Single-photon emission CT with CT scintigraphy with radiolabeled white blood cells might be another useful diagnostic modality in the evaluation of CIED-associated endocarditis and septic embolism.[27]

At the time of device removal, culture of the generator pocket site and lead tips can aid in

Table 2
Classification of cardiac implantable electronic device infections

Classification	Definition
Early postimplantation inflammation	Erythema affects the generator implantation incision site, without purulent exudate, dehiscence, fluctuance, or systemic signs of infection, occurring within 30 d of implantation; there is an allergic reaction to local dressing/skin preparation included in this group; close observation may be required, but antimicrobial therapy is not necessarily indicated. A small localized area of erythema (<1 cm) and/or purulence associated with a suture (stitch abscess) is included in this group, and this should resolve with removal of the suture and a short course of antimicrobial therapy, if clinically indicated.
Uncomplicated generator pocket infection	There is absence of symptoms or signs of systemic infection AND negative blood cultures WITH the following: 1. Spreading cellulitis affecting the generator site AND/OR 2. Incision site purulent exudate (excluding simple stitch abscess) AND/OR 3. Wound dehiscence AND/OR 4. Erosion through the skin with exposure of the generator or leads AND/OR 5. Fluctuance (abscess) or fistula formation
Complicated generator pocket infection	There is a generator pocket infection (as previously outlined) WITH the following: 1. Evidence of lead or endocardial involvement AND/OR 2. Systemic signs or symptoms of infection AND/OR 3. Positive blood cultures
Lead infection	
Definite	There are symptoms or signs of systemic infection AND the following: 1. Echocardiography consistent with vegetation attached to the leads AND presence of major Duke microbiological criteria OR 2. Culture, histology, or molecular evidence of infection on explanted lead
Possible	There are symptoms or signs of systemic infection AND the following: 1. Echocardiography consistent with vegetation attached to leads BUT no major Duke microbiological criteria present OR 2. Major Duke microbiological criteria present BUT no echocardiographic evidence of lead vegetation
Device-associated native or prosthetic valve endocarditis	The Duke criteria for definite endocarditis are satisfied with echocardiographic evidence of valve involvement in patients with CIED.

Summary of classification as proposed by the joint Working Party project, on behalf of the British Society of Antimicrobial Chemotherapy, British Heart Rhythm Society, British Cardiovascular Society, British Heart Valve Society, and British Society for Echocardiography.

Data from Sandoe JA, Barlow G, Chambers JB, et al. Guidelines for the diagnosis, prevention and management of implantable cardiac electronic device infection. Report of a joint Working Party project on behalf of the British Society for Antimicrobial Chemotherapy (BSAC, host organization), British Heart Rhythm Society (BHRS), British Cardiovascular Society (BCS), British Heart Valve Society (BHVS) and British Society for Echocardiography (BSE). J Antimicrob Chemother 2015;70(2):334–5; with permission.

identifying causative organisms and guiding antibiotic therapy. In the absence of frank pus, pocket tissue culture during surgical removal might be more effective than pocket swab culture for the identification of pathogenic organisms.[28] Although culture of lead tips is recommended, it must be realized that contamination of leads can occur with extraction through an infected pocket. Contamination of leads likely explains negative blood cultures and the lack of systemic signs or symptoms of infection in some patients with uncomplicated pocket infection and positive lead tip cultures.[1]

MANAGEMENT

Early superficial or incisional inflammation of the pocket site without signs suggestive of device involvement, no fluctuance, discharge, or dehiscence, does not necessarily require removal. An empirical 7- to 10-day course of antimicrobial therapy with staphylococcal coverage can be attempted with close follow-up for clinical improvement.[1,5] If there are signs of persistent inflammation despite such a trial, generator involvement is likely.

Confirmed infection of a CIED requires prompt removal of the entire system (generator and leads)

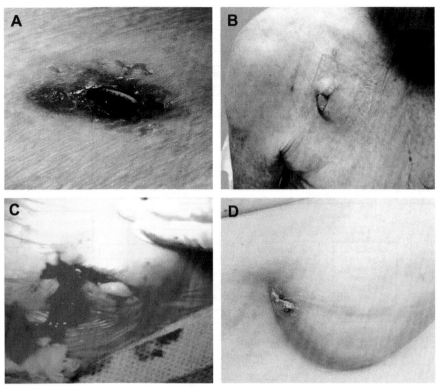

Fig. 2. Adherence between the device and skin with overt perforation of the device (*A*) and leads (*B*) representing pocket infection. Pus at the site of surgical incision during device removal (*C*). Adherence between a subcutaneous ICD generator and skin with imminent perforation (*D*).

in combination with antimicrobial therapy (**Fig. 3**). Antibiotics should be initiated after obtaining at least 2 sets of independent blood cultures. Initial therapy should include broad-spectrum antibiotics with staphylococcal coverage, which could be tailored according to culture results and organism sensitivities. Because of the high incidence of oxacillin-resistant staphylococcus species, vancomycin should be administered as the initial therapy. Infections due to oxacillin-susceptible staphylococcal species can be treated with cefazolin or nafcillin alone with discontinuation of vancomycin. Vancomycin should be continued in patients who are not candidates for beta-lactam antibiotic therapy and those with infections due to oxacillin-resistant staphylococci.[1,5]

Data to guide optimal duration of antibiotic therapy are lacking. The duration of antimicrobial therapy is recommended to be 10 to 14 days after CIED removal for an uncomplicated pocket infection or device erosion.[1,5] After CIED removal, therapy can be switched to an oral agent once speciation and susceptibility results have been obtained. At least 2 weeks of intravenous antibiotic therapy following device removal is required for patients with blood stream

infection. Persistent bacteremia (>24 hours) after device removal warrants a minimum of 4 weeks of antibiotic therapy, even if TEE is negative for endocarditis. The duration of antimicrobial therapy should be at least 4 to 6 weeks if endocardial infection is confirmed.[1,29]

Conservative therapy without complete system removal is associated with unacceptably high recurrence rates of infection.[6,30] Device or lead erosion with exposure of the system through the skin should be treated as an infection with required removal. Pre-erosion associated with skin inflammation or granulation might also be a manifestation of infection requiring explantation.[5] Lead removal can most commonly be performed transvenously and is the preferred approach in most cases. CIED infection is the most common indication of transvenous lead extraction with high success rates of complete system removal.[31] Transvenous lead extraction should be performed in high-volume centers, by experienced operators, with the presence of surgical backup.[31] The size of vegetation identified by echocardiography might influence the method of lead extraction, with larger vegetation requiring surgical extraction. Open surgical removal should be considered for large lead-associated

A

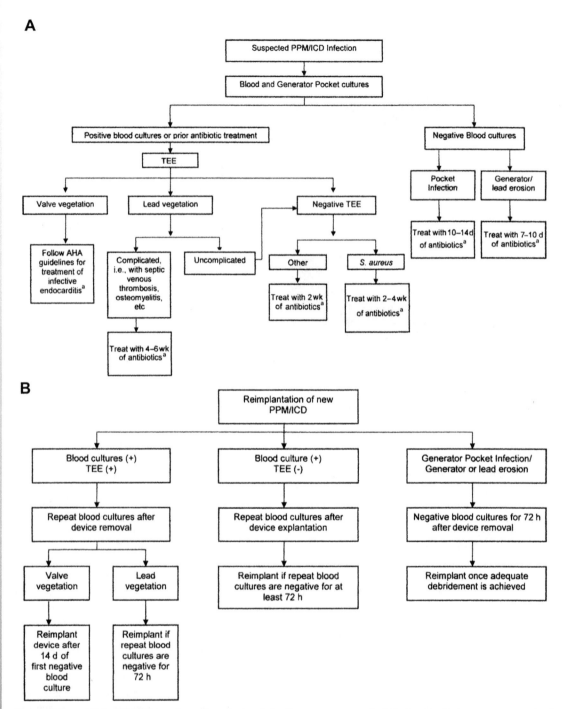

Fig. 3. Mayo Clinic algorithm of cardiac device infection management: (*A*) Approach to management of adults with PPM/ICD infection. (*B*) Guidelines for reimplantation of new device in patients with PPM/ICD infection. [a]Duration of antibiotics should be counted from the day of device explantation. AHA, American Heart Association. (*From* Sohail MR, Uslan DZ, Khan AH, et al. Management and outcome of permanent pacemaker and implantable cardioverter-defibrillator infections. J Am Coll Cardiol 2007;49(18):1857; with permission.)

vegetation (>20 mm) and when valve surgery might be indicated for other reasons.[5]

The risks and benefits of reimplantation need to be assessed very carefully for patients with CIED infection. Up to one-third of patients might not require reimplantation, as clinical circumstances might have changed since the initial implant.[6] Data to define the optimal time for reimplantation are lacking. The timing of reimplantation can be influenced by the causative organism, the severity of the infection, and the clinical indication for CIED (eg, pacemaker dependence). In complex CIED infection, safe reimplantation can be considered when blood cultures are confirmed negative (for at least 72 hours). For patients with transvenous ICD infections requiring reimplantation who do not have pacing indications, strong consideration should be given to implantation of a subcutaneous ICD (S-ICD).[32] Implantation of a leadless pacemaker might be considered for pacemaker patients with prior pocket infections, especially in those who do not require maintenance of atrioventricular synchrony.[33] If another transvenous device is necessary, implantation should be performed on the contralateral side from the infected device.

PREVENTION OF CARDIAC IMPLANTABLE ELECTRONIC DEVICE INFECTION
Preoperative Prevention

Preoperative risk assessment should begin with identification of higher-risk patients and the institution of appropriate steps to minimize the risk. Fever within 24 hours before a CIED implant is associated with an increased risk of infection.[9] Strong consideration should be made to delaying elective implantation in the setting of fever until an underlying infection is either ruled out or appropriately managed.

Postoperative pocket hematomas are associated with a significantly higher risk of infection.[18,34] Therefore, special consideration must be taken into perioperative management of patients who might be at an increased bleeding risk (eg, patients taking antiplatelet agents and/or oral anticoagulants). With data suggesting that bridging anticoagulation (with heparin or low-molecular-weight heparin) is associated with an unacceptably high incidence of bleeding, there has been a strong push to avoid this practice when possible.[35] In patients taking vitamin K antagonists (VKAs) with a high risk of thromboembolism, continuation of VKA has been associated with a marked decrease in the incidence of pocket hematoma when compared with bridging anticoagulation with heparin.[36,37] With regard to direct oral anticoagulants (DOACs), the current data are limited to recommend a best standard of care. Current practice generally includes stopping DOACs 24 to 48 hours before the procedure and restarting them within 24 to 48 hours afterward (depending on the thromboembolic risk) without bridging.[38,39] The results of ongoing randomized trials will assess the relative risk and benefit of uninterrupted versus interrupted DOAC at the time of CIED implant.[40] Dual antiplatelet therapy can increase the estimated odds of bleeding by 5.0 (95% CI, 3.0–8.3).[35] Consideration should be given to delaying elective CIED implantation until dual antiplatelet therapy is no longer indicated.[12] However, when clinically necessary, and with appropriate intraoperative care, CIED implantation can be performed safely in patients on uninterrupted dual antiplatelet therapy.[41]

Operative Prevention

Meticulous attention to the sterile technique should be used by physicians and any support staff involved in device implantation. Preoperative antiseptic preparation of the skin at the implant site should be performed. Preoperative skin cleansing with chlorhexidine-alcohol has been shown to be more protective than povidone-iodine for the prevention of superficial and deep surgical wound infections[42]; however, no differences in the antiseptic effects of these two agents were reported in one series of CIED implantation.[43] An ongoing clinical trial is comparing the effectiveness of these two agents for prevention of infection in patients undergoing biventricular device implantation.[44]

Before the implant of any foreign device, systemic antibiotic prophylaxis is generally recommended. Antibiotic prophylaxis within 1 hour before CIED implantation is effective at reducing surgical site infection.[45,46] Dosing regimens commonly include intravenous administration of a first-generation cephalosporin, such as cefazolin 1 to 2 g. In the case of cephalosporin allergy or in patients with a documented history of colonization with methicillin-resistant staphylococci, vancomycin 1 g intravenously can be administered within 1 to 2 hours of the surgical incision. In the case of allergy to cephalosporins and vancomycin, daptomycin, clindamycin, or linezolid are alternative options.[1]

Besides systemic antibiotic prophylaxis, many implanting physicians use accompanying strategies to lessen the infectious risk. One such strategy is irrigation of the pocket before closure. No difference in CIED infection rate was shown in a single center experience between clindamycin and saline solution irrigation.[47] Another study showed that topical antibiotics (povidone-iodine or neomycin) applied after closure of the surgical incision did not significantly reduce CIED infection, in combination with preprocedural intravenous antibiotics.[48]

Randomized trials have demonstrated that catheter-associated infections can be reduced by rifampin/minocycline-coated catheters.[49] A recently explored approach to the prevention of

CIED infection has been the placement of the CIED in a minocycline/rifampin-eluting antibacterial envelope that slowly releases antibiotics into the generator pocket over a 7-day period.[50] Although now approved by the Food and Drug Administration, large multicenter prospective randomized trials are still lacking; however, some studies have shown a clinical benefit by reducing infection rates in high-risk patients with ICDs or biventricular ICDs undergoing an upgrade or early (within 2 weeks) pocket re-exploration.[19]

Postoperative Prevention

Empirical postoperative antibiotic therapy is not generally recommended, though continues to be used in many centers. Practice guidelines advocate early patient follow-up in a clinic setting as well as thorough patient education to achieve early identification of CIED-related infectious complications and appropriate wound healing.[1] As early reoperation is a significant risk for CIED infection, postoperative hematomas should only be evacuated if it is feared that excessive skin tension is affecting wound healing or if there is impending wound dehiscence.[14] Needle aspiration is discouraged in order to avoid the risk of introducing skin flora into the pocket and the subsequent risk of infection. Antimicrobial prophylaxis for the prevention of CIED infection is not necessary for dental or other invasive procedures not directly related to device manipulation.[1]

EMERGING CONSIDERATIONS

Leadless pacemakers have been developed to decrease complications associated with traditional transvenous systems. Leadless pacemakers are expected to reduce the risk of CIED infection because of the small size, lack of proximity/communication to a cutaneous incision, and late encapsulation of the device.[51] In recent registries, leadless pacemakers have shown an exceedingly low infection rate (<1%).[52] In the recently published postapproval registry that tracked 795 patients, sepsis was reported in only 1 instance within 48 hours of the implant procedure and was successfully treated using intravenous antibiotics, without the need for device removal.[52] Leadless pacemakers offer an alternative option for patients with severe device infection, especially in those with blocked venous access or for those who are pacemaker dependent.[53]

The S-ICD was developed to offer adequate protection from sudden cardiac death without the risks/complications of transvenous leads.[54] The concept of the S-ICD is particularly attractive for patients with limited or no vascular access, in those who are at high risk or who have had prior intravascular infections, and in younger patients. In the pooled analysis of the IDE (Investigational Device Exemption) study and the EFFORTLESS (Evaluation oF FactORs ImpacTing CLinical Outcome and Cost EffectiveneSS) registry superficial/incision infection treated conservatively occurred in 0.3% of patients and infection requiring device removal or revision occurred in 1.7% of patients.[55] There was no evidence that patients implanted with the S-ICD after transvenous ICD explantation for infection were more likely to experience a subsequent reinfection.[32] Guidelines for the management of transvenous cardiac rhythm device infection do not apply to the S-ICD, as the consequences of infection and failure of conservative management are less concerning. Device infection and erosion can sometimes be treated successfully with antibiotics and pocket/electrode revision; however, if S-ICD removal is required, this is a less morbid procedure, as the S-ICD system lacks an intravascular component.[56] S-ICD should be considered in patients who are at high risk of infection and have no pacing indications.

REFERENCES

1. Baddour LM, Epstein AE, Erickson CC, et al. Update on cardiovascular implantable electronic device infections and their management: a scientific statement from the American Heart Association. Circulation 2010;121(3):458–77.
2. Voigt A, Shalaby A, Saba S. Continued rise in rates of cardiovascular implantable electronic device infections in the United States: temporal trends and causative insights. Pacing Clin Electrophysiol 2010;33(4): 414–9.
3. Greenspon AJ, Patel JD, Lau E, et al. 16-year trends in the infection burden for pacemakers and implantable cardioverter-defibrillators in the United States 1993 to 2008. J Am Coll Cardiol 2011; 58(10):1001–6.
4. Da Costa A, Lelièvre H, Kirkorian G, et al. Role of the preaxillary flora in pacemaker infections: a prospective study. Circulation 1998;97(18):1791–5.
5. Sandoe JA, Barlow G, Chambers JB, et al. Guidelines for the diagnosis, prevention and management of implantable cardiac electronic device infection. Report of a joint working party project on behalf of the British Society for Antimicrobial Chemotherapy (BSAC, host organization), British Heart Rhythm Society (BHRS), British Cardiovascular Society (BCS), British Heart Valve Society (BHVS) and British Society for Echocardiography (BSE). J Antimicrob Chemother 2015;70(2):325–59.
6. Sohail MR, Uslan DZ, Khan AH, et al. Management and outcome of permanent pacemaker and implantable cardioverter-defibrillator infections. J Am Coll Cardiol 2007;49(18):1851–9.

7. Bongiorni MG, Tascini C, Tagliaferri E, et al. Microbiology of cardiac implantable electronic device infections. Europace 2012;14(9):1334–9.

8. Lekkerkerker JC, van Nieuwkoop C, Trines SA, et al. Risk factors and time delay associated with cardiac device infections: Leiden device registry. Heart 2009;95(9):715–20.

9. Klug D, Balde M, Pavin D, et al. Risk factors related to infections of implanted pacemakers and cardioverter-defibrillators: results of a large prospective study. Circulation 2007;116(12):1349–55.

10. Johansen JB, Jørgensen OD, Møller M, et al. Infection after pacemaker implantation: infection rates and risk factors associated with infection in a population-based cohort study of 46299 consecutive patients. Eur Heart J 2011;32(8):991–8.

11. Kirkfeldt RE, Johansen JB, Nohr EA, et al. Complications after cardiac implantable electronic device implantations: an analysis of a complete, nationwide cohort in Denmark. Eur Heart J 2014;35(18):1186–94.

12. Padfield GJ, Steinberg C, Bennett MT, et al. Preventing cardiac implantable electronic device infections. Heart Rhythm 2015;12(11):2344–56.

13. Uslan DZ, Sohail MR, St Sauver JL, et al. Permanent pacemaker and implantable cardioverter defibrillator infection: a population-based study. Arch Intern Med 2007;167(7):669–75.

14. Romeyer-Bouchard C, Da Costa A, Dauphinot V, et al. Prevalence and risk factors related to infections of cardiac resynchronization therapy devices. Eur Heart J 2010;31(2):203–10.

15. Palmisano P, Accogli M, Zaccaria M, et al. Rate, causes, and impact on patient outcome of implantable device complications requiring surgical revision: large population survey from two centres in Italy. Europace 2013;15(4):531–40.

16. Prutkin JM, Reynolds MR, Bao H, et al. Rates of and factors associated with infection in 200 909 Medicare implantable cardioverter-defibrillator implants: results from the National Cardiovascular Data Registry. Circulation 2014;130(13):1037–43.

17. Sridhar AR, Lavu M, Yarlagadda V, et al. Cardiac implantable electronic device-related infection and extraction trends in the U.S. Pacing Clin Electrophysiol 2017;40(3):286–93.

18. Polyzos KA, Konstantelias AA, Falagas ME. Risk factors for cardiac implantable electronic device infection: a systematic review and meta-analysis. Europace 2015;17(5):767–77.

19. Mittal S, Shaw RE, Michel K, et al. Cardiac implantable electronic device infections: incidence, risk factors, and the effect of the AigisRx antibacterial envelope. Heart Rhythm 2014;11(4):595–601.

20. Nielsen JC, Gerdes JC, Varma N. Infected cardiac-implantable electronic devices: prevention, diagnosis, and treatment. Eur Heart J 2015;36(37):2484–90.

21. Leung S, Danik S. Prevention, diagnosis, and treatment of cardiac implantable electronic device infections. Curr Cardiol Rep 2016;18(6):58.

22. Chamis AL, Peterson GE, Cabell CH, et al. Staphylococcus aureus bacteremia in patients with permanent pacemakers or implantable cardioverter-defibrillators. Circulation 2001;104(9):1029–33.

23. Athan E, Chu VH, Tattevin P, et al. Clinical characteristics and outcome of infective endocarditis involving implantable cardiac devices. JAMA 2012;307(16):1727–35.

24. Cahill TJ, Prendergast BD. Infective endocarditis. Lancet 2016;387(10021):882–93.

25. Downey BC, Juselius WE, Pandian NG, et al. Incidence and significance of pacemaker and implantable cardioverter-defibrillator lead masses discovered during transesophageal echocardiography. Pacing Clin Electrophysiol 2011;34(6):679–83.

26. Granados U, Fuster D, Pericas JM, et al. Diagnostic accuracy of 18F-FDG PET/CT in infective endocarditis and implantable cardiac electronic device infection: a cross-sectional study. J Nucl Med 2016;57(11):1726–32.

27. Erba PA, Sollini M, Conti U, et al. Radiolabeled WBC scintigraphy in the diagnostic workup of patients with suspected device-related infections. JACC Cardiovasc Imaging 2013;6(10):1075–86.

28. Dy Chua J, Abdul-Karim A, Mawhorter S, et al. The role of swab and tissue culture in the diagnosis of implantable cardiac device infection. Pacing Clin Electrophysiol 2005;28(12):1276–81.

29. Baddour LM, Wilson WR, Bayer AS, et al. Infective endocarditis in adults: diagnosis, antimicrobial therapy, and management of complications: a scientific statement for healthcare professionals from the American Heart Association. Circulation 2015;132(15):1435–86.

30. Margey R, McCann H, Blake G, et al. Contemporary management of and outcomes from cardiac device related infections. Europace 2010;12(1):64–70.

31. Bongiorni MG, Kennergren C, Butter C, et al. The European Lead Extraction ConTRolled (ELECTRa) study: a European Heart Rhythm Association (EHRA) registry of transvenous lead extraction outcomes. Eur Heart J 2017;38(40):2995–3005.

32. Boersma L, Burke MC, Neuzil P, et al. Infection and mortality after implantation of a subcutaneous ICD after transvenous ICD extraction. Heart Rhythm 2016;13(1):157–64.

33. Chang PM, Doshi RN. Implantation of a leadless cardiac pacemaker for recurrent pocket infections. HeartRhythm Case Rep 2016;2(4):339–41.

34. Essebag V, Verma A, Healey JS, et al. Clinically significant pocket hematoma increases long-term risk of device infection: BRUISE CONTROL INFECTION study. J Am Coll Cardiol 2016;67(11):1300–8.

35. Bernard ML, Shotwell M, Nietert PJ, et al. Meta-analysis of bleeding complications associated with cardiac rhythm device implantation. Circ Arrhythm Electrophysiol 2012;5(3):468–74.

36. Cheng A, Nazarian S, Brinker JA, et al. Continuation of warfarin during pacemaker or implantable cardioverter-defibrillator implantation: a randomized clinical trial. Heart Rhythm 2011;8(4):536–40.

37. Birnie DH, Healey JS, Wells GA, et al. Pacemaker or defibrillator surgery without interruption of anticoagulation. N Engl J Med 2013;368(22):2084–93.

38. Essebag V, Proietti R, Birnie DH, et al. Short-term dabigatran interruption before cardiac rhythm device implantation: multi-centre experience from the RE-LY trial. Europace 2017;19(10):1630–6.

39. Leef GC, Hellkamp AS, Patel MR, et al. Safety and efficacy of rivaroxaban in patients with cardiac implantable electronic devices: observations from the ROCKET AF trial. J Am Heart Assoc 2017;6(6) [pii:e004663].

40. Essebag V, Healey JS, Ayala-Paredes F, et al. Strategy of continued vs interrupted novel oral anticoagulant at time of device surgery in patients with moderate to high risk of arterial thromboembolic events: the BRUISE CONTROL-2 trial. Am Heart J 2016;173:102–7.

41. Dreger H, Grohmann A, Bondke H, et al. Is antiarrhythmia device implantation safe under dual antiplatelet therapy? Pacing Clin Electrophysiol 2010; 33(4):394–9.

42. Darouiche RO, Wall MJ Jr, Itani KM, et al. Chlorhexidine-alcohol versus povidone-iodine for surgical-site antisepsis. N Engl J Med 2010;362(1):18–26.

43. Da Costa A, Tulane C, Dauphinot V, et al. Preoperative skin antiseptics for prevention of cardiac implantable electronic device infections: a historical-controlled interventional trial comparing aqueous against alcoholic povidone-iodine solutions. Europace 2015; 17(7):1092–8.

44. Comparison of alcoholic chlorhexidine 2% versus alcoholic povidone iodine for infections prevention with cardiac resynchronization therapy device implantation (CHLOVIS). Available at: https://clinicaltrials.gov/ct2/show/NCT01841242. Accessed June 18, 2017.

45. de Oliveira JC, Martinelli M, Nishioka SA, et al. Efficacy of antibiotic prophylaxis before the implantation of pacemakers and cardioverter-defibrillators: results of a large, prospective, randomized, double-blinded, placebo-controlled trial. Circ Arrhythm Electrophysiol 2009;2(1):29–34.

46. Darouiche R, Mosier M, Voigt J. Antibiotics and antiseptics to prevent infection in cardiac rhythm management device implantation surgery. Pacing Clin Electrophysiol 2012;35(11):1348–60.

47. Lakshmanadoss U, Nuanez B, Kutinsky I, et al. Incidence of pocket infection postcardiac device implantation using antibiotic versus saline solution for pocket irrigation. Pacing Clin Electrophysiol 2016; 39(9):978–84.

48. Khalighi K, Aung TT, Elmi F. The role of prophylaxis topical antibiotics in cardiac device implantation. Pacing Clin Electrophysiol 2014;37(3):304–11.

49. León C, Ruiz-Santana S, Rello J, et al. Benefits of minocycline and rifampin-impregnated central venous catheters. A prospective, randomized, double-blind, controlled, multicenter trial. Intensive Care Med 2004;30(10):1891–9.

50. Bloom HL, Constantin L, Dan D, et al. Implantation success and infection in cardiovascular implantable electronic device procedures utilizing an antibacterial envelope. Pacing Clin Electrophysiol 2011; 34(2):133–42.

51. Ritter P, Duray GZ, Steinwender C, et al. Early performance of a miniaturized leadless cardiac pacemaker: the Micra Transcatheter Pacing study. Eur Heart J 2015;36(37):2510–9.

52. Roberts PR, Clementy N, Al Samadi F, et al. A leadless pacemaker in the real-world setting: the micra transcatheter pacing system post-approval registry. Heart Rhythm 2017;14(9):1375–9.

53. Kypta A, Blessberger H, Kammler J, et al. Leadless cardiac pacemaker implantation after lead extraction in patients with severe device infection. J Cardiovasc Electrophysiol 2016;27(9):1067–71.

54. Weiss R, Knight BP, Gold MR, et al. Safety and efficacy of a totally subcutaneous implantable-cardioverter defibrillator. Circulation 2013;128(9):944–53.

55. Burke MC, Gold MR, Knight BP, et al. Safety and efficacy of the totally subcutaneous implantable defibrillator: 2-year results from a pooled analysis of the IDE study and EFFORTLESS Registry. J Am Coll Cardiol 2015;65(16):1605–15.

56. Brouwer TF, Driessen AHG, Olde Nordkamp LRA, et al. Surgical management of implantation-related complications of the subcutaneous implantable cardioverter-defibrillator. J Am Coll Cardiol 2016;2(1): 89–96.

Venous System Interventions for Device Implantation

Jose M. Marcial, MD, Seth J. Worley, MD, FHRS*

KEYWORDS

- Subclavian occlusion • Venoplasty • Upgrade • Biventricular • Occlusion • Stenosis • His pacing
- Focused force venoplasty

KEY POINTS

- The 2017 Heart Rhythm Society (HRS) Expert Consensus Statement recognizes subclavian venoplasty (SV) as a safe and effective lead management option when venous access becomes an issue due to occlusion of the desired access point.
- Peripheral vein venography, sonography, CT scan, and so forth overestimate the severity of the obstruction. Contrast injection at the site of occlusion (local venogram) frequently delineates a path to the central circulation.
- Compared with progressively larger dilators, SV improves the quality of venous access, providing the unrestricted catheter manipulation critical to both His bundle pacing and left ventricular lead implantation.
- SV preserves venous access and reduces lead burden by decreasing the need to tunnel or implant a new system on the contralateral side.
- By acquiring the tools and following a consistent step-by-step approach, implanting physicians can easily add SV to lead management options.

Video content accompanies this article at http://www.cardiacep.theclinics.com.

INTRODUCTION

Subclavian vein stenosis/occlusion is an important clinical problem. As indications for cardiovascular implantable electronic devices (CIEDs) expand and patients with existing CIED leads require the addition or replacement of leads, implanting physicians increasingly need to navigate these venous occlusions.[1–8] Moreover, subclavian obstructions can significantly impair the possibilities of achieving cardiac resynchronization by preventing placement of a left ventricular (LV) lead.[9,10] Even if vascular access is gained using progressively larger dilators, catheter manipulation is

Conflict of Interest: None (J.M. Marcial). Royalties from Merit Medical and Pressure Products for the sale of the Worley LV lead implant tools. Compensation from Medtronic, Abbott, and Biotronik for teaching the "Interventional Approach to LV lead Implantation" using the Worley tools and techniques. Neither Merit Medical nor Pressure products sell a balloon for venoplasty. The author does not receive direct or indirect compensation from Merit Medical for the sale of the accessories (catheters, wires, and contrast injection system) discussed in this article. The author has no overt or covert financial interest in promoting the use of subclavian venoplasty to obtain and/or improve venous access (S.J. Worley).
Department of Medicine, Division of Cardiology, Cardiac Arrhythmia Center, Medstar Heart and Vascular Institute, Medstar Washington Hospital Center, 110 Irving Street Northwest, Washington, DC 20010, USA
* Corresponding author. Department of Medicine, Division of Cardiology, Cardiac Arrhythmia Center, Medstar Heart and Vascular Institute, Medstar Washington Hospital Center, 110 Irving Street Northwest, Suite 5A-12, Washington, DC 20010.
E-mail address: seth@mcworley.com

Card Electrophysiol Clin 10 (2018) 163–177
https://doi.org/10.1016/j.ccep.2017.11.017
1877-9182/18/© 2017 The Author(s). Published by Elsevier Inc. This is an open access article under the CC BY-NC-ND license (http://creativecommons.org/licenses/by-nc-nd/4.0/).

frequently impaired by the residual stenosis. Restricted catheter manipulation impairs LV lead placement and His bundle pacing. Crossing intraluminal occlusions followed by subclavian venoplasty (SV) has been demonstrated a safe alternative.[11–16] Furthermore, SV may be preferable to using a contralateral access approach, the supraclavicular approach,[17,18] or powered/mechanical sheath extraction, with extraction posing additional risks.[19–23] The technique of SV should thus become an integral part of the core armamentarium of the implanting physician.

EPIDEMIOLOGY

The incidence of subclavian vein stenosis after device implantations varies widely in the literature, ranging from 30% to 50%.[1,2,6,24–26] One group prospectively studied venography at 6 months postimplantation in 202 patients and identified greater than moderate stenosis in 51%.[27] Previous use of transvenous temporary leads, LV ejection fraction less than 40%, and advanced age (>65 years) were found to be independent risk factors for a higher incidence of venous occlusion. Another group performed consecutive venography on 40 patients and found significant stenosis in 23% at a mean postprocedure follow-up of 4 months.[25] Most of the patients in these studies were asymptomatic. The lack of symptoms was felt to be secondary to the collateral venous circulation that developed as the stenosis progressed.

PATHOPHYSIOLOGY OF SUBCLAVIAN OCCLUSIONS

Studies have described subclavian venous thrombosis of both an early[25] (within 6 months) and late[26] (at 6 years) progression. Late thrombosis is most often asymptomatic and is a result of chronic fibrosis around the device leads, which allows time for concurrent collateralization. Autopsies have demonstrated inflammatory and fibrotic changes that occur at the endothelial-lead interface and at the insertion site of the leads in the vein.[28] Dense fibrotic lesions are most likely to be found in anatomic sites like the lead insertion point, venous bifurcation sites, and the costoclavicular space. In a large series of more than 300 patients who underwent SV, obstructions were seen to be peripheral (subclavian/distal innominate) in 61%, central (innominate/superior vena cava [SVC]) in 17%, and both central and peripheral in 22.1% of cases.[12] Endothelial injury and repetitive mechanical trauma at bifurcation sites or where bony compression occurs may account for these findings.

SAFETY AND EFFICACY OF SUBCLAVIAN VENOPLASTY

The largest series reporting the use of SV for lead implantation included 373 cases over an 11-year period.[12] Successful access was achieved in 371 of 373, with no adverse clinical outcome, no distal embolization, no venous disruption, and no acute damage to the leads. The same group subsequently extended the results to 488 SV procedures performed from January 27, 2004, to November 20, 2014, via an electronic health record query. There were no acute clinical events in the cohort. Contrast extravasation was common during crossing of total occlusions and was observed with balloon ruptures on 3 occasions, but none was clinically significant. Questioning whether the pressure and mechanical stress to which existing leads are subjected during SV affect long-term lead performance, the group also looked for damage to existing leads becoming manifest over 12 months after venoplasty. Of the initial 488 patients, 20 were lost to follow-up. In the remaining 468 patients, there were 2 atrial lead dislodgements and 1 insulation defect found in a preexisting atrial lead. The atrial lead dislodgements were detected at 3 months and 5 months post SV, respectively, whereas the insulation defect was detected at 9 months. When compared with a cohort who had lead replacement without SV, there was no evidence to suggest that SV caused delayed lead damage. In an attempt to acquire additional safety data, an email survey of 23 centers performing SV was conducted in 2015. All centers contacted responded. There was a mean of 19.4 cases ± 12.7 cases per center with no center reporting an adverse event. Thus, it seems that SV not only is safe but also does not pose any danger to existing leads.

Operative lead management should include SV as a means to conserve venous access and assist in optimal lead placement. Because of the extensive fibrous tissue surrounding the leads (**Fig. 1**), venoplasty is an intrinsically safe

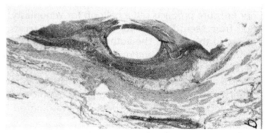

Fig. 1. Example of the dense fibrous tissue that develops around the pacing lead.

procedure and should be considered fibroplasty as opposed to venoplasty. The safety experience described by Worley and colleagues,[12] however, applies to patients with chronic leads (>2 years) where venoplasty was performed to add a lead(s). When SV is compared with the use of progressively larger dilators, venoplasty is faster and there are problems with dilators: catheters remain difficult to manipulate throughout the procedure, the more central stenosis at the SVC–right atrium (RA) junction is not dilated, and a false sense of safety is created. There are some situations where venoplasty may not be advisable, such as at eccentric occlusions along the SVC (**Fig. 2**) and for a swollen arm developing within the first several months of implant, indicative of early progression of thrombosis. In the latter situation, fibrous tissue has not yet developed and larger balloons are required, increasing the likelihood of venous disruption. In addition, there is little evidence that venoplasty for a swollen arm produces lasting patency, and spontaneous collateral vein development usually results in long-term clinical resolution of arm swelling. Spittel and colleagues[3] reported early success with venoplasty in the treatment of 2 patients with symptomatic venous stenosis. In view of these risks, however, conservative options, including watchful waiting for collateral vessels to develop, seems a reasonable alternative.

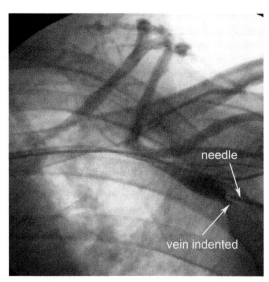

Fig. 3. Venous access as contrast is injected into a peripheral vein. The occlusion along with collateral veins are apparent. The vein is entered peripheral to the occlusion. When the needle is inserted into the vein as contrast is flowing, the vein can be seen to indent, confirming where the needle enters the vein. When crossing an occlusion, it is important to enter the vein as far peripheral to the occlusion as possible.

Ji and colleagues[23] were able to evaluate the utility of SV at their hospital, wherein only some of the implanting physicians decided to learn and adopt the SV technique; 41 patients with subclavian vein occlusion were scheduled for the addition of a lead(s); implanters who adopted the SV technique performed 18 cases and implanters who did not adopt the SV technique performed 23 cases. When implanting physicians were competent in the venoplasty technique, procedure times were shorter (2:31 hours for the venoplasty competent operators compared with 3:28 hours for operators who were not venoplasty competent). When the implanting physicians were venoplasty competent, implants were more frequently successful: there were 5 implant failures in the 23 cases (21.5%) resulting from inability to gain venous access when the implanter was not venoplasty competent. On the other hand, there were no implant failures in the 18 cases when the implanter was venoplasty competent.[23]

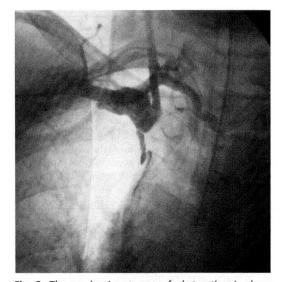

Fig. 2. The predominant area of obstruction is along the lateral wall SVC rather than within the subclavian innominate vein. Although a wire was easily advanced into the RA, venoplasty was not performed because of the lack tissue surrounding the obstruction and the catastrophic consequences of any SVC tear.

Step-by-Step Approach to Subclavian Venoplasty

Steps	Description	Additional Comments
Step 1	In patients with previous leads, because of the possibility of subclavian obstruction, the authors start venous access with a 15-cm stiffened dilator micropuncture kit (**Box 1**) rather than using the 18-gauge needle and wire that come with the sheath.	
Step 2	Perform peripheral venogram using a routine intravenous line. Although the contrast is flowing, enter the vein with the needle as far peripheral to the occlusion as possible (**Fig. 3**; Videos 1–3) without regard to the location of the rib. Unlike traditional axillary vein access, the needle should enter the body at a shallow angle of approximately 30°.	The key to success is to enter the vein peripheral to the occlusion at a shallow angle (30° to the skin). To this end, it is best to puncture the vein while contrast is flowing to confirm where the needle enters the vein (see Videos 1–3). To achieve the proper angle and vein entry site, it is usually necessary to insert the needle into the skin lateral to the pocket and tunnel the wire into the pocket. If the needle enters the vein at the site of occlusion, it is difficult to advance the wire and any opening through which to advance the wire will be lost. Do not be concerned if it seems like there is a total occlusion, the peripheral venogram usually overestimates the severity of the obstruction (**Fig. 4**, Video 4).
Step 3	Carefully advance the wire into the vein up to the site of obstruction. It is important to not disrupt the site of obstruction with the needle or the wire.	
Step 4	Carefully advance the 5F dilator or stiffened dilator/5F catheter over the wire (see Videos 1 and 2; Video 5). The tip of the dilator should not be pushed beyond the tip of the wire. The goal is the get the tip of the dilator/catheter a few millimeters peripheral to the obstruction.	
Step 5	Attach a contrast injection system with hemostatic Y-adapter to the hub of the dilator/catheter (**Figs. 5** and **6**). An injection system similar to that shown in **Fig. 5**A can be assembled from spare parts available in most laboratories or purchased more cost effectively as a kit (see **Box 1**).	
Step 6	Insert a 0.035-in or 0.018-in nitinol angled polymer tip hydrophilic wire (glide wire) into the hemostatic valve. Nitinol angled polymer tip hydrophilic wires are available from several vendors (see **Box 1**). In some cases, the 0.035-in wire is too large to cross the obstruction.	The 0.018-in nitinol polymer tip hydrophilic wire is superior to a 0.014-in angioplasty wire because the angioplasty wire is stainless steel, which is easily bent whereas the nitinol 0.018-in wire retains its shape.
Step 7	Attach a torque device to the proximal end of the wire 5 cm–10 cm from where it enters the hemostatic valve (see **Fig. 5**C).	
Step 8	Close the hemostatic valve.	
Step 9	Use puffs of contrast and the torque device to direct the wire across the occlusion (see Videos 1 and 5).	In many cases the glide wire crosses the occlusion. If not the 5F dilator/micropuncture catheter is replaced with a braided angled hydrophilic catheter (see **Box 1**) to provide direction and support for the wire.

(continued on next page)

Steps	Description	Additional Comments

Step 10	If the wire alone cannot be advanced across the obstruction, replace the 5F dilator/5F micropuncture catheter with an angled 4 or 5F braided catheter with hydrophilic coating (see **Box 1**).	As detailed in **Box 1**, the angle and length of the tip as well as the braid in the walls of the catheter are critical, and substitution is not advised. The angled-tip catheter is used to inject contrast and aim the wire toward an opening (see Video 2). A variety of hydrophilic exchange catheters are available but a braided catheter is preferred because of greater pushability and torque capability compared with nonbraided catheters (eg, Terumo Glidecath). The catheter is stiff enough to be pushed into the occlusion followed by the wire (see Video 3). On occasion, advancing the catheter with puffs of contrast without a wire can be more effective than blindly trying to follow a wire (Video 6).
Step 11	When a wire cannot be advanced through the occlusion, retained wire lead removal followed by venoplasty is an option if one of the leads is movable within the fibrous adhesions (Video 7). Retained wire lead removal can be accomplished via (1) wire under the insulation technique, (2) wire in the stylet lumen with femoral removal, (3) over the wire removal of an LV pacing lead.	
Step 12	Confirm that the wire has entered the heart. Advance the wire until the tip enters either the pulmonary artery or the inferior vena cava. If the wire does not advance into the pulmonary artery or inferior vena cava, do not proceed.	Confirm in the right anterior oblique and left anterior oblique projections that the wire follows the lead(s) to the SVC or PA.
Step 13	Exchange the glide wire for an Amplatz Extra Stiff wire using a braided 4 or 5F hydrophilic catheter.	The glide wire used to cross the occlusion often does not provide sufficient support to advance the balloon through the obstruction (see Video 4).
Step 14	Advance a 6-mm or 9-mm × 4-cm ultranoncompliant balloon (lumen diameter .035-in) over the Amplatz Extra Stiff wire (see **Box 1**) to just beyond the SVC-innominate junction. Use a 9-mm balloon if the plan is to add 2 leads or there is elastic recoil after 6-mm balloon inflation.	
Step 15	If the ultranoncompliant balloon does not track to the SVC-innominate junction, first try predilating with the lower profile 4-mm × 4-cm noncompliant balloon (see **Box 1**). If the 4-mm balloon does not advance, move to a .018-in lumen lower profile balloon using the braided catheter to replace the 0.035-in Amplatz wire with a 0.018-in extrastiff wire (eg, V-18 Control Wire). Predilate with the .018-in lumen low-profile balloon (eg, Sterling Balloon). Once dilated, use the catheter to replace the .018-in wire with the .035-in Amplatz wire and finish dilating with the 6-mm or 9-mm ultranoncompliant balloon.	If the 4-mm balloon does not advance, switch to a .018-in lumen lower-profile balloon using the braided catheter to replace the 0.035-in Amplatz wire with a 0.018-in extrastiff wire (eg, V-18 Control Wire). Predilate with the .018-in lumen low-profile balloon (eg, Sterling Balloon). Once dilated, use the catheter to replace the .018-in wire with the .035-in Amplatz wire and finish dilating with the 6-mm or 9-mm ultranoncompliant balloon

(*continued on next page*)

Steps	Description	Additional Comments
	(continued)	
Step 16	Always perform the first inflation at or central to the SVC-innominate junction because a stenosis is often present but not recognized on the venogram. The profile of the balloon increases after the first inflation–deflation cycle (called winging), making it impossible to advance to the SVC-innominate junction.	Initially, the authors did not dilate at the SVC-innominate junction but when advancing the sheath was tried, a stenosis requiring additional venoplasty was found in approximately 20% of cases. Because the profile of the balloon increases after the first inflation–deflation cycle (called winging), the balloon used for the more apparent peripheral stenosis did not advance through the central stenosis.
Step 17	Inflate the balloon to the rated burst pressure (RBP) indicated on the balloon package (26 atm–30 atm for the peripheral balloons listed in **Box 1** and 18 atm–20 atm for the low-profile peripheral balloon (ie, Sterling Balloon).	
Step 18	Keep the balloon inflated until the pressure is stable at RBP and there is no residual waist. If the waist is not eliminated, use focused force venoplasty (**Fig. 7**).	
Step 19	Deflate the balloon by applying negative pressure to the inflation device.	
Step 20	Once the contrast is evacuated from the balloon, withdraw the balloon until the tip reaches the former tail position (head to tail overlap).	Do not withdraw the balloon until the contrast is evacuated from the balloon (**Fig. 8**).
Step 21	Continue overlapping inflations until the tail of the balloon is visible in the pocket.	The recommendation to continue until the tail is visible in the pocket frequently produces concern but is essential and does not seem to cause excessive bleeding. If bleeding is a problem, it is easily addressed with a hemostatic suture.
Step 22	Advance a long (25-cm) sheath over the wire. Always use a long sheath after venoplasty. If it is not very easy to advance the sheaths, there is excessive elastic recoil. If elastic recoil is present, it is worth taking the time to upsize to a 9-mm diameter balloon.	The other explanation for difficulty advancing the sheath is a residual peripheral stenosis from failure to inflate the balloon with the tail visible in the pocket as recommended.
Step 23	If 2 leads are needed, advance 2 Amplatz Extra Stiff wires into the long sheath and withdraw the sheath retaining the 2 wires.	

BALLOON OPTIONS

Coronary balloons are too small, in both length and diameter, for SV. With a 0.035-in wire across the obstruction, it makes sense to start with a .035-in lumen balloon (see **Box 1**). With retained wire lead removal and when the stenosis is tight enough to require a 0.018-in wire, predilate with a .018-in lumen ultra–low-profile balloon (eg, Sterling). As indicated in **Box 1**, the recommended balloon diameter is 6 mm or 9 mm and length 4 cm to 6 cm. The 9-mm balloon is useful if there is excess elastic recoil or if the intent is to add 2 leads. Alternatively, elastic recoil may be addressed with focused force venoplasty (see **Fig. 7**). If a 9-mm diameter balloon is not available for adding 2 leads, the stenosis can be redilated with the 6-mm balloon when the first long sheath (with dilator) is in place. The recommended balloons are 75 cm to 80 cm in length, thus requiring only a standard-length wire.

Box 1
Annotated list of equipment for crossing and dilating a subclavian obstruction/occlusion

Contrast injection system

Attached the dilator from a 5F sheath or the 5F catheter of the micropuncture system. Contrast injection with the tip of the dilator/catheter at the site of occlusion often identifies an opening through which to advance a wire. The Y-adapter with rotating hemostatic valve allows the wire to be advanced through the dilator/catheter to cross the occlusion: contrast injection system Worley Advanced Kit 1 CAK 1 (comes with contrast bowl and labels) (order # K12-WORLEY1, Merit Medical)

Dilator from a 5F sheath vs stiffened micropuncture

Prior adopting the micropuncture kit with stiffened radiopaque dilator, the dilator from 5F sheath was advanced over the 0.035-in J wire. Conversion to the stiffened micropuncture kit was precipitated by

1. Difficulty advancing a 0.035-in wire into the vein for initial venous access (easier using a 0.018-in wire)
2. Difficulty advancing the dilator over the wire (not stiff enough)
3. Difficulty visualizing the tip of the dilator to be certain it was in the vein (not radiopaque)

The authors now use 5F 15-cm micropuncture kit with stiffened radiopaque dilator for initial venous access. The 21-gauge needle and angled-tip 0.018-in nitinol wire can make venous access easier. Compared with standard micropuncture, the stiffened dilator (indicated by the S in the order number) provides the support required to advance over the wire through scar tissue. Being radiopaque makes it is easier to be certain the tip is in the vein. The 15-cm length (usually 10 cm) makes it more likely that the tip reaches beyond the stenosis. Catheter = 5F × 15-cm; wire = 0.018-in × 60-cm nitinol with platinum tip; needle = 21G (order # S-MAK501N15BT)

Wires for crossing subclavian obstructions

Angled polymer jacketed nitinol wires with a hydrophilic coating (also known as glide wires) work well for crossing subclavian obstructions. These wires are available from multiple vendors with slightly different names. In general, 0.014-in angioplasty wires are not helpful because they are constructed from stainless steel, which is easily deformed whereas nitinol wires tend to retain their shape.

1. 0.035-in × 180-cm angled-tip (not straight) wires available from multiple vendors, including Merit Medical Laureate wire (order # LWSTDA35180, Merit Medical)
2. 0.018-in × 180-cm angled-tip (not straight) wire available from multiple vendors, including Merit Medical Laureate wire (order # LWSTDA18180, Merit Medical)

Wires for retained wire lead removal

For the wire under the insulation/wire in the stylet lumen and over the wire removal of most LV leads use a polymer jacketed extra support wire (eg, Choice PT Extra Support or Acuity Whisper Extra Distal Support [Boston Scientific])

Medtronic LV leads have a 0.018-in lumen, which allows removal over a more supportive wire (eg, V-18 Control Wire (polymer jacketed 200-cm Boston Scientific).

Torque device (also known as steering handle) for directing the angled-tip glide wire

A torque device is used to direct the tip of glide wire (caution: 1 size may not work for all wires) (A) Torque device for 0.014 in–0.018-in wires. (B) Torque device for 0.025 in–0.038-in wires.

Catheters used to (1) exchange from glide to Amplatz Extra Stiff wire and (2) cross a difficult subclavian obstruction/total occlusion.

1. Catheters for wire exchange

The glide wire used to cross the occlusion frequently does not provide sufficient support to advance the balloon. The glide wire must be exchanged for an extra support wire (Amplatz Extra Support). For wire exchange, a 4F/5F braided catheter with hydrophilic coating works best. The braid and hydrophilic coating are essential. Similar catheters without metal braid (eg, Terumo Glidecath) may not have adequate stability to be advanced over the wire into the central circulation. Although the 5F is most commonly used, occasionally a tight stenosis requires downsizing to 4F. An alternative is the straight catheter when the glide wire advances to the central circulation without the need for an angled-tip catheter.

2. Catheters for crossing difficult occlusions

To cross a totally occluded subclavian, a properly shaped, angled-tip, braided catheter with a hydrophilic coating is essential. The length and angle of the tip are critical; slight variations are surprisingly important. The catheter is used in 2 ways: (1) to better direct and provide support for the glide wire; the braided catheter provides support to push the wire into the occlusion; once the wire advances the catheter is worked up to the tip of the wire, and (2) with puffs of contract without a wire to navigate through collaterals and tortuosity; I have the most experience with the 5F version of the catheters listed; similar catheters without metal braid (eg, Terumo Glidecath) do not have adequate torque control or support:

1. 5F Impress KA2 Hydrophilic Angiographic Catheter 5F 65-cm (order # 56538KA2-H, Merit Medical)

2. 4F Impress KA2 Hydrophilic Angiographic Catheter 4F 65-cm (order # 46538KA2-H, Merit Medical)

J-tip extra stiff support wire to replace the glide wire

Note: Not all Amplatz Extra Stiff wires are created equal! For example, both the Boston Scientific and Cook are labeled "Amplatz Extra Stiff"; the floppy distal section of the Boston Scientific J-tip Amplatz is too long to be useful for providing support in the coronary sinus. To advance a balloon, either wire is satisfactory; for simplicity of inventory, order the Cook J-tip Amplatz 0.035-in × 180-cm (THSCF-35-180-3-AES, order # G03565).

Balloons for SV when a 0.035-in wire is advanced across the obstruction

A 0.035-in glide wire is usually used to cross the obstruction, thus a balloon with a 0.035-in lumen is required. If a .014/.018-in wire is across the obstruction see balloons for retained wire lead removal below.

1. To add 1 lead, use a 6-mm diameter × 4-cm balloon with a shaft length 75-cm. Example, CONQUEST (Kevlar), order # CQ-7564, Bard Peripheral Vascular Ultra-Noncompliant: wire lumen 0.035-in, over the wire, RBP 30 atm.

2. To add 2 leads or if there is elastic recoil, use a 9-mm × 4-cm balloon with a shaft length 75-cm balloon, Bard Peripheral Vascular Ultra-Noncompliant: wire lumen 0.035-in, over the wire, RBP 26 atm. Order # CQ-7594, Bard Peripheral Vascular.

3. When the balloons (discussed previously) do not advance across the obstruction predilate with (1) Cordis Powerflex Pro OTW Balloon (0.035-in wire lumen) 4-mm × 40-mm balloon shaft length 80 cm; order # 4400404S or (2) exchange the 0.035-in wire for 0.018-in extra support wire (V-18 Control Wire) and predilate with a low profile peripheral balloon (eg, Sterling Balloon [discussed later]).

Balloons for SV when a 0.014-in/0.018-in wire is advanced or introduced by the retained wire lead removal technique

If a .018-in lumen balloon is advanced over a .014-in wire, once the tip of the balloon is in the central circulation, the 0.0014-in wire should be exchanged for a more supportive .018-in wire, for example, V-18 Control Wire (discussed previously). To adequately dilate the obstruction, the 0.018-in lumen balloon frequently needs to be replaced with an ultranoncompliant .035-in lumen balloon (discussed previously). After initial dilation use a 4F/5F hydrophilic catheter to exchange the 0.018-in for a 0.035-in Amplatz wire. Boston Scientific Sterling OTW (0.018-in wire lumen) Balloon Catheter: 6-mm × 40-mm balloon; shaft length 80-cm (UPN # H74939032604080, catalog # 39,032–60,408).

FOCUSED FORCE VENOPLASTY

Approximately 3% of cases require focused force venoplasty for a stenosis (see **Fig. 7**) refractory to an ultranoncompliant balloon (RBP 30 atm). Focused force can also be attempted when there is excessive elastic recoil (ie, when it remains difficult to manipulate the catheter after initial balloon dilation despite no visible waist). To apply focused force, remove the balloon, advance a long 5F sheath or a 6F multipurpose guide (nondiagnostic catheter) over the Amplatz wire, advance a second Amplatz wire through the sheath/guide, remove the

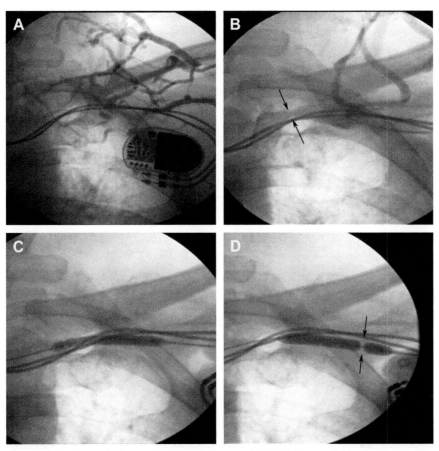

Fig. 4. Crossing a subclavian occlusion and performing venoplasty. (*A*) The peripheral venogram reveals extensive collaterals, suggesting total occlusion. (*B*) Injection at the site of occlusion through the dilator from a 5F sheath (local venogram) reveals a stenosis (*arrrows*) not a total occlusion through which the wire is easily advanced. (*C*) A 6-mm by 4-cm noncompliant balloon is inflated at the site of occlusion seen on the venogram. (*D*) The balloon is inflated more peripherally, revealing a stenosis (*arrows*) not appreciated on either the peripheral or local venogram.

sheath/guide and advance the balloon over 1 of the wires. The balloon is then inflated to RBP against the wire beside the balloon. The stiff wire beside the balloon pressed against the fibrous tissue is more aggressive then the balloon alone. The procedure is also referred to as the poor man's cutting balloon. The authors have not observed lead damage with focused force venoplasty.

FACTORS THAT MAKE A SUBCLAVIAN OCCLUSION DIFFICULT TO CROSS

An attempt at venous access in a patient with in situ lead(s) before a venogram is often successful. If there is an obstruction, however, the initial blind attempt(s) can disrupt the venous anatomy making it impossible to cross the occlusion.

If the artery is entered inadvertently the subsequent hematoma compresses the vein, making access even more difficult. If a still image of the venogram or ultrasound is started with, it is not clear where the needle enters the vein relative to the obstruction. If the needle enters the vein at the site of occlusion, the wire does not advance and/or an existing opening is obscured.

COMBINING RETAINED WIRE LEAD REMOVAL AND VENOPLASTY

In some cases, it may be impossible to cross a total subclavian obstruction. If 1 of the leads is mobile within the fibrous adhesions, retained wire lead removal followed by venoplasty can be used instead of extraction. When a lead is

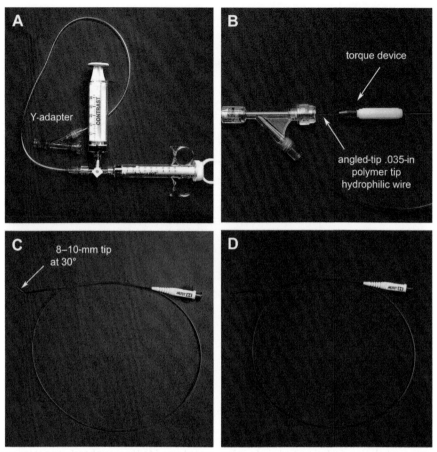

Fig. 5. Equipment used to cross and dilate a subclavian obstruction. (*A*) The contrast injection system (Worley Advanced Kit 1 CAK 1 [includes contrast bowl and labels], order # K12-WORLEY1, Merit Medical). (*B*) The .035-in × 180-cm angled polymer tip hydrophilic (Laureate wire, order # LWSTDA35180, Merit Medical) is advanced through the hemostatic valve of the Y-adapter. A torque device is essential for directing the wire through the opening observed with local contrast injection. (*C*) The 5F braided angled-tip hydrophilic catheter (5F 65-cm Impress KA2 Hydrophilic Angiographic Catheter, order # 56538KA2-H, Merit Medical) is used to direct a wire through an occlusion (crossing catheter). The wire braid in the catheter provides torque control and pushability that are important for crossing difficult obstructions. The length (6–8 mm) and angle (30°) of the tip are also important. In my experience, similar catheters with a longer tip or more acute angle are less effective. (*D*) The 4F braided straight catheter (65 cm; Impress Straight Hydrophilic Angiographic Catheter, order # 46538STS-H, Merit Medical) used to exchange an existing wire for a more supportive wire over which to advance the balloon. The authors find that a braided hydrophilic catheter advances through an obstruction when a nonbraided catheter of the same French size does not advance. (*Courtesy of* Merit Medical, South Jordan, UT; with permission.)

"extracted" for venous access, the fibrous adhesions encasing the lead are pulverized by the mechanical/powered sheaths to provide sufficient lumen to add a lead(s). Because of the risks involved, SVC extraction with powered/mechanical sheaths requires termination of the procedure to arrange for operating room backup. When the lead can be used to get a wire into the central circulation, venoplasty is a safer alternative to pulverization. The wire under the insulation technique is one of several methods

whereby a lead can be sacrificed to introduce a wire into the central circulation (**Fig. 9**; see Video 7). Whether a lead can be advanced back into the circulation with a wire attached depends on the following: (1) the surface characteristic of the pacing lead insulation (ie, silicone, polyurethane, or copolymer hybrid); (2) the characteristics of the fibrous binding (ie, thickness, elasticity, density, and adhesion of the lead); (3) the length of the fibrous binding surrounding the lead (ie, left greater than right);

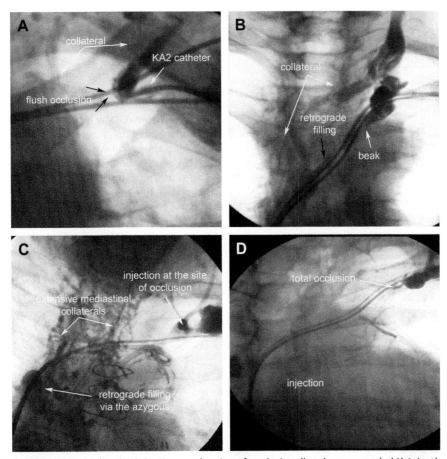

Fig. 6. Subclavian occlusion despite injection at the site of occlusion (local venogram). (*A*) Injection with the angled tip hydrophilic braided crossing catheter (see **Fig. 5C**) at the site of obstruction reveals that the subclavian is flush occluded. Despite this the obstruction was crossed using the KA2 catheter and glide wire. The KA2 was advanced into the RA, the hydrophilic wire exchanged for an extra support wire and venoplasty performed. (*B*) Injection at the site of occlusion reveals near-total occlusion; however, contrast is seen to taper to a beak shaped. Directing the wire into the beak with the KA2 is associated with a good chance of successful crossing of the occlusion. Retrograde filling of contrast is also observed and is associated with successful crossing. The KA2 and glide wire were used to successfully cross the occlusion. (*C*) There is total occlusion at the site of injection though the dilator from a 5F sheath. There is retrograde filling via collateral to the azygous vein. A beak at the site of occlusion suggests that crossing the occlusion is possible. Surprisingly, a .035-in angled polymer tip hydrophilic wire was easily passed through the occlusion without the need for the KA2. The glide wire was exchanged for a .035-in superstiff wire using the 4F braided hydrophilic exchange catheter (see **Fig. 5D**) but the 6-mm diameter balloon did not advance through the occlusion. The .035-in wire was exchanged for a .018-in wire and a 6-mm × 4-cm low-profile balloon was advanced through the occlusion and venoplasty performed. (*D*) Total occlusion without a beak is seen with contrast injection at the site of occlusion. There is no retrograde filling of the innominate. Femoral access and injection at the site where the lead enters the SVC revealed flush occlusion. The obstruction could not be crossed.

(4) the diameter of the wire attached to the lead because a larger wire is less likely to fit in the fibrous sleeve beside the pacing lead than a smaller wire; and (5) the friction generated between the surface of the wire and the fibrous binding. A wire with a polymer jacket (ie, the black coating on a glide wire) has a lower coefficient of friction than a standard hydrophilic wire. Polymer jacketed wires are commonly referred to simply as hydrophilic, which can cause confusion.

When the lead does not advance back into the central circulation, access can be salvaged by cutting off the connector pin end and inserting the wire into the stylet lumen. The lead is then extracted from below with a loop snare pulling

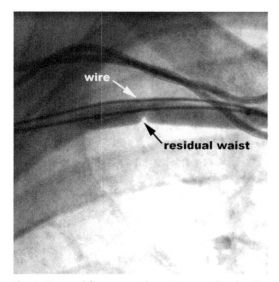

Fig. 7. Focused force venoplasty. See text for details.

the lead and wire into the central circulation (**Fig. 10**). Modern LV pacing leads can frequently be removed over a wire. Without venoplasty, however, the fibrous adhesions make it difficult/impossible to use the retained wire to add a lead. When the LV lead is movable but the wire does not exit the tip, it can be snared and removed from below pulling the wire into the central circulation. Pulling the lead from below can also be useful when the insulation bunches up (ie, accordion effect). Combining femoral lead removal of an existing lead with venoplasty can avoid the need for surgical backup and is a particularly attractive alternative in patients with prior sternotomy. For example, if there is an existing active fixation atrial lead in a patient with prior open heart surgery, the lead can be used for access, as illustrated in **Fig. 10**. Conversely, retained wire femoral

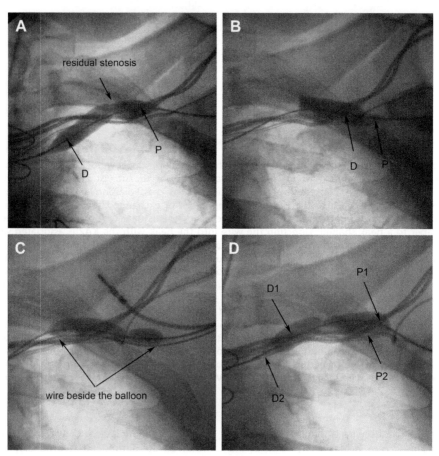

Fig. 8. Difficult subclavian obstruction with extensive elastic recoil. (*A*) The balloon is inflated with a residual waist. The distal (D) and proximal (P) markers on the balloon catheter are separated by 4 cm. (*B*) The balloon is withdrawn before the contrast is fully removed. The proximal (P) and distal (D) markers on the balloon are closer together indicating that the tip of the balloon is folded back on itself making it larger and more difficult to remove. (*C*) After the balloon is readvanced a wire is advanced beside the balloon and the balloon inflated against the wire (focused force venoplasty). (*D*) A second balloon is advanced beside the first and both balloons inflated simultaneously. D1 and P1 are the distal and proximal markers, respectively, on the first balloon. D2 and P2 are the distal and proximal markers, on the second balloon.

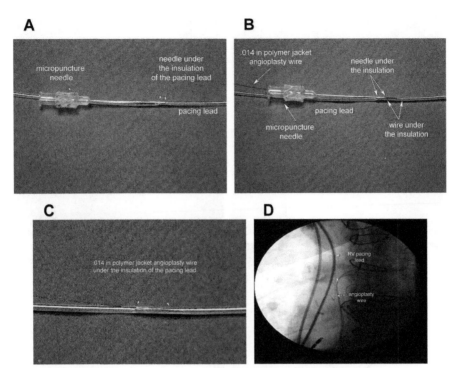

Fig. 9. Wire under the insulation technique for retained wire lead removal followed by venoplasty. (*A*) The tip of the micropuncture needle is inserted under the insulation of the pacing lead. (*B*) A polymer jacketed extrastiff .014-in wire is advanced through the micropuncture needle between the insulation and the outer conductor of the pacing lead. (*C*) The needle is removed with the wire under the insulation. (*D*) The pacing lead is advanced back into the circulation with the wire attached.

extraction of an old passive fixation atrial lead in a patient without previous open heart surgery could result in perforation at the site of attachment of the tip of the lead to the myocardium.

SUBCLAVIAN VENOPLASTY: QUALITY OF VENOUS ACCESS, LEAD BURDEN, AND PRESERVATION OF VENOUS ACCESS

The 2017 HRS Expert Consensus statement[29] includes SV as an option when venous access becomes an issue due to occlusion of the desired access point. The discussion does not address the quality of venous access provided by SV compared with progressively larger dilators. Restricted catheter manipulation from residual stenosis compromises the implanters ability to implant leads, particularly evident with His bundle pacing and LV lead implantation.

In addition, the Consensus Statement suggests that venoplasty adds to overall lead burden by leaving redundant lead(s) behind. This is not the case when venoplasty is used for access in the absence of redundant leads or when used in conjunction with the retained wire lead removal. Because of the risk and

logistics associated with extraction, many implanting physicians, when faced with a subclavian obstruction, implant an entirely new system on the contralateral side. Adding SV as an option certainly preserves venous access and likely reduces lead burden even when performed with a redundant lead, for example, upgrade from pacemaker to ICD. With regard to preservation of venous access, the expert consensus seems to equate SV to contralateral lead implantation with tunneling across the chest. Unlike tunneling, SV preserves venous access. SV should be the standard of care for access in most patients with venous occlusion without redundant leads. Recognizing that extraction, unlike SV, results in (1) procedural delay while operating room backup is arranged, (2) early reopening of the pocket with increased risk of infection, (3) higher expense, and (4) increased risk of minor and major complications, which calls into question the use of extraction as the first-line approach to device upgrades for patients with venous occlusion and redundant leads, even when performed in experienced centers. Centers experienced in extraction can easily add SV to their lead management options.

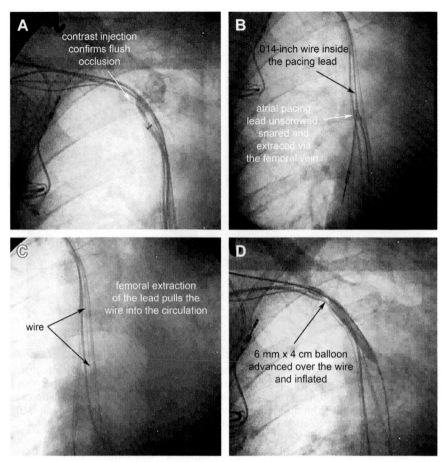

Fig. 10. Retained wire femoral lead removal followed by venoplasty in a case of total occlusion that could not be crossed. (*A*), femoral access and contrast injection confirms that the right innominate is flush occluded at the SVC. It was not possible to advance a wire from either direction despite using the braided angled hydrophilic catheter (KA2). (*B*) The suture sleeve of the active fixation atrial lead was released and the screw retracted in an unsuccessful attempt to use the wire under the insulation technique to advance a wire into the circulation. Subsequently the IS-1 connector was removed and a 300-cm 014-in angioplasty wire advanced through the stylet lumen to the tip of the lead. A 25-mm loop snare (6F × 100-cm snare catheter + a loop 25-mm diameter 120-cm in length One Snare, order # ONE2500, Merit Medical) was advanced through a long sheath over the tip and closed on the body of the atrial lead containing the angioplasty wire. (*C*) The atrial lead was extracted via the femoral vein pulling the angioplasty wire into the circulation. The .014-in angioplasty wire was exchanged for a .035-in superstiff wire using the 4F braided hydrophilic exchange catheter (see **Fig. 5D**). (*D*) A 6 mm × 4 cm noncompliant balloon was advanced to the subclavian-SVC junction and inflated to the RBP of the balloon. Overlapping balloon inflations were performed until the tail of the balloon was seen in the pocket on the final inflation.

SUPPLEMENTARY DATA

Supplementary data related to this article can be found online at https://doi.org/10.1016/j.ccep.2017.11.017.

REFERENCES

1. Sticherling C, Chough SP, Baker RL, et al. Prevalence of central venous occlusion in patients with chronic defibrillator leads. Am Heart J 2001;141(5): 813–6.

2. Lickfett L, Bitzen A, Arepally A, et al. Incidence of venous obstruction following insertion of an implantable cardioverter defibrillator. A study of systematic contrast venography on patients presenting for their first elective ICD generator replacement. Europace 2004;6(1):25–31.

3. Spittell PC, Vlietstra RE, Hayes DL, et al. Venous obstruction due to permanent transvenous pacemaker electrodes: treatment with percutaneous transluminal balloon venoplasty. Pacing Clin Electrophysiol 1990;13(3):271–4.

4. Spittell PC, Hayes DL. Venous complications after insertion of a transvenous pacemaker. Mayo Clin Proc 1992;67(3):258–65.

5. Oginosawa Y, Abe H, Nakashima Y. The incidence and risk factors for venous obstruction after implantation of transvenous pacing leads. Pacing Clin Electrophysiol 2002;25(11):1605–11.

6. Haghjoo M, Nikoo MH, Fazelifar AF, et al. Predictors of venous obstruction following pacemaker or implantable cardioverter-defibrillator implantation: a contrast venographic study on 100 patients admitted for generator change, lead revision, or device upgrade. Europace 2007;9(5):328–32.

7. Bulur S, Vural A, Yazıcı M, et al. Incidence and predictors of subclavian vein obstruction following biventricular device implantation. J Interv Card Electrophysiol 2010;29(3):199–202.

8. Bracke F, Meijer A, Van Gelder B. Venous occlusion of the access vein in patients referred for lead extraction: influence of patient and lead characteristics. Pacing Clin Electrophysiol 2003;26(8):1649–52.

9. Poole JE, Gleva MJ, Mela T, et al. Complication rates associated with pacemaker or implantable cardioverter-defibrillator generator replacements and upgrade procedures: results from the REPLACE registry. Circulation 2010;122(16):1553–61.

10. Duray GZ, Israel CW, Pajitnev D, et al. Upgrading to biventricular pacing/defibrillation systems in right ventricular paced congestive heart failure patients: prospective assessment of procedural parameters and response rate. Europace 2008;10(1):48–52.

11. McCotter CJ, Angle JF, Prudente LA, et al. Placement of transvenous pacemaker and ICD leads across total chronic occlusions. Pacing Clin Electrophysiol 2005;28(9):921–5.

12. Worley SJ, Gohn DC, Pulliam RW, et al. Subclavian venoplasty by the implanting physicians in 373 patients over 11 years. Heart Rhythm 2011;8(4):526–33.

13. Worley SJ. Implant venoplasty: dilation of subclavian and coronary veins to facilitate device implantation: indications, frequency, methods, and complications. J Cardiovasc Electrophysiol 2008;19(9):1004–7.

14. Worley SJ, Gohn DC, Pulliam RW. Over the wire lead extraction and focused force venoplasty to regain venous access in a totally occluded subclavian vein. J Interv Card Electrophysiol 2008;23(2):135–7.

15. Baerlocher MO, Asch MR, Myers A. Successful recanalization of a longstanding complete left subclavian vein occlusion by radiofrequency perforation with use of a radiofrequency guide wire. J Vasc Interv Radiol 2006;17(10):1703–6.

16. Worley SJ, Gohn DC, Pulliam RW. Excimer laser to open refractory subclavian occlusion in 12 consecutive patients. Heart Rhythm 2010;7(5):634–8.

17. Antonelli D, Freedberg NA, Rosenfeld T. Lead insertion by supraclavicular approach of the subclavian vein puncture. Pacing Clin Electrophysiol 2001; 24(3):379–80.

18. Fox DJ, Petkar S, Davidson NC, et al. Upgrading patients with chronic defibrillator leads to a biventricular system and reducing patient risk: contralateral LV lead placement. Pacing Clin Electrophysiol 2006; 29(9):1025–7.

19. Jones SO, Eckart RE, Albert CM, et al. Large, single-center, single-operator experience with transvenous lead extraction: outcomes and changing indications. Heart Rhythm 2008;5(4):520–5.

20. Byrd CL, Wilkoff BL, Love CJ, et al. Clinical study of the laser sheath for lead extraction: the total experience in the United States. Pacing Clin Electrophysiol 2002;25(5):804–8.

21. Wilkoff BL, Byrd CL, Love CJ, et al. Pacemaker lead extraction with the laser sheath: results of the pacing lead extraction with the excimer sheath (PLEXES) trial. J Am Coll Cardiol 1999;33(6):1671–6.

22. Venkataraman G, Hayes DL, Strickberger SA. Does the risk-benefit analysis favor the extraction of failed, sterile pacemaker and defibrillator leads? J Cardiovasc Electrophysiol 2009;20(12):1413–5.

23. Ji SY, Gundewar S, Palma EC. Subclavian venoplasty may reduce implant times and implant failures in the era of increasing device upgrades. Pacing Clin Electrophysiol 2012;35(4):444–8.

24. Stoney WS, Addlestone RB, Alford WC, et al. The incidence of venous thrombosis following long-term transvenous pacing. Ann Thorac Surg 1976; 22(2):166–70.

25. Antonelli D, Turgeman Y, Kaveh Z, et al. Short-term thrombosis after transvenous permanent pacemaker insertion. Pacing Clin Electrophysiol 1989;12(2): 280–2.

26. Goto Y, Abe T, Sekine S, et al. Long-term thrombosis after transvenous permanent pacemaker implantation. Pacing Clin Electrophysiol 1998;21(6): 1192–5.

27. Da Costa SS, Scalabrini Neto A, Costa R, et al. Incidence and risk factors of upper extremity deep vein lesions after permanent transvenous pacemaker implant: a 6-month follow-up prospective study. Pacing Clin Electrophysiol 2002;25(9):1301–6.

28. Robboy SJ, Harthorne JW, Leinbach RC, et al. Autopsy findings with permanent pervenous pacemakers. Circulation 1969;39(4):495–501.

29. Kusumoto FM, Schoenfeld MH, Wilkoff BL, et al. 2017 HRS expert consensus statement on cardiovascular implantable electronic device lead management and extraction. Heart Rhythm 2017; 14(12):e503–51.

Moving?

Make sure your subscription moves with you!

To notify us of your new address, find your **Clinics Account Number** (located on your mailing label above your name), and contact customer service at:

Email: journalscustomerservice-usa@elsevier.com

800-654-2452 (subscribers in the U.S. & Canada)
314-447-8871 (subscribers outside of the U.S. & Canada)

Fax number: 314-447-8029

Elsevier Health Sciences Division
Subscription Customer Service
3251 Riverport Lane
Maryland Heights, MO 63043

*To ensure uninterrupted delivery of your subscription, please notify us at least 4 weeks in advance of move.

Printed and bound by CPI Group (UK) Ltd, Croydon, CR0 4YY

03/10/2024

01040304-0019